The Adult with Down Syndrome

A New Challenge for Society

Edited by

Jean A. Rondal PhD(Psy), DLing
University of Liège, Belgium

Alberto Rasore-Quartino MD(MedGenClinPed)
Ospedali Galliera, Genova, Italy

and

Salvatore Soresi DPsy
University of Padua, Italy

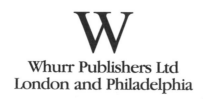

W

Whurr Publishers Ltd
London and Philadelphia

© 2004 Whurr Publishers Ltd
First published 2004
by Whurr Publishers Ltd
19b Compton Terrace
London N1 2UN
England

British Library Cataloguing in Publication Data
A catalogue record for this book is available from the British Library.

ISBN 1 86156 397 3

Typeset by Adrian McLaughlin, a@microguides.net
Printed and bound in the UK by Athenæum Press Ltd, Gateshead

Contents

Acknowledgements

The contributions to this volume are elaborations of invited presentations from the Second International Symposium on Down Syndrome organized under the auspices of the Secretary of State for Health and Social Security of the Republic of San Marino, with the Patronage of the European Down Syndrome Association. The Symposium took place in San Marino, 9–11 May 2002. We are grateful to the Republic of San Marino for helping in the preparation of the event and for insuring the free use of its Congress facilities. Particular thanks are due to Dott. Sante Canducci, Secretary of State for Health and Social Security of the San Marino Republic, Dott. Dario Manzaroli, Director of the Hospital Services of San Marino, Dott.ssa Emma Rossi, Director of the Services of Minors of the Republic of San Marino, Professor Filiberto Bernardi, President of ASDEI and Gabriele Merli, President of Associazione Trisomia 21 Rimini.

Regarding the preparation of the book manuscript, we are indebted to a number of collaborators, among them prominently Anastasia Piat-Di Nicolantonio. Last, but not least, our gratitude goes to the fine team at Whurr Publishers for hosting us in their prestigious series and helping in every way possible in the realization of the book.

Jean-Adolphe Rondal
Alberto Rasore-Quartino
Salvatore Soresi

Preface

Substantial gains in life span expectancy in Down syndrome over the last decades have resulted in markedly increased figures of adults and ageing people with the condition in our societies.

Some prospective statistics suggest that within the next 40 or 50 years, there will be two or three times as many Down syndrome adults as there are today. Given these indications, it is imperative for our societies to study carefully the practical implications of such a state of affairs, and set up and encourage systematic research on the particular biomedical and psychosocial aspects of augmented longevity in Down syndrome people.

This book constitutes a first attempt at summarizing a large amount of verified information on what it may be like to be an adult and then ageing as a person with Down syndrome. It is divided into four sections. Section I contains one chapter devoted to the epidemiology of Down syndrome in the first decades of the third millennium. Section II deals with a series of biomedical issues, from genetics and endocrinology to heart defects, thyroid problems, auditory deficiencies, coeliac disease and atlantoaxial instability. Some of these problems are already apparent at younger ages (even congenitally) and their consequences may extend over the life span. They need to be addressed from the first months or years as stressed in the devoted chapters. Two chapters in Section II deal with ageing in people with Down syndrome. There is a statistical likelihood of precocious ageing in these people for a complex of reasons, which are poorly understood as yet. Some of them are documented in Chapter 11. Chapter 12 is devoted to Alzheimer disease in Down syndrome. An as yet undefined proportion of Down syndrome persons present with a brain degenerative condition close or similar to Alzheimer disease beyond 40 years of age. Chapter 13 examines the facts and the myths surrounding the use of pharmacological agents and vitamins and minerals with persons with Down syndrome in order to alleviate some common disorders (e.g. thyroid problems, coeliac disease, blood disorders and malignancies) or to improve cognitive functioning (e.g. Sicca cell therapy, 5-hydroxytriptamine, dimethylsulphoxide, and more recently, piracetam).

Section III deals with cognition (particularly memory and language aspects) in adult and ageing years. Basic research points towards additional difficulties in shorter- and longer-term memories. It is less clear whether additional language difficulties are the rule in Down syndrome adults advancing in age. Such difficulties do not appear to be widely spread and marked until at least 50 years of age. Systematic data to assess the decline hypothesis are missing beyond that age. For those persons with Down syndrome exhibiting a degenerative process of the Alzheimer type, language degeneration seems to occur, even when good language levels existed prior to the start of the pathological process.

Section IV is devoted to several important issues related to sexual behaviour and contraception in Down syndrome adults, the role of siblings in helping Down syndrome adults when parents are no longer able to do so or are no longer there, professional orientation and work experiences of persons with Down syndrome in the open society. Two chapters (22 and 23) deal more particularly with the subject of continued rehabilitation in adults and ageing Down syndrome persons. Important intervention perspectives still exist at these ages, which have not been exploited on a large basis so far.

This book is only a beginning. We need much more information and research on almost every one of the topics introduced. There are a number of further questions regarding the life and problems of adults and older people with Down syndrome on which next to nothing is known at present. It is hoped that the book will stimulate more researchers and research agencies to address those issues that concern thousands of persons in the world and confront our ability and willingness as societies to do more than pay lip service to these people.

Jean-Adolphe Rondal
Alberto Rasore-Quartino
Salvatore Soresi

Contributors

G. Albertini, San Raffaele Pisana Clinic, Health Care and Rehabilitation Centres, Roma

G. Annerén, Department of Genetics, Uppsala University

G. Assenza, Istituto di Clinica Pediatrica, Università La Sapienza, Roma

X. Altafaj, Department of Physiology and Pharmacology, University of Cantabria, Santander

C. Baamonde, Department of Physiology and Pharmacology, University of Cantabria, Santander

C. Baccichetti, Dipartimento di Pediatrica, Ospedali di Padova

R. Benavides-Piccione, Department of Physiology and Pharmacology, University of Cantabria, Santander

M. Bonamico, Istituto di Clinica Pediatrica, Università La Sapienza, Roma

M. Carbone, Istituto di Clinica Pediatrica, Università di Siena

A. Contardi, Associazione Italiana Persone Down, Roma

L. Cottini, Dipartimento di Psicologia, Università d'Urbino

J. DeFelipe, Cajal Institute, Madrid

D. Devenny, Institute for Basic Research in Developmental Disabilities, New York

M. Dierssen, Cajal Institute, Madrid

M. Digilio, Istituto di Clinica Pediatrica, Università La Sapienza, Roma

L. Diociaiuti, Istituto di Clinica Pediatrica, Università Cattolica, Roma

P. Drigo, Dipartimento di Pediatrica, Ospedali di Padova

A. Egeo, Divisione di Neonatologia, Ospedali Galliera, Genova

G. Elston, Cajal Institute, Madrid

X. Estivill, Department of Physiology and Pharmacology, University of Cantabria, Santander

D. Fabris Monterumici, Dipartimento de Pediatrica, Ospedali di Padova

M. Ferri, Istituto di Clinica Pediatrica, Università La Sapienza, Roma

R. Ferri, Oasi Maria SS., Troina

C. **Fillat**, Department of Physiology and Pharmacology, University of Cantabria, Santander

J. **Flórez**, Department of Physiology and Pharmacology, University of Cantabria, Santander

H. **Goldstein**, Department of Preventive Medicine, Copenhagen University

J. **Gustafsson**, Department of Genetics, Uppsala University

C. **Jarrold**, Department of Psychology, University of Bristol

C. **Jenkins**, Department of Psychology, University of Portsmouth

E. **Kida**, Institute for Basic Research in Developmental Disabilities, New York

P. **Kittler**, Institute for Basic Research in Developmental Disabilities, New York

S. **Krinsky-McHale**, Institute for Basic Research in Developmental Disabilities, New York

J. **MacDonald**, Department of Psychology, University of Paisley

P. **Mariani**, Istituto di Clinica Pediatrica, Università La Sapienza, Roma

B. **Marino**, Istituto di Clinica Pediatrica, Università La Sapienza, Roma

M. **Martínez de Lagran**, Department of Physiology and Pharmacology, University of Cantabria, Santander

C. **Martínez-Cué**, Genomic Regulation Center, Barcelona

P. **Mastroiacovo**, International Center on Birth Defects, Roma

M. **Mazzocco**, Divisione di Neonatologia, Ospedali Galliera, Genova

M. **Medicina**, Institute of Otorhino-Laryngoiatry, University of Genova

S. **Miano**, Oasi Maria SS., Troina

F. **Mileto**, Istituto di Clinica Pediatrica, Università La Sapienza, Roma

Å. **Myrelid**, Department of Genetics, Uppsala University

A. **Moretti**, Centro Cepim/Unidown, Genova

A. **Mura**, Department of Surgical Specialties, Ospedali Galliera, Genova

R. **Nenna**, Istituto di Clinica Pediatrica, Università La Sapienza, Roma

L. **Nota**, Dipartimento di Psicologia dello Sviluppo, Università di Padova

J. **Perera**, Centro Principe de Asturias, Palma de Mallorca

A. **Rasore-Quartino**, Divisione di Neonatologia, Ospedali Galliera, Genova

C. **Romano**, Oasi Maria SS., Troina

J.A. **Rondal**, Secteur de Psycholinguistique, Université de Liège

A. **Rosano**, Istituto Italiano di Medicina Sociale, Roma

P. **Scartezzini**, Divisione di Neonatologia, Ospedali Galliera, Genova

M. **Sliwinski**, Department of Psychology, Syracuse University

S. **Soresi**, Dipartimento di Psicologia dello Sviluppo, Università di Padova

F. **Veglia**, Istituto di Psicologia, Università di Torino

S. **Vicari**, Ospedale Pediatrico Bambino Gèsu, Roma

K. **Wisniewski**, Institute for Basic Research in Developmental Disabilities, New York

SECTION I
EPIDEMIOLOGY

Chapter 1
Epidemiology of Down syndrome in the third millennium

P. Mastroiacovo, L. Diociaiuti, A. Rosano

Introduction

Over the last two decades, Down syndrome (DS) epidemiology in Europe and other countries has been influenced by three main factors that have determined a significant modification of incidence and prevalence:

- Changes in the distribution of maternal reproductive age
- The number of terminations of pregnancy after a prenatal diagnosis
- The decreased mortality in the early years of life and then a prolonged survival of persons with DS

This chapter presents data on the incidence of DS in Europe showing the influence of these factors, recent data on survival and main causes of mortality. Finally, in the absence of data on the whole population prevalence of DS, there is an exercise to estimate the prevalence in Italy.

Incidence

The real incidence of DS, as well as of other congenital anomalies, is actually unknown since all the conceived zygotes should be evaluated and counted.

Usually the best estimate of the incidence has been the 'birth prevalence': number of affected newborns (liveborns + stillborns) out of total number of newborns (x 1,000 or x 10,000) in a specific population and period of time.

Since the introduction of prenatal diagnosis and termination of pregnancies the concept of 'perinatal prevalence' should be introduced as the best estimate of the incidence.

Perinatal prevalence includes in the numerator:

1. Foetuses terminated during pregnancy after prenatal diagnosis, any gestational age
2. Stillborns and liveborns

and in the denominator it includes:

1. All stillborns and liveborns
2. All terminated pregnancies after prenatal diagnosis of DS
3. All terminated pregnancies after prenatal diagnosis for any other conditions

It should be noted that for some congenital disorders, such as DS and many other chromosomal anomalies, the perinatal prevalence is 'naturally' higher than birth prevalence since a proportion of foetuses, terminated after prenatal diagnosis would have been lost to a spontaneous abortion (Morris et al., 1999). So, perinatal prevalence and birth prevalence are not comparable. For example, time trend analysis based earlier on birth prevalence and then on perinatal prevalence will show a 'naturally' false increase. Similarly, comparison between a population where terminations of pregnancy are not allowed (only birth prevalence can be estimated) and a population where there is a high proportion of terminations of pregnancy (perinatal prevalence), is not sound.

Birth prevalence of Down syndrome in Europe

We are interested in knowing the birth prevalence of DS for two main reasons:

- To know the risk of having a child with DS
- To know how many children with DS are actually born in a population

The risk of having a child with DS is well known. It is similar in all studied populations (Carothers et al., 1999) and the best estimates have been given by Bray et al. (1998). Table 1.1 shows these data. They represent the risk of having a child with DS at birth (26–42 weeks of gestation). The risk of finding a DS foetus at 12–25 weeks of gestation through prenatal diagnosis is higher.

The next paragraphs concentrate on the 'observed' birth prevalence in some European countries.

Birth prevalence in recent years (1995–1999)

Table 1.2 gives the birth prevalence observed in the period 1995–1999 in some European countries as indicated by the existing birth defects registries at regional or national level (Eurocat Report 8, 2002; ICBDMS Annual Reports 1997–2001).

Table 1.1 Risk of Down syndrome at birth by maternal age (Bray et al., 1998)

Maternal age (y)	Risk 1 in	Rate x 1,000	CI 90% inf	CI 90% sup
16	1493	0.67	0.65	0.72
17	1486	0.67	0.65	0.73
18	1476	0.68	0.66	0.73
19	1462	0.68	0.66	0.73
20	1445	0.69	0.67	0.74
21	1423	0.70	0.68	0.75
22	1395	0.72	0.70	0.76
23	1359	0.74	0.72	0.78
24	1315	0.76	0.74	0.80
25	1259	0.79	0.77	0.83
26	1193	0.84	0.82	0.88
27	1115	0.90	0.87	0.93
28	1025	0.97	0.95	1.01
29	926	1.08	1.04	1.12
30	821	1.22	1.17	1.26
31	714	1.40	1.33	1.45
32	608	1.64	1.56	1.70
33	508	1.97	1.86	2.03
34	416	2.40	2.26	2.47
35	336	2.97	2.79	3.06
36	268	3.72	3.50	3.83
37	211	4.73	4.46	4.85
38	164	6.06	5.72	6.22
39	127	7.82	7.39	8.05
40	97	10.15	9.58	10.49
41	75	13.24	12.45	13.76
42	57	17.31	16.22	18.11
43	43	22.67	21.12	23.93
44	33	29.70	27.50	31.65
45	25	38.89	35.80	41.84
46	19	50.83	46.48	55.24
47	14	66.26	60.23	72.69
48	8	110.97	100.05	124.01
50	6	142.13	127.61	159.87

CI = confidence interval, inf = inferior limit, sup = superior limit

The range is wide: between 5.6 per 10,000 births in Hungary and 21.6 in Dublin. The wide range is due to various reasons: the legislation and extent of terminations of pregnancies, the frequency of total births by maternal age (mainly over 35 years) and the completeness of the reporting. The extent of terminations of pregnancy and the proportion of total births from mothers aged 35 years or more are given in Table 1.2. The completeness of reporting is difficult to estimate.

Table 1.2 Birth prevalence in some European registries in the 5-year period 1995–1999 (data from Eurocat Report 8 and ICBDMS Annual Reports 1997–2001)

Registries	Birth prevalence crude rate x 10,000	Total birth by 35+ year mothers (%)	Termination of pregnancy (%)
Hungary	5.6	7.5	67
Antwerp (Belgium)	5.8	9.7	44
England and Wales	6	10.2	55
Czech Republic	6.2	7.9	57
Southern Portugal	6.2	11.3	17
Barcelona (Spain)	6.3	22.1	69
Strasbourg (France)	7.1	12.5	67
Vaud (Switzerland)	7.1	15.8	71
Styria (Austria)	7.6	9.9	43
Campania (Italy)	7.7	12.4	43
Tuscany (Italy)	7.7	18	55
Northeast (Italy)	7.9	17.7	50
Central East France	7.9	18.6	60
Paris (France)	8	23.9	76
Hainaut (Belgium)	8.1	10.9	56
Emilia Romagna (Italy)	8.8	17	18
Saxony-Anhalt (Germany)	9.1	14.3	49
Northern Netherlands	10.2	14.1	31
Mersey (UK)	10.3	13.2	43
Norway	10.4	12.1	12
Wales (UK)	10.6	14.9	43
Glasgow (UK)	10.7	14.3	37
Finland	11	9.3	51
North Thames West (UK)	11.9	11	50
Asturias (Spain)	12.7	18.2	38
Basque Country (Spain)	13.9	23.8	53
Dublin (Ireland)	21.3	18.7	0

Time trend

Time trend has been extensively analysed in the reports of the two main organizations acting in the field of birth defects epidemiology: EUROCAT and ICBDMS (Eurocat Report 8, 2002; ICBDMS Annual Reports 1997–2001).

In Table 1.3 we present the changes observed between the most recent 5-year period (1995–1999) and the oldest 5-year periods available.

The observed decreases in birth prevalence are due mainly to the extent of terminations of pregnancy (e.g. Emilia Romagna in Italy). The observed increases are due to the increase of maternal age over 35 years (e.g. Dublin in Ireland). The precise impact of terminations of pregnancy after prenatal diagnosis should, however, be analysed on standardized rates by maternal age, which is not possible with the available published

Table 1.3 Change in the birth prevalence in some European registries. The oldest 5-year period available is compared with the latest period 1995–1999, the same for all registries (Data from Eurocat Report 8 and ICBDMS Annual Reports 1997–2001)

Registries	Period	Oldest period available	1995–1999	Change (%)
Hungary	1974–1979	8.9	5.6	−37§
Czech Republic	1974–1979	8.4	6.2	−26§
England and Wales	1974–1979	7.0	6.1	−13§
Central East France	1974–1979	11.3	7.8	−31§
Emilia Romagna (Italy)	1974–1979	21.6	8.8	−59§
Norway	1974–1979	9.8	10.4	+6
Strasbourg (France)	1980–1984	9.4	7.1	−24§
Northeast (Italy)	1980–1984	13.9	7.9	−43§
Paris (France)	1980–1984	11.5	8	−30§
Hainaut (Belgium)	1980–1984	8.8	8.1	−8
Saxony-Anhalt (Germany)	1980–1984	8.5	9.1	+7
Northern Netherlands	1980–1984	9.8	10.2	+4
Spain	1980–1984	14.4	10.7	−26§
Glasgow (UK)	1980–1984	9.8	10.7	+9
Dublin (Ireland)	1980–1984	18.2	21.3	+17§
Styria (Austria)	1986–1990	8.6	7.6	−11
Vaud (Switzerland)	1989–1993	9.3	7.1	−24§
Antwerp (Belgium)	1990–1994	10.9	5.8	−46§
Southern Portugal	1990–1994	8.6	6.2	−28
Campania (Italy)	1990–1994	10.0	8.2	−18§
Tuscany (Italy)	1990–1994	9.8	7.7	−21§
Asturias (Spain)	1990–1994	11.8	12.7	+8
Basque Country (Spain)	1990–1994	13.1	13.9	+6
Barcelona (Spain)	1992–1996	8.6	6.3	−26§

§ = statistically significant ($p < 0.01$)

data. Moreover a precise analysis is hampered by the change of completeness of reporting over the years.

Survival

The survival of persons with DS has progressively increased from 1955 to today (Table 1.4). The best improvement has been observed in the first year of life. For example the cohort of children born in the early 1950s had a 1-year survival of 50%; recently this figure has increased to 90%. The main factor for this improvement has been the medical treatment of infections (pneumonia and gastroenteritis) and the surgical treatment of congenital heart diseases.

In various countries we can now predict a survival at 5 years of around 85%. After this period, mortality is not high and the median survival (the age at which 50% of subjects are expected to die), according to the Baird and Sadovnick (1987) life table, is estimated to be 58 years.

Table 1.4 Survival rates at 1 and 5 years of children with Down syndrome. Year identifies the mean year of birth of the studied cohort

Author	Year	No	Country	1-y	5-y
Record and Smith, 1955	1948	252	UK	44%	40%
Carter, 1958	1951	725	UK	43%	40%
Collmann and Stoller, 1964	1953	729	Australia	53%	49%
Fabia and Drolette, 1970	1959	2,421	USA	71%	65%
Baird and Sadovnick, 1987	1967	600	Canada	88%	81%
Fryers and Mackay, 1979	1970	50	UK	83%	77%
Masaki et al., 1981	1971	1,052	Japan	95%	87%
Mulcahy, 1979	1977	231	Australia	81%	75%
Frid et al., 1999	1977	219	Sweden	85%	–
Malone, 1988	1981	149	Australia	97%	89%
Bell et al., 1989	1981	366	Australia	88%	81%
Mastroiacovo et al., 1992	1982	917	Italy	84%	76%
Mikkelsen et al., 1990	1982	278	Denmark	80%	74%
Hayes et al., 1997	1985	389	Ireland	88%	82%
Leonard et al., 2000	1988	440	Australia	92%	87%
Castilla et al., 1998	1991	360	S. America	74%	–
Mastroiacovo, 2002	1990	2,013	Italy	88%	82%
Leonard et al., 2000	1989	129	Australia	92%	86%
Nembhard et al., 2001	1996	456	USA	92%	–

Mortality

The leading causes of death among people with DS are congenital heart disease and pneumonia. Table 1.5 shows the underlying causes of death compiled by the US Center for Disease Control and Prevention National Center for Health Statistics for 1983–1997 (Yang et al., 2002).

Table 1.5 Diseases associated with death of persons with Down syndrome, not reciprocally exclusive and not only causes of death (Yang et al., 2002)

Disease	Proportion
Aspiration, pneumonia, influenza	29%
Congenital heart defects	28%
Seizure disorders	9%
Ischaemic heart disease	7%
Infectious and parasitic diseases	7%
Diseases of pulmonary circulation	6%
Other congenital anomalies	3%
Dementia	6%
Hypothyroidism	3%
Diabetes	3%
Leukaemia	2%
Other malignancy	2%
Sudden infant death syndrome	0.2%

Congenital heart disease (CHD) is the principal factor influencing survival in the first year of life. In the Hijii et al. study (1997), the 24-year survival rate was 92.2% in the group without CHD, and 74.6% in the group with CHD.

The CHD subjects who underwent surgical correction presented a 24-year survival similar to the non-CHD subjects (87.8%), while those with CHD who did not undergo surgery presented a 41.4% survival rate.

Prevalence of Down syndrome in the general population

In the absence of specific surveys on the prevalence of DS in the general population in Europe, we have estimated the prevalence of DS subjects in Italy today. This is mainly an exercise and a rough estimation. We have:

1. Estimated the birth prevalence rates between 1930 and 1978 using the so-called biological rates (see Table 1.1) and the distribution of total births by maternal age (ISTAT, 1986), assuming no relevant influence of prenatal diagnosis and ToP
2. Used the birth prevalence rates given by the Italian birth defects registry from 1978 up to 1999 (ICBDMS 1978–1999 Annual reports). The figures in 1978–1979 were identical to those estimated by the biological rates; after this period, the figures were lower because of the increasing extent of terminations of pregnancy after prenatal diagnosis (see Figure 1.1)
3. Used the life table published by Baird and Sadovnick (1988) assuming that the survival at 1 year was 30% for the cohort of persons born in 1930 and 88% in 1987 (as observed) with an increase in survival of 1%

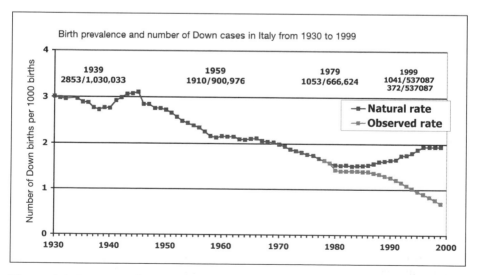

Figure 1.1 Estimates of Down syndrome subjects in Italy from 1930 to 2000. Source: Mastroiacovo (ICBDMS)

each year. So, for example, in 1960 we estimated a survival at 1 year of 60% and in 1980 of 80%. Actually, as shown in Table 1.4, in Italy we estimated a survival at 1 year of 84% for a cohort born around 1982

4. Used the Italian age distribution in the general population (ISTAT, 2001)
5. Estimated, using the data above, the dynamic and age structure of Down population from 1930 to 1999

The main results of this exercise are given in Table 1.6. It can be seen that in Italy:

1. The total number of persons with DS is around 38,000; that means 1 in 1,500 persons in the Italian population
2. The highest prevalence is in the 15–44 years age group, 1 in 900–1000 persons
3. 61% of persons with DS are more than 25 years of age

Table 1.6 Estimated prevalence of Down syndrome subjects in Italy (1999) and their age distribution

Age interval (years)	Number	Proportion %	Prevalence
0–6	2,346	6.1	1 in 1,367
6–14	4,495	11.8	1 in 1,030
15–24	7,335	19.2	1 in 967
25–44	17,857	46.8	1 in 987
45+	5,589	14.7	1 in 4,391
Total	**38,122**	**100**	**1 in 1,511**

The most important point of this exercise is that it can be applied to other populations if appropriate assumptions are used.

References

Baird PA, Sadovnick AD (1987) Life expectancy in Down syndrome. J Pediatr 110: 849.

Baird PA, Sadovnick AD (1988) Life expectancy in Down syndrome adults. Am J Hum Genet 43: 239.

Baird PA, Sadovnick AD (1989) Life tables for Down syndrome. Hum Genet 82: 291.

Bell JA, Pearn JH, Firman D (1989) Childhood deaths in Down's syndrome. Survival curves and causes of death from a total population study in Queensland, Australia, 1976 to 1985. J Med Genet 26: 764

Bray I, Wright DE, Davies C, Hook EB (1998) Joint estimation of Down syndrome risk and ascertainment rates: a meta-analysis of nine published data sets. Prenat Diagn 18: 9.

Carothers AD, Hecht CA, Hook EB (1999) International variation in reported live-birth prevalence rates of Down syndrome, adjusted for maternal age. J Med Genet 36: 386.

Carter CO (1958) A life table for Mongols with the causes of death. J Ment Defic Res 2: 64.

Castilla EE, Rittler M, Dutra MdG, Lopez-Camelo JS, Campana H, Paz JE, Orioli IM, ECLAMC-Downsurv Group (1998) Survival of children with Down syndrome in South America. Am J Med Genet 79: 108.

Collmann RD, Stoller A (1964) A life table for Mongols in Victoria, Australia. J Ment Defic Res 7: 53.

Eurocat Report 8. University of Ulster 2002 www.eurocat.ulster.ac.uk

Fabia J, Drolette M (1970) Life tables up to age 10 for mongols with and without congenital heart defect. J Ment Defic Res 14: 235.

Frid C, Drott P, Lundell B, Rasmussen F, Anneren G (1999) Mortality in Down's syndrome in relation to congenital malformations. J Intellect Disab Res 43: 234.

Fryers T, Mackay RI (1979) Down syndrome: prevalence at birth, mortality and survival. A 17-year study. Early Hum Dev 3: 29.

Hayes C, Johnson Z, Thornton L, Fogarty J, Lyons R, O'Connor M, Delany V, Buckley K (1997) Ten-year survival of Down syndrome births. Int J Epid 26: 822

Hijii T, Fukushige J, Igarashi H, Takahashi N, Ueda K (1997) Life expectancy and social adaptation in individuals with Down syndrome with and without surgery for congenital heart disease. Clin Pediatr 36: 327.

ICBDMS Annual Report 1997–2001, ICBD Roma www.icbd.org.

ISTAT Sommario di statistiche storiche 1926–1985, pp. 42–3. Ed. ISTAT, 1986.

ISTAT Popolazione residente per sesso, età e regione al 1° gennaio 1999. Ed. ISTAT, Roma, 2001

Leonard S, Bower C, Petterson B, Leonard H (2000) Survival of infants born with Down's syndrome: 1980–1996. Paediatr Perinat Epidemiol 14: 163.

Malone Q (1988) Mortality and survival of the Down's syndrome population in Western Australia. J Ment Defic Res 32: 59.

Masaki M, Higurashi M, Iijima K, Ishikawa N, Tanaka F, Fujii T, Kuroki Y, Matsui I, Iiinuma K, Matsuo N, Takeshita K, Hashimoto S (1981) Mortality and survival for Down syndrome in Japan. Am J Hum Genet 33: 629.

Mastroiacovo P, Bertollini R, Corchia C (1992) Survival of children with Down syndrome in Italy. Am J Med Genet 42: 208.

Mastroiacovo P (2002) Personal communication.

Mikkelsen M, Poulsen H, Nielson KG (1990) Incidence, survival and mortality in Down syndrome in Denmark. Am J Med Genet Supp 7: 75.

Morris JK, Wald NJ, Watt HC (1999) Fetal loss in Down syndrome pregnancies. Prenat Diagn 19: 142.

Mulcahy MT (1979) Down's syndrome in Western Australia: mortality and survival. Clin Genet 16: 103.

Nembhard WN, Waller DK, Sever LE, Canfield MA (2001) Patterns of first-year survival among infants with selected congenital anomalies in Texas, 1995–1997. Teratology 64: 267.

Record RG, Smith A (1955) Incidence, mortality and sex distribution of mongoloid defectives. Br J Prev Soc Med 9: 10.

Yang Q, Rasmussen SA, Friedman JM (2002) Mortality associated with Down's syndrome in the USA from 1983 to 1997: a population-based study. The Lancet 359: 1019.

SECTION II
GENETIC, BIOLOGICAL, MEDICAL AND PHARMACOLOGICAL ISSUES

Chapter 2
Genotype–phenotype neural correlates in trisomy 21

M. Dierssen, R. Benavides-Piccione, C. Martínez-Cué, X. Estivill, C. Baamonde, C. Fillat, M. Martínez de Lagrán, X. Altafaj, J. Flórez, G. Elston, J. DeFelipe

Down syndrome (DS) is the most common genetic cause of mental handicap, affecting 1 in 1,000 newborn children in Europe (Hassold and Jacobs, 1984; Mastroiacovo, 2002). Subjects with DS show several CNS abnormalities. At a gross morphological level, DS brains are smaller than normal, and the depth and number of sulci are reduced. Neuronal density is decreased in distinct regions, including the cochlear nuclei, cerebellum, hippocampus, basal forebrain, the granular layers of the neocortex and areas of the brainstem; abnormal neuronal morphology is observed, especially in the neocortex (reviewed in Flórez, 1992). More recently, smaller overall brain volumes with disproportionately smaller cerebellar and frontal lobe volumes have been reported (Pinter et al., 2001). Some of these alterations may be related to an abnormal development of the nervous system during pre- and post-natal life. In foetuses, a reduction in the width of the cortex and abnormal cortical lamination patterns, altered dendritic arbors and dendritic spines, altered electrophysiological properties of membranes, reduced synaptic density and abnormal synaptic morphology have been described (Becker et al., 1986, 1993; Marin-Padilla, 1976; Suetsugu and Mehraein, 1980; Takashima et al., 1981; Ferrer and Guillota, 1990).

Defining how an extra copy of all or part of chromosome 21 (HSA21) results in the phenotype of DS is a specific case of the more general problem of explaining how chromosomal imbalance produces abnormalities in morphology and function. No single mechanism can explain the deleterious consequences of aneuploidy and, therefore, there is no simple solution to counteract its phenotypic impact. While some loci may have a greater phenotypic effect, it is the cumulative effect of imbalance of many genes that determines the overall phenotype. Two hypotheses have been proposed to explain the DS phenotype:

1. The amplified developmental instability hypothesis (Shapiro, 1999, 2001) suggests that the DS phenotype is the result of a non-specific disturbance of chromosome balance, resulting in a disruption of homeostasis
2. The gene dosage hypothesis proposes that DS phenotypes may stem directly from the cumulative effect of overexpression of specific chromosome 21 gene products or indirectly through the interaction of these HSA21 genes products with the whole genome, transcriptome or proteome

Evidence from different murine models points to specific genes affecting phenotypes rather than the non-specific effect of the amount of extra genetic material (see Pritchard and Kola, 1999, for review).

Based on the analysis of human individuals with segmental trisomy 21, it has been proposed that genetic loci situated in the DS critical region (DSCR) could harbour genes with major effect. However, the resolution of this approach is limited by the high phenotypic variation among DS individuals, and, to date, no convincing evidence exists of association between any particular phenotypic trait and overexpression of a specific HSA21 gene. The availability of the DNA sequence of HSA21 (Hattori et al., 2000), will have an immediate impact on the study of the genetic aspects of DS by providing a comprehensive catalogue of the genes on HSA21. However, the functions of most of these genes remain largely unknown, as does their contribution, if any, to the DS phenotype. Even knowing the molecular defect, it is difficult to decipher the complex pathophysiology of the disease, the developmental consequences of the trisomy and the impact on behaviour and cognitive function. Thus we are now facing a new era, the postgenomics, in which the goal will be to identify protein function and the physiological role of gene products. The generation of animal models that provide ready access to cells and tissues from different developmental stages of the disease is a powerful tool to help us understand the role of individual genes in DS and some of the clinical alterations observed in DS.

Various approaches have been used to study the consequences of increased gene dosage in DS and to investigate phenotype–genotype relationships of HSA21 genes in mice:

1. Transgenic animals overexpressing single or combinations of genes
2. Transgenic mice with large foreign DNA pieces introduced on yeast artificial chromosomes (YACs) or bacterial artificial chromosomes in mice

3. Mouse models that carry all or part of MMU16 which has regions of
conserved homology with HSA21

The use of transgenesis for modelling Down syndrome

The use of transgenic techniques to model human disease has led to
major advances in our understanding of pathogenic mechanisms, but has
also highlighted the limitations of conventional transgenic methodology
for the production of accurate animal models, and the difficulties associated with modelling human pathophysiology in mice. Important issues
are the use of the same genetic background (Gerlai, 1996), but also a
good phenotypic characterization, based on standardized protocols
(Crawley and Paylor, 1997; Rogers et al., 1997).

Although overexpressing a single gene will not be a model of DS, the
value of single gene transgenesis is to identify genes related to specific
pathophysiological features. The development and analysis of transgenic
mice that overexpress single genes, either with their own genomic
regions for gene regulation and expression, or with heterologous pro-
moter sequences that drive the expression of the genes in specific tissues,
permits, to some extent, the study of the contribution of each gene to the
phenotype. The gene content of HSA21 has been estimated as 225 genes
and 59 pseudogenes. Of these, 127 correspond to known genes (Hattori
et al., 2000). However, to date only a few HSA21 encoded genes have
been used to make transgenic mice (see Kola and Hertzog, 1997;
Pritchard and Kola, 1999 for review). The selection of candidate genes is
done on the basis of their location in the chromosomal region that has
been considered critical for the development of the syndrome, the previous knowledge of the functions of the proteins that they encode, or their
spatiotemporal pattern of expression.

Mouse trisomies

Orthologous genes are frequently linked in similarly conserved chromosomal segments in the mouse and human genomes (Mouse Genome
Database: http://www.informatics.jax.org). For this reason, aneuploidy for
regions of the mouse genome that are conserved on human chromosomes can serve to study the concerted effect of over- (or under-)
expression of multiple genes. HSA21 shows conserved syntenies to
mouse chromosomes 16, 17 and 10 (Hattori et al., 2000). Comparative
mapping between mice and humans has revealed that HSA21 shares a
large region of genetic homology with MMU16. Based on this rationale,
mice trisomic for MMU16 have been extensively used as a model for
DS. The trisomy models have the advantage that they overexpress the

orthologues of multiple genes located on HSA21, which permits the study of how arrays of genes interact to control each other at the level of transcription. Hence their power lies in modelling and characterizing the syndrome (or a part of it) and in testing therapeutic strategies.

The first mice used had the complete MMU16 in three copies (Ts16 mice). However, more recently, two partial trisomic mice have been generated named Ts65Dn (Davisson et al., 1990) and Ts1CjE (Sago et al., 1998). Using double heterozygosity for homobrachial Robertsonian chromosomes, murine trisomies can be produced at reasonably high frequencies. When male mice with balanced bilateral Robertsonian translocations of MMU16 (e.g. the fusion of MMU16 with another chromosome) are mated with normal females, approximately one-third of the progeny surviving to 15 days gestation have trisomy 16 (Ts16), whereas two-thirds are euploid (Gearhart et al., 1986). These mice exhibit some characteristics of DS, but their value is limited by several factors. First, Ts16 mice die *in utero*. This inability to survive is an insurmountable obstacle to the study of many of the major features that occur as part of the DS phenotype postnatally (e.g. mental handicap, thyroid disturbances) or even much later in life (e.g. Alzheimer's disease neuropathology). In addition, MMU16 contains a large number of genes whose human counterparts are located on chromosomes other than HSA21 (3, 16, 22) and several genes located on the distal end of the long arm of HSA21 which are thought to be essential for the DS phenotype are not located on MMU16. Thus, Ts16 mice are not trisomic for some HSA21 genes and are at a dosage imbalance for other genes not implicated in the pathogenesis of DS.

In spite of all these shortcomings, the Ts16 model has the advantage over other MMU16-related models (see below) in that the mice show characteristic cardiac as well as craniofacial and ocular malformations, much more like those observed in individuals with DS (Oster-Granite, 1986). With regard to the heart, the trisomy produces endocardial cushion defects (Miyabara et al., 1984) and vascular malformations related to the embryonic aortic arch system. Delays are also found in the development of the sphenoid, mandible and maxilla, as well as distortions of the cervical vertebrae and alterations in the development of the inner ear. Significant and complex alterations are observed in the morphogenesis and neurochemistry of the brain, as well as in the properties of the cultured neurons (Coyle et al., 1991; Oster-Granite and Lacey-Casem, 1995). Common alterations have been also described in the development of the cerebellum, hippocampus, cortical plate and ocular structures including a reduction of periorbital connective tissue and micro-ophthalmia (Grausz et al., 1991). Finally, morphogenetic abnormalities have been described during embryonic development of the Ts16 neocortex (Haydar et al., 2000); these depend on altered proliferative characteristics during Ts16 neurogenesis, resulting in a delay in the generation of neocortical neurons, and on a deficit in founder cells, leading to proportional reduction in the overall number of neurons (Haydar et al., 2000). Many of the features described are qualitatively similar to those appearing in individuals with DS.

Recently, three viable models bearing an extra copy of a part of MMU16 have been produced: Ts65Dn mice contain three copies of MMU16 from *App* to *Mx1*, Ts1Cje mice have three copies from *Sod1* to *Mx1* and Ms1Ts65 from *App* to *Sod1*. These mice show some of the DS phenotypes, mostly learning and behavioural abnormalities.

Ts65Dn partial trisomy model

The generation by Davisson et al. (1990) of a partial trisomy 16 mouse, the Ts(17[16])65Dn or Ts65Dn model, that includes most of the MMU16 region homologous to HSA21 (from *App* to *Mx1*) but lacks the remaining approximately 40% of HSA21 genes, represents a major advance in mouse models. This model is viable and a high percentage of the mice reach old age. Production of adult mice trisomic for specific segments was based on two facts:

- Mice heterozygous for reciprocal translocation chromosomes, where the translocation chromosomes are small, can produce progeny trisomic for the small translocation product
- Mice trisomic for small chromosomal segments usually survive to adulthood

Reciprocal translocations were induced by irradiating the testes of DBA/2J mice. The males were mated immediately to C57BL/6J females to recover radiation damage induced in spermatids and spermatozoa. F1 progeny from these matings were screened for chromosomal aberrations in females (peripheral lymphocytes) and males (testis).

Several translocations involving MMU16 can be produced with translocation breakpoints spaced along the entire length of the chromosome since Ts65Dn has the distal tip (16C4–> ter) of MMU16 with centromeric material from MMU17. Mice carrying chromosomal aberrations were mated to B6 mice to determine whether they were fertile and to recover the translocation products. Female mice heterozygous for reciprocal translocations, in which one translocation product is very small, often produce offspring trisomic for the genetic segments contained in the small marker chromosome. Stocks for the translocations were maintained by mating the carriers to B6 or a B6 X C3H/HeJ (B6C3H) F1 hybrid. The fact that the Ts65Dn are on a segregating background involving two inbred strains, adds variability to the phenotype. However, behavioural effects found in these mice have been quite robust and findings across laboratories show considerable agreement.

Although many overexpressed genes in Ts65Dn are homologous to those included in the DSCR, these mice do not show many of the gross abnormalities frequently observed in DS, such as cardiac valvular congenital abnormalities (Montero et al., 1996); however, analogous effects on craniofacial structures have been reported in Ts65Dn mice (Richtsmeier et al., 2000). Ts65Dn thymuses exhibit greater programmed cell death activity than controls, and Ts65Dn thymocytes are highly susceptible to programmed cell death induced by LPS and dexamethasone (Paz-Miguel et al., 1999). Thymus abnormalities are probably caused by *Sod1* hyperexpression, in that reactive oxygen intermediate generation is enhanced in thymocytes and clearly correlates with apoptosis. Ts65Dn mice also exhibit other features comparable to those found in DS.

Cognitive and motor function

Cognitive deficits have been consistently demonstrated in the Ts65Dn model, including spatial learning that requires the integration of visual and spatial information (Escorihuela et al., 1995; Reeves et al., 1994), as well as working memory and long-term memory (Escorihuela et al., 1998). However, extensive training may facilitate the achievement of levels of performance as high as in control mice. Other behavioural anomalies are also present in Ts65Dn mice. They show consistent hyperactivity, reduced attention levels (Escorihuela et al., 1995; Reeves et al., 1994; Coussons-Read and Crnic, 1996; Holtzman et al., 1996), and reduced responsiveness to nociceptive stimuli (Martínez-Cué et al., 1999).

The motor impairments in the Ts65Dn mice are controversial. Costa et al. (1999) found mild to severe motor dysfunction, with the most evident impairments related to equilibrium and motor coordination, a finding which agrees with reported clinical observations made on individuals with DS. In contrast, Baxter et al. (2000, see below) report no impairment on a variety of motor tests, in spite of the finding of cerebellar abnormalities in the Ts65Dn mice. Recently, spontaneous and persistent stereotypic behaviour was found to be part of the behavioural phenotype of the Ts65Dn (Lewis et al., 1999). The molecular basis for these anomalies is not clear.

There have been few therapeutic attempts on the Ts65Dn mice. However, recently, the effects of enriched environment applied to pups for 7 weeks after weaning upon behavioural and cognitive performances have been assessed in the partially trisomic Ts65Dn mice (Martínez-Cué et al., 2002). Environmental enrichment induced a slight but significant improvement of performance in Ts65Dn females but deteriorated performance in Ts65Dn male mice in the Morris water maze, indicating that gender is a factor that plays a modulatory role in the influence of this treatment (Martínez-Cué et al., 2002).

Neurochemical and anatomical studies

Neurochemical studies have revealed functional abnormalities in the central noradrenergic system in the cerebral cortex and hippocampus but not in the cerebellum. In these regions, basal as well as stimulated production of cyclic AMP (cAMP) was reduced (Dierssen et al., 1996, 1997), and this reduction in adenyl cyclase efficacy may account for the disturbed cognitive achievement seen in Ts65Dn mice. Abnormal patterns of phospholipase C functioning in several brain areas of the Ts65Dn mice have also been detected. Adenyl cyclase and phospholipase C signalling pathways are also severely disturbed in the brain of DS and Alzheimer's disease patients, though the response of DS brains to serotonergic and cholinergic stimulation was significantly depressed, and that of Alzheimer's disease brains was only to cholinergic stimulation (Ruiz de Azúa et al., 2001). These findings further strengthen the validity of this aneuploid mouse as a model for DS.

Stereological morphometric studies have also demonstrated minor irregularities in some regions of the hippocampus of Ts65Dn mice, including reductions in the volume of CA2 and in the neuronal density in the dentate gyrus (Insausti et al., 1998). Holtzman et al. (1996) have found an age-related degeneration of septohippocampal cholinergic neurons and astrocytic hypertrophy, which are Alzheimer's like changes also found in DS individuals. These investigators found that basal forebrain cholinergic neurons were normal at weaning, but had significant loss by 6 months of age that was also evident at later ages. Granholm et al. (2000) showed that these neurons were normal in number and size up to 4 months of age but were significantly reduced in number and size by 6 months of age and thereafter. In addition, a decline in performance on a spatial reversal task corresponded to the loss in cholinergic phenotype in medial septal neurons.

A significantly lower number (30%) of asymmetrical synapses (presumptive excitatory synapses) was detected in the temporal cortex of Ts65Dn mice without difference in symmetrical synapses (presumptive inhibitory synapses). However, the mean synaptic apposition lengths of both asymmetrical and symmetrical synapses were significantly larger in Ts65Dn mice (15% and 11%, respectively), suggesting that excitatory synapses are preferentially affected in Ts65Dn mice and that there is an attempt to compensate for the deficit of asymmetrical synapses by increasing the contact zone area of existing synapses (Kurt et al., 2000). Finally, high-resolution magnetic resonance imaging and histological analysis revealed neuroanatomical parallels between DS and Ts65Dn cerebellum (Baxter et al., 2000). Cerebellar volume is reduced in Ts65Dn mice due to a reduction of both the internal granular layer and the molecular layer, with a parallel reduction in granule cell numbers.

Ts1Cje murine model

A second partial trisomy 16 model has recently been developed, termed Ts1Cje mouse (Sago et al., 1998). This model is trisomic for a smaller region of MMU16 from *Sod1* to *Mx1*. The Ts1Cje mouse was derived during *Sod1* gene targeting and involves an MMU12:16 reciprocal translocation and thus has a diploid chromosome number. Heterozygous *Sod1* mutant mice were found to segregate aberrantly when crossed to wild type animals. FISH studies of the heterozygous *Sod1* mutants revealed a translocation between MMU16 proximal to *Sod1* and the very distal region of MMU12. The balanced carriers for the translocation designated Ts(12;16)1Cje have one each of the normal chromosomes MMU12 and MMU16 in addition to the 12^{16} and 16^{12} translocation chromosomes. Partial trisomy of the distal region of MMU16, the Ts1Cje mouse, is generated when a gamete carrying MMU12^{16} and MMU16 combines with a normal gamete carrying MMU12 and MMU16. In addition, few if any of the telomeric genes on MMU12 were missing from the 12^{16} chromosome. Therefore Ts1Cje appears to be trisomic only for the segment of the distal region of MMU16, but because the *Sod1* allele on MMU12 is disrupted by the neomycine resistance sequence, the Ts1Cje animals are not functionally trisomic for *Sod1*.

Ts1Cje mice survive to adulthood and present no apparent limb or facial malformations or other dysmorphic features. Contrary to Ts65Dn, Ts1Cje mice do not show hyperactivity, but rather they are hypoactive. They do not display stereotypic behaviour and their learning deficits are less severe. They perform efficiently in the Morris water maze when the platform is visible, but they show impairment in the hidden platform and probe tests, and in the reverse platform test (Sago et al., 1998). In fact, the learning impairment in Ts1Cje mice is less severe than that found in Ts65Dn animals, but stronger than in the Ms1Ts65 or in the YAC152Ftel transgenic mice that contain YACs a genomic fragment to which *Dyrk1A* was found to map. Ts1Cje mice do not demonstrate the neuronal atrophy found in Ts65Dn, suggesting that the region from *App* to *Sod1* is required for this neuropathological trait. The only known genes in these regions are *App*, associated with Alzheimer's disease and *Grik1*, whose product, the GluR5 kainate receptor regulates synaptic transmission.

Ms1Ts65

To assess the contribution of the segment of MMU16 from proximal to *App* to *Sod1* to the phenotype of Ts65Dn, a new partial trisomic model has recently been generated (Sago et al., 1998) that has three copies of the region covering *App* to *Sod1*. It is called Ms1Ts65. Since the impact of mouse strain on the effects of a transgene or a segmental trisomy can be substantial, the comparison between the three existing segmental trisomic models has been carried out on the same genetic background. Ms1Ts65 mice present a much less severe phenotypic impact than the longer segmental trisomies. The results showed no visible platform deficits on the Morris maze of any of the trisomics. Thus, the phenotype of the Ts65Dn appears to be lessened by the addition of another strain (CD-1) to the background. Results on the hidden platform and reversal phases of the Morris maze task show increasing deficits as the size of the trisomic segment increases, i.e. the Ts65Dn mice are impaired compared to diploid controls on more measures than the Ts1Cje mice, who are in turn less impaired than the Ms1Cje mice. In other words, the Morris maze deficit does not appear to track with either of the smaller segments of the MMU16 region. Nor did activity, as the Ts1Cje mice were hypoactive, but the MS1Ts65 mice were not hyperactive. Thus, it is clear that genes from both sub-regions must interact to produce the phenotype of the Ts65Dn mouse.

Finally, a new strategy has been reported that involves the transference of a human chromosome into mice, through the mouse germ line (Tomizuca et al., 1997). These mice carry all or part of HSA21 as a freely segregating extra chromosome. To produce these 'transchromosomal' animals, a selectable marker is placed into HSA21 and the chromosome is transferred from a human somatic cell line into mouse ES cells using irradiation microcell-mediated chromosome transfer. Transchromosomal ES cells containing different HSA21 regions ranging in size from 50 to approximately 0.2 Mb are then used to create chimeric mice. These mice maintain HSA21 sequences and express HSA21 genes in multiple tissues (Hernández et al., 1999), and could be particularly useful for modelling human aneuploidy syndromes and to provide a qualitatively different approach for the study of the pathology of trisomy 21. Recently (Inoue et al., 2000), a chimeric mouse carrying an HSA21 has been generated. In this mouse specific cardiovascular malformations and delayed cardiomyocyte differentiation were observed; these were restored following the deletion of a specific region of HSA21.

Environmental enrichment effects in the Ts65Dn mouse

Early studies of the intact brain using Golgi impregnated material, attempted to correlate changes in dendritic spine morphology with development, enriched environment and ageing, with the rationale being that these conditions may exert major changes in brain structure and function (Rosenzweig et al., 1972; Volkmar and Greenough, 1972). These studies correlated experience with an increase in the spine density, as well as in the complexity of dendritic arborization and in the length of cortical dendrites. In our experimental design, euploid, non-trisomic mice exposed to an enriched environment presented an increase in the dendritic complexity and the number of spines. The differences with previously published work may be due to the species differences, since there are no previous data in the literature on this particular aspect in mice. Alternatively, the methodology used in the present experiments, which allows the visualization and quantification of the whole dendritic tree, may also account for the described differences, since previous studies used Golgi staining, a technique that does not allow quantitative analysis.

Exposure to an enriched environment (EE) enhances performance in learning, memory and visual acuity tasks, suggesting that circuits are modified in order to optimize multiple levels of information processing and storage (Fernández-Teruel et al., 1997; Prusky et al., 2000). Our previous study showed that exposure to complex environments has the capacity to modulate behaviour and spatial memory of Ts65Dn and euploid mice (Martinez-Cué el al., 2002). However, these functional effects are shown not to be correlated with modifications in the morphology of the pyramidal neurons, either in the dendritic arborization or in the number of spines in the EE trisomic mice (Dierssen et al., 2003). On the contrary, the euploid mice presented an increase in their arbor complexity and spine number that may account for the better performance observed in some behavioural tasks (Dierssen et al., 2003; Martínez-Cué et al., 2002). These results suggest that the molecular pathways that mediate neuronal reinforcement in the early stages of pruning might be affected by the partial trisomy of MMU16, resulting in different behavioural and cognitive abilities. However, it is interesting to note that, despite the marked differences in the number of spines found in the dendritic arbors of pyramidal cells in the different experimental groups, the distribution of the spines throughought their arbors remains remarkably similar (Eslton and DeFelipe, 2002). The mechanisms that determine spine distribution are controversial. However, in the cortex, it has been suggested that processes leading to shrinkage and elongation of dendritic spines are controlled locally, while processes leading to formation of novel spines may represent extension of local biochemical events or may be engineered centrally, through messages arriving from the soma, where a global increase in dendritic spine density is seen following a nuclear message (phosphorylation of CREB). Recently it has been documented that the levels of neurotrophic factors such as BDNF are increased in the central nervous system in response to increased environmental complexity (Torasdotter et al., 1998; Pham et al., 1999; Falkenberg et al., 1992; Ickes et al., 2000). These neurotrophic factor levels are altered in Ts65Dn mice, with an impact on the survival of the basal prosencephalon cholinergic nucleus (Cooper et al., 2001). However, other candidate molecules are implicated in the mechanism that guides morphological restructuring, synaptogenesis and synaptic weighing. These control the plastic changes induced by environmental enrichment in the CNS (Rampon et al., 2000), and may also be affected in this DS model. Thus, the behavioural consequences of enrichment observed in the Ts65Dn mice may not be dependent on the structural reorganization of the pyramidal cells of the frontal cortex. Since stable long-term changes in spines have been related to the formation of stable memories, it might be argued that the less stable behavioural effects of environmental enrichment could be dependent on more transient effects on functional synaptic mechanisms. However, we cannot discard the possibility that other cortical areas could be affected by the exposure to an enriched environment in these mice.

Conclusions

Down syndrome is a paradigmatic complex disease and the mechanism by which it produces phenotypic abnormalities is not understood. Despite intense investigation of the pathology, biochemistry and physiology of DS, it is still not known how the individual genes on HSA21, either singly or in concert produce the alterations associated with the trisomy. Several useful mouse models of DS have been generated, and new strategies are being initiated. The identification of a growing number of HSA21 genes will undoubtedly lead to the generation of many new single-gene transgenic models. In the YAC/BAC/PAC transgenics, the approach is rather different and involves the utilization of several overlapping or contiguous YACs that can cover a significant part of the genome. In a strategy termed 'in vivo libraries', large fragments of the genome can be propagated in vivo. These latter two approaches overcome some of the limitations of single-gene transgenics since the models generated harbour the introduced sequences at a low-copy number, similar to DS, and the regulatory elements that control the normal gene expression are present. Finally, the mouse trisomies constitute animal models for DS with different degrees of phenotypic impact, but they do not permit the role of each gene in the pathophysiology of the disease to be deciphered. Most likely, the strategies of crossing the trisomic models with knockout models, or antisense technology will shed light on the role of single genes in a trisomic environment. The models described herein, are the best available at the present for evaluating the efficacy of different pharmacological, genetic or environmental therapeutic strategies. To understand the molecular pathogenesis of DS, an overall analysis and comparative study of the existing models should be considered, but for this, mice should be of the same genetic background, and experimental protocols for the characterization and description of the phenotype of the models generated must be standardized and cover every aspect of mouse neurological, behavioural, biochemical and histopathological features.

Acknowledgments

This work was supported in part by grants of CEC/BIOMED2 (BMH4-CT98-3039), CICYT (SAF99-0092-CO2-01), FIS 00/0795, DGCYT PM99-0105, Jerôme Lejeune Foundation and Fundación Marcelino Botín.

Bibliography

Baxter LL, Moran TH, Richtsmeier JT, Troncoso J, Reeves R (2000) Discovery and genetic localization of Down syndrome cerebellar phenotypes using the Ts65Dn mouse. Hum Mol Genet 9: 195–202.

Becker LE, Armstrong DL, Chan F (1986) Dendritic atrophy in children with Down's syndrome. Ann Neurol 20: 520–6.

Becker LE, Mito T, Takashima S, Onodera K, Friend WC (1993) Association of phenotypic abnormalities of Down syndrome with an imbalance of genes on chromosome 21. APMIS Suppl 40: 57–70.

Calamandrei G, Alleva E, Cirulli F, Queyras A, Volterra V, Capirci O, Vicari S, Giannotti A, Turrini P, Aloe L (2000) Serum NGF levels in children and adolescents with either Williams syndrome or Down syndrome. Dev Med Child Neurol 42: 746–50.

Cooper JD, Salehi A, Delcroix JD, Howe CL, Belichenko PV, Chua-Couzens J, Kilbridge JF, Carlson EJ, Epstein CJ, Mobley WC (2001) Failed retrograde transport of NGF in a mouse model of Down's syndrome: reversal of cholinergic neurodegenerative phenotypes following NGF infusion. Proc Natl Acad Sci USA 98: 10439–44.

Costa AC, Walsh K, Davisson MT (1999) Motor dysfunction in a mouse model for Down syndrome. Physiol Behav 68: 211–20.

Coussons-Read ME, Crnic LS (1996) Behavioral assessment of the Ts65Dn mouse, a model for Down syndrome: altered behavior in the elevated plus maze and open field. Behav Genet 26: 7–13.

Coyle JT, Oster-Granite ML, Reeves R, Hohmann C, Corsi P, Gearhart J (1991) Down syndrome and the trisomy 16 mouse: impact of gene imbalance on brain development and aging. Res Publ Assoc Res Nerv Ment Dis 69: 85–99.

Crawley J, Paylor R (1997) A proposed test battery and constellations of specific behavioral paradigms to investigate the behavioral phenotypes of transgenic and knockout mice. Horm Behav 31: 197–211.

Davisson MT, Schmidt C, Akeson EC (1990) Segmental trisomy for murine chromosome 16: a new system for studying Down syndrome. In D Patterson and CJ Epstein (eds) Molecular Genetics of Chromosome 21 and Down syndrome. New York: Wiley-Liss, pp. 263–80.

Dierssen M, Benavides-Piccione R, Martínez-Cué C, Estivill X, Flórez J, Elston GN, DeFelipe J (2003) Alterations of neocortical pyramidal cell phenotype in the TS65DN mouse model of Down syndrome: effects of environmental enrichment. Cerebral Cortex, in press.

Dierssen M, Vallina IF, Baamonde C, Lumbreras MA, Martínez-Cué C, Calatayud SG, Flórez J (1996) Impaired cyclic AMP production in the hippocampus of a Down syndrome murine model. Dev Brain Res 95: 122–4.

Dierssen M, Vallina IF, Baamonde C, García-Calatayud S, Lumbreras MA, Flórez J (1997) Alterations of central noradrenergic transmission in Ts65Dn mouse, a model for Down syndrome. Brain Res 749: 238–43.

Dorsey SG, Bambrick LL, Balice-Gordon RJ, Krueger BK (2002) Failure of brain-derived neurotrophic factor-dependent neuron survival in mouse trisomy 16. J Neurosci 22: 2571–8.

Elston GN, DeFelipe J (2002) Alterations of neocortical pyramidal cell phenotype in the Ts65Dn mouse model of Down syndrome: effects of environmental enrichment. Cerebral Cortex, submitted.

Escorihuela RM, Fernández-Teruel A, Vallina IF, Baamonde C, Lumbreras MA, Dierssen M, Tobeña A, Flórez J (1995) Behavioral assessment of Ts65Dn mice: a putative DS model. Neurosci Lett 199: 143–6.

Escorihuela RM, Vallina IF, Martínez-Cué C, Baamonde C, Dierssen M, Tobeña A, Flórez J, Fernández-Teruel A (1998) Impaired short- and long-term memory in Ts65Dn mice, a model for DS. Neurosci Lett 247: 171–4.

Falkenberg T, Mohammed AK, Henriksson B, Persson H, Winblad B, Lindefors N (1992) Increased expression of brain-derived neurotrophic factor mRNA in rat hippocampus is associated with improved spatial memory and enriched environment. Neurosci Lett 138: 153–6.

Fernández-Teruel A, Escorihuela RM, Castellano B, Gonzalez B, Tobena A (1997) Neonatal handling and environmental enrichment effects on emotionality, novelty/reward seeking, and age related cognitive and hippocampal impairmentes: focus on the Roman rat lines. Behav Genet 27: 513–26.

Ferrer I, Gullotta F (1990) Down's syndrome and Alzheimer's disease: dendritic spine counts in the hippocampus. Acta Neuropathol (Berl) 79: 680–5.

Flórez J (1992) Neurologic abnormalities. In SM Pueschel, JK Pueschel (eds) Biomedical Concerns in Persons with Down Syndrome. Baltimore: Paul H Brookes Pub Co, pp. 159–73.

Gearhart JD, Davisson MT, Oster-Granite ML (1986) Autosomal aneuploidy in mice: generation and developmental consequences. Brain Res Bull 16: 789–801.

Gerlai R (1996) Gene targetting studies of mammalian behavior: is it the mutation or the background phenotype? Trends Neurosci 19: 177–81.

Globus A, Rosenzweig MR, Bennett EL, Diamond MC (1973) Effects of differential experience on dendritic spine counts in rat cerebral cortex. J Comp Physiol Psychol 82: 175–81.

Granholm A-CE, Sanders LA, Crnic LS (2000) Loss of cholinergic phenotype in basal forebrain coincides with cognitive decline in a mouse model of Down's syndrome. Exptl Neurol 161: 647–63.

Grausz H, Richtsmeier JT, Oster-Granite ML (1991) Morphogenesis of the brain and craniofacial complex in trisomy 16 mice. In: CJ Epstein (ed.) The Morphogenesis of Down Syndrome. New York: Wiley-Liss, pp. 169–88.

Hassold T, Jacobs P (1984) Trisomy in man. Ann Rev Genet 18: 69–97.

Hattori M, Fujiyama A, Taylor TD, Watanabe H, Yada T, Park HS, Toyoda A, Ishii K, Totoki Y, Choi DK, Soeda E, Ohki M, Takagi T, Sakaki Y, Taudien S, Blechschmidt K, Polley A, Menzel U, Delabar J, Kumpf K, Lehmann R, Patterson D, Reichwald K, Rump A, Schillhabel M, Schudy A (2000) The DNA sequence of human chromosome 21. The chromosome 21 mapping and sequencing consortium. Nature 405(6784): 311–19.

Haydar TF, Nowakowsky RS, Yarowsky PJ, Krueger BK (2000) Role of founder cell deficit and delayed neuronogenesis in microcephaly of the trisomy 16 mouse. J Neurosci 20: 4156–64.

Hernández D, Mee PJ, Martin JE, Tybulewicz VL, Fisher EM (1999) Transchromosomal mouse embryonic stem cell lines and chimeric mice that contain freely segregating segments of human chromosome 21. Hum Mol Genet 8: 923–33.

Holtzman DM, Santucci D et al. (1996) Developmental abnormalities and age-related neurodegeneration of a mouse model of Down syndrome. Proc Natl Acad Sci USA 93: 13333–8.

Ickes BR, Pham TM, Sanders LA, Albeck DS, Mohammed AH, Granholm AC (2000) Long-term environmental enrichment leads to regional increases in neurotrophin levels in rat brain. Exp Neurol 164: 45–52.

Inoue T, Shinohara T, Takehara S, Inoue J, Kamino H, Kugoh H, Oshimura M (2000) Specific impairment of cardiogenesis in mouse ES cells containing a human chromosome 21. Biochem Biophys Res Commun 273(1): 219–24.

Insausti AM, Megías M, Crespo D, Cruz-Orive LM, Dierssen M, Vallina IF, Insausti R, Flórez J (1998) Hippocampal volume and neuronal number in Ts65Dn mice: a murine model of Down syndrome. Neurosci Lett 253: 1–4.

Kola I, Hertzog P (1997) Animal models in the study of the biological function of genes on HSA21 and their role in the pathophysiology of Down syndrome. Hum Mol Genet 6: 1713–27.

Kurt MA, Davies DC, Kidd M, Dierssen M, Florez J (2000) Synaptic deficit in the temporal cortex of partial trisomy 16 (Ts65Dn) mice. Brain Res 858(1): 191–7.

Lewis MH, Powell SB, Turner CA, Newman HA, Bugenhagen P, Gendreau P, Crnic L (1999) Spontaneous stereotypy in an animal model of Down syndrome (Ts65Dn mice). Society for Neuroscience Abstracts 25: 849.

Marin-Padilla M (1976) Pyramidal cell abnormalities in the motor cortex of a child with Down's syndrome: A Golgi study. J Comp Neurol 167: 63–81.

Martínez-Cué C, Baamonde C, Vallina IF, Lumbreras MA, Dierssen M, Flórez J (1999) Reduced responsiveness of Ts65Dn mice to pain. Neuroreport 10: 1119–22.

Martínez-Cué C, Baamonde C, Lumbreras M, Paz J, Davisson MT, Schmidt C, Dierssen M, Flórez J (2002) Differential effects of environmental enrichment on behavior and learning of male and female Ts65Dn mice, a model for Down syndrome. Behav Brain Res 134: 185–200.

Mastroiacovo P (2002) Epidemiology of Down syndrome in the third millenium. 2nd International conference EDSA 'The Adult with Down Syndrome. A new Challenge for Society', San Marino.

Miyabara S, Sugihara H, Yonemitsu N, Yun K (1984) Comparative study of phenotypic expression of mice trisomy 16 by different female strains: attempt at an animal model for human trisomy 21. Cogn Anomal 24: 283–92.

Montero JJ, Flórez J, Baamonde C, Vallina IF, García-Calatayud S, Dierssen M (1996) Valoración ecográfica mediante doppler pulsado de la función cardíaca en el ratón Ts65Dn, un modelo murino de síndrome de Down. Rev Síndrome Down 13: 31–2.

Oster-Granite ML (1986) The neurobiologic consequences of autosomal aneuploidy in mice and men. Brain Res Bull 16: 767–71.

Oster-Granite ML, Lacey-Casem ML (1995) Neurotransmitter alterations in the trisomy 16 mouse: a genetic model system for studies of Down syndrome. Ment Retard Develop Dis Res Rev 1: 227–36.

Paz-Miguel JE, Flores R, Sanchez-Velasco P, Ocejo-Vinyals G, Escribano de Diego J, Lopez de Rego J, Leyva-Cobian F (1999) Reactive oxygen intermediates during programmed cell death induced in the thymus of the Ts(1716)65Dn mouse, a murine model for human Down's syndrome. J Immunol 163: 5399–410.

Pham TM, Ickes B, Albeck D, Soderstrom S, Granholm AC, Mohammed AH (1999) Changes in brain nerve growth factor levels and nerve growth factor receptors in rats exposed to environmental enrichment for one year. Neuroscience 94: 279–86.

Pinter JD, Eliez S, Schmitt JE, Capone GT, Reiss AL (2001) Neuroanatomy of Down's syndrome: a high-resolution MRI study. Am J Psychiatry 58: 1659–65.

Pritchard MA, Kola I (1999) The 'gene dosage effect' hypothesis versus the 'amplified developmental instability' hypothesis in Down syndrome. J Neural Transm Supp 57: 293–303.

Prusky GT, Reidel C, Douglas RM (2000) Environmental enrichment from birth enhances visual acuity but not place learning in mice. Behav Brain Res 114: 11–15.

Rampon C, Jiang CH, Dong H, Tang YP, Lockhart DJ, Schultz PG, Tsien JZ, Hu Y (2000) Effects of environmental enrichment on gene expression in the brain. Proc Natl Acad Sci USA 97: 12880–4.

Reeves RH, Yao J, Crowley MR, Buck S, Zhang X, Yarowsky P, Gearhart JD, Hilt DC (1994) Astrocytosis and axonal proliferation in the hippocampus of S100b transgenic mice. Proc Natl Acad Sci USA 91: 5359–63.

Richtsmeier JT, Baxter L, Reeves R (2000) Parallels of craniofacial development in Down syndrome and Ts65Dn mice. Develop Dynam 217: 137–45.

Rogers DC, Fisher EM, Brown SD, Peters J, Hunter AJ, Martin JE (1997) Behavioral and functional analysis of mouse phenotype: SHIRPA, a proposed protocol for comprehensive phenotype assessment. Mamm Genome 8: 711–13.

Rozenzweig MR, Bennett EL, Diamond MC (1972) Brain changes in relation to experience. Sci Am 226: 22–9.

Ruiz de Azúa I, Lumbreras MA, Zalduegui A, Baamonde C, Dierssen M, Florez J, Salles J (2001) Reduced phospholipase C-beta activity and isoform expression in the cerebellum of TS65Dn mouse: a model of Down syndrome. J Neurosci Res 66: 540–5.

Sago H, Carlson EJ, Smith D, Kilbridge J, Rubin EM, Mobley W, Epstein CJ, Huang T (1998) Ts1Cje, a partial trisomy 16 mouse model for Down syndrome, exhibits learning and behavioral abnormalities. Proc Natl Acad Sci USA 95: 6256–61.

Shapiro BL (1999) The Down syndrome critical region. J Neural Transm Suppl 57: 41–60.

Shapiro BL (2001) Developmental instability of the cerebellum and its relevance to Down syndrome. J Neural Transm Suppl 61: 11–34.

Siarey RJ, Stoll J, Rapoport SI, Galdzicki Z (1997) Altered long-term potentiation in the young and old Ts65Dn mouse, a model for Down syndrome. Neuropharmacol 36: 1549–54.

Smith DJ, Zhu Y, Zhang J, Cheng JF, Rubin EM (1995) Construction of a panel of transgenic mice containing a contiguous 2-Mb set of YAC/P1 clones from HSA21q22.2. Genomics 27: 425–34.

Smithies O, Kim H-S (1994) Targeted gene duplication and disruption for analyzing quantitative genetic traits in mice. Proc Natl Acad Sci USA 91: 3612–15.

Suetsugu M, Mehraein P (1980) Spine distribution along the apical dendrites of the pyramidal neurons in Down's syndrome. A quantitative Golgi study. Acta Neuropathol (Berl) 50: 207–10.

Sumarsono SH, Wilson TJ, Tymms MJ, Venter DJ, Corrick CM, Kola R, Lahoud MH, Papas TS, Seth A, Kola I (1996) Down's syndrome-like skeletal abnormalities in Ets2 transgenic mice. Nature 379: 534–7.

Takashima S, Becker LE, Armstrong DL, Chan F (1981) Abnormal neuronal development in the visual cortex of the human fetus and infant with Down's syndrome. A quantitative and qualitative Golgi study. Brain Res 225: 1–21.

Tomizuca K, Yoshida H, Uejima H, Kugoh H, Sato K, Ohguma A, Hayasaka M, Hanaoka K, Oshimura M, Ishida I (1997) Functional expression and germline transmission of a human chromosome fragment in chimaeric mice. Nature Genet 16: 133–43.

Torasdotter M, Metsis M, Henriksson BG, Winblad B, Mohammed AH (1998) Environmental enrichment results in higher levels of nerve growth factor mRNA in the rat visual cortex and hippocampus. Behav Brain Res 93: 83–90.

Volkmar FR, Greenough WT (1972) Rearing complexity affects branching of dendrites in the visual cortex of the rat. Science 176: 1145–7.

Whitaker-Azmitia PM, Wingate M, Borella A, Gerlai R, Roder J, Azmitia EC (1997) Transgenic mice overexpressing the neurotrophic factor S-100 beta show neuronal cytoskeletal and behavioral signs of altered aging proccesses: implications for Alzheimer's disease and Down's syndrome. Brain Res 776: 51–60.

Yang XW, Model P, Heintz N (1997) Homologous recombination based modification in *Escherichia coli* and germline transmission in transgenic mice of a bacterial artificial chromosome. Nature Biotechnol 15: 859–65.

Zapata A, Capdevila JL, Tarrason G, Adan J, Martínez JM, Piulat J, Trullás R (1997) Effects of NMDA-R1 antisense oligodeoxynucleotide administration: behavioral and radioligand binding studies. Brain Res 745: 114–20.

Chapter 3
The pathogenesis of congenital heart disease in Down syndrome: a molecular approach and a promising candidate gene

P. Scartezzini, A. Egeo, M. Mazzocco,
A. Rasore-Quartino

Congenital heart disease (CHD) affects 0.5–0.8% live births and is the leading non-infectious cause of death in children (Hoffman, 1995). Like most complex genetic traits in humans, the causes of CHD are yet poorly understood and difficult to determine. The process of heart formation requires the fine integration of several molecular and morphogenetic events and must involve the action of a large number of genes. The study of chromosomal disorders and autosomal dominant syndromes associated with specific anomalies of heart development is an essential step to identifying genes involved in the pathogenesis of CHD.

Down syndrome (DS), affecting 1 in 700 live births, is one of the most common chromosomal disorders and a major cause of mental handicap and CHD in humans (Epstein, 1986). CHD affects over 40% of DS newborns and represents the most dramatic feature of the clinical picture. Endocardial cushion defects (ECD) (atrioventricular canal defects and atrioventricular septal defects) are the typical forms of CHD found in DS patients (Marino et al., 1990a, 1990b). Interestingly, about 60% of the cases of ECD are associated with DS (Carmi et al., 1992). Such a high incidence strongly suggests that genes mapping to chromosome 21 could be involved in specific aspects of heart morphogenesis and that their abnormal expression in chromosome 21 trisomic cells could disturb specific molecular mechanisms of heart development.

Several genes have been identified so far, that play a crucial role in cardiogenesis. Their function has been related to specific stages of heart development, including the formation of the primitive heart tube, cardiac looping and chamber formation (Srivastava and Olson, 2000). None of these genes, however, maps to chromosome 21, although it is possible that specific interaction with genes mapping to chromosome 21, may affect their function.

Identifying genes mapping to chromosome 21, that are expressed in the developing heart, will provide clues to understand the molecular mechanisms that lead to DS-CHD.

A crucial step toward the identification of candidate genes for DS-CHD was the phenotypic, cytogenetic and molecular characterization of several patients with partial trisomy 21. This approach led to the identification of a 5 Mb region in 21q22.2–21q22.3 encompassing D21S3 to PFKL, which appears to be strongly associated with the presence DS-CHD (Barlow et al., 2001). This candidate region excludes both the region surrounding D21S55 (Down syndrome critical region), which is thought to contain candidate genes for several anomalies present in DS (Korenberg et al., 1994), and the telomeric region, containing the collagen VI genes (Klewer et al., 1998).

The complete sequencing of human chromosome 21 (Hattori et al., 2000) has shown that the region between D21S3 and PFKL contains about 60 known or predicted genes. The functional characterization of these genes will be a crucial step towards the identification of genes involved in the pathogenesis of DS-CHD.

Identification of gene mapping to chromosome 21 within the DS-CHD region

In recent years, we have addressed our research activity to the identification of genes located within the DS-CHD region and expressed in the foetal heart. We focused our efforts on a region of about 1 kb surrounding the HMG14 gene. As a start point we performed direct cDNA selection using a chromosome 21 YAC clone spanning the region of interest, and a cDNA mixture synthesized from foetal heart poly [A+] RNA. Among several cDNA clones isolated, four were confirmed to map to chromosome 21 within the DS-CHD region. These partial cDNA clones were used as probes to screen tissue-specific cDNA libraries to obtain full-length cDNA. The new chromosome 21 genes identified were named DSCR2, WDR9, WRB and SH3BGR (Vidal-Taboada et al., 1998a). Their chromosomal localization is shown in Figure 3.1.

DSCR2 (chromosome 21 leucine-rich protein, c21-LRP) is widely expressed, with higher levels in testis and in the human leukaemic T cell line, Jurkat (Vidal-Taboada et al., 2000). DSCR2 encodes a protein of 288 amino acids, which could play a role in cell proliferation (Vidal-Taboada et al., 1998b).

The WDR9 (WD Repeat 9) gene is organized in 41 exons and 40 introns, spanning 125 Kb between DSCR2 and HMG14 and is expressed in several human and mouse tissues and cell lines (Ramos et al., 2002). The WDR9 mRNA has a size of 13 kb and codes for a protein of 2269 amino acids containing several WD repeats.

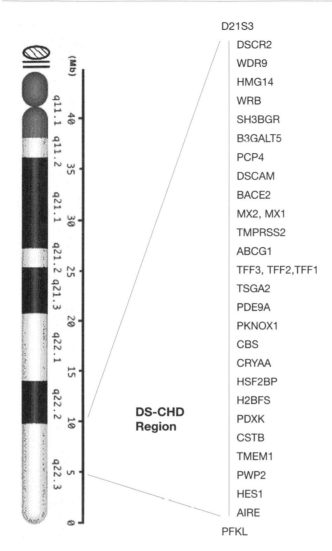

D21S3
DSCR2
WDR9
HMG14
WRB
SH3BGR
B3GALT5
PCP4
DSCAM
BACE2
MX2, MX1
TMPRSS2
ABCG1
TFF3, TFF2,TFF1
TSGA2
PDE9A
PKNOX1
CBS
CRYAA
HSF2BP
H2BFS
PDXK
CSTB
TMEM1
PWP2
HES1
AIRE
PFKL

DS-CHD
Region

Figure 3.1 Schematic representation of genes mapping to the Down syndrome congenital heart disease minimal region.

WRB (tryptophan-rich basic protein) gene maps close to HMG14. WRB appears to be expressed in all the human tissues analysed and encodes a basic protein of 174 amino acids containing a highly conserved coiled coil domain (Egeo et al., 1998a).

The SH3BGR gene maps about 100 kb telomeric to WRB and is organized in seven exons and six introns that span about 65 kb of genomic sequence. Interestingly, SH3BGR transcripts have been detected only in human foetal and adult heart and skeletal muscle (Scartezzini et al., 1997). This highly specific expression pattern suggested SH3BGR as a promising candidate gene for DS-CHD. Therefore we focused our efforts to characterize further the SH3BGR gene.

Spatio-temporal expression profile of SH3BGR during mouse development

As a first step, we analysed the spatio-temporal expression profile of SH3BGR during mouse development using the murine orthologue (Sh3bgr) as a probe (Egeo et al., 2000). Whole mount *in situ* hybridization was used to analyse mouse embryos between 7.5 (E7.5) and 10.5 (E10.5) days of gestational age. This is the crucial period of heart morphogenesis, i.e. when the cells of the precardiogenic mesoderm form the primitive cardiac tube, which, through the looping process, leads to the formation of the heart. The expression in the developing heart structures is an essential requirement for consideration of a chromosome 21 gene as a candidate for DS-CHD. Our experiments clearly showed that SH3BGR is already expressed in the cells of the precardiogenic mesoderm at E7.5 (Figure 3.2A). Subsequently, from E8.5 to E10.5, namely during the period when the tubular heart undergoes rightward looping, SH3BGR is highly expressed in the developing heart. Moreover, the presence of SH3BGR transcripts is restricted to heart structures and no signal is detectable in the other embryonal tissues, including branchial arches (Figures 3.2B–D).

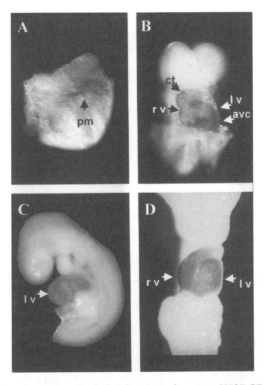

Figure 3.2 Whole mount *in situ* hybridization showing SH3BGR expression during early mouse development at the following stages: A: E7.75; B: E8.5; C: E9.5; D: E10.5. pm: precardiogenic mesoderm; ct: conotruncus; avc: atrioventricular canal; rv: right ventricle; lv: left ventricle (Egeo et al., 2000).

The following developmental stages were analysed for SH3BGR expression using *in situ* hybridization on tissue sections. SH3BGR transcripts are present through the myocardium from E11.5 to newborn and high levels of expression persist in the adult heart.

From E12.5, SH3BGR transcripts are detectable in skeletal muscle and in the smooth muscle of the oesophagus, gut and urinary bladder. In contrast SH3BGR is not expressed in other types of smooth muscle, including vascular and bronchial smooth muscle.

The analysis of spatio-temporal expression, demonstrating that SH3BR is selectively transcribed in early stages of mouse heart development, strongly support a role of this gene in heart morphogenesis and suggests that SH3BGR may be a promising candidate gene for DS-CHD.

Moreover, due to its expression in skeletal muscle and developing gut wall, SH3BGR could be involved in the pathogenesis of muscular hypotonia and gastrointestinal anomalies, that affect 90% and 5–7% DS patients respectively. Recently, our results have been confirmed by two independent groups that have defined the expression pattern of nearly all the murine orthologues of the genes located on human chromosome 21 (Reymond et al., 2002 ; Gitton et al., 2002).

Cellular localization of the SH3BGR protein

To further characterize the functional role of SH3BGR, we have analysed the cellular localization of the encoded protein. SH3BGR codes for a protein of 176 amino acids, which is characterized by the presence of a highly conserved N-terminal domain and by a C-terminal domain highly enriched in glutamic acid residues (Scartezzini et al., 1997). The N-terminal domain is predicted to assume a thioredoxin-like fold and contain a conserved proline-rich motif, which could mediate protein–protein interaction.

To analyse the subcellular localization, the SH3BGR full-length cDNA was cloned in EGFP plasmid and the DNA construct was transfected in C2C12 cells. The SH3BGR protein is located to the cytoplasm and its localization is not modified by C2C12 differentiation and formation of myotubes (Figure 3.3).

SH3BGR belongs to a new human gene family: the SH3BGR gene family

After the identification and characterization of SH3BGR, we identified three new human genes, SH3BGRL (Egeo et al., 1998b), SH3BGRL2 (Mazzocco et al., 2002) and SH3BGRL3 (Mazzocco et al., 2001) mapping to chromosome Xq13.3, 6q13–15 and 1p36.1 respectively. These genes encode small proteins, which show a high homology to the N-terminal region of the SH3BGR protein, but completely lack the C-terminal glutamic acid-rich region. Different to SH3BGR, the other genes belonging to

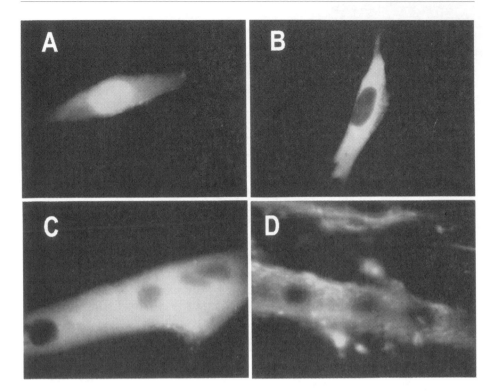

Figure 3.3 Cellular localization of the SH3BGR encoded protein in wild type (wt) and differentiating C2C12 cells. A: control GFP; B: wt C2C12 cells; C: C2C12 after 3 days of differentiation; D: C2C12 after 6 days of differentiation. The SH3BGR protein clearly localizes to cytoplasm.

the SH3BGR family are expressed in almost all the tissues examined, and the encoded proteins were detected both in the cytoplasm and in the nucleus of cultured cells. The proline-rich motif is highly conserved in all the proteins of the SH3BGR family. Therefore, these proteins could compete for binding to target proteins, and a dosage imbalance of SH3BGR protein could disturb specific biological processes in chromosome 21 trisomic cells.

Future research

The aims of future research include defining the specific function of SH3BGR in myocardial and muscular cells and determining the effects of overexpression using transgenic mouse models. The identification and functional characterization of genes involved in the pathogenesis of CHD in DS will provide important insights into the molecular mechanisms of heart development and congenital heart disease that affect both DS and non-DS newborns.

References

Barlow GM, Chen X-N, Shi ZY, Celle L, Spinner N, Zackai E, Lyons GE, Mjaatvedt C, Pettenati MJ, Van Riper AJ, Vekemans M, Korenberg JR (2001). Down syndrome congenital heart disease: a narrowed region and a candidate gene. Genetics in Medicine 3(2): 91–101.

Carmi R, Boughman JA, Ferencz C (1992) Endocardial cushions defect: further studies of isolated versus syndromic occurrence. Am J Med Genet 43: 569–75.

Egeo A, Mazzocco M, Sotgia F, Arrigo P, Bergonon S, Oliva R, Nizetic D, Rasore-Quartino A, Scartezzini P (1998a) Identification and characterization of a new human cDNA from chromosome 21q22.3 encoding a basic nuclear protein. Hum Genet 102: 289–93.

Egeo A, Mazzocco M, Arrigo P, Vidal-Taboada JM, Oliva R, Pirola B, Giglio S, Rasore-Quartino A, Scartezzini P (1998b) Identification and characterization of a new human gene encoding a small protein with high homology to the proline-rich region of the SH3BGR gene. Biochem Biophys Res Commun 247: 302–6.

Egeo A, Di Lisi R, Sandri C, Mazzocco M, Lapide M, Schiaffino S, Scartezzini P (2000) Developmental expression of the SH3BGR gene, mapping to Down syndrome heart critical region. Mech Dev 90(2): 313–16.

Epstein CJ (1986) Down syndrome (trisomy 21). In CR Scriver, AL Beaudet, WS Sly, D Valle (eds) The Metabolic and Molecular Bases of Inherited Disease. New York: McGraw-Hill, pp. 749–94.

Gitton Y, Dahmane N, Balk S, Altaba AR, Neidhardt G, Scholtze M, Hermann BG, Kahlem P, Benkahla A, Schrinner S, Yildirimman R, Herwig R, Lehrach H, Yaspo ML (2002) A gene expression map of human chromosome 21 orthologues in the mouse. Nature 420: 586–90.

Hattori M, Fujiyama A, Taylor TD, Watanabe H, Yada T, Park HS, Toyoda A, Ishii K, Totoki Y, Choi DK, Groner Y, Soeda E, Ohki M, Takagi T, Sakaki Y, Taudien S, Blechschmidt K, Polley A, Menzel U, Delabar J, Kumpf K, Lehmann R, Patterson D, Reichwald K, Rump A, Schillhabel M, Schudy A, Zimmermann W, Rosenthal A, Kudoh J, Schibuya K, Kawasaki K, Asakawa S, Shintani A, Sasaki T, Nagamine K, Mitsuyama S, Antonarakis SE, Minoshima S, Shimizu N, Nordsiek G, Hornischer K, Brant P, Scharfe M, Schon O, Desario A, Reichelt J, Kauer G, Blocker H, Ramser J, Beck A, Klages S, Hennig S, Riesselmann L, Dagand E, Haaf T, Wehrmeyer S, Borsym K, Gardiner K, Nizetic D, Francis F, Lehrach H, Reinhardt R, Yaspo ML (2000) The DNA sequence of human chromosome 21. Nature 405: 311–19.

Hoffman JIE (1995) Incidence of congenital heart disease: I. Postnatal incidence. Periatr Cardiol 16: 103–13.

Klewer SE, Krob SL, Kolker SJ, Kitten GT (1998) Expression of type VI collagen in the developing mouse heart. Dev Dyn 211(3): 248–55.

Korenberg JR, Chen XN, Shipper R, Sun Z, Gonsky R, Gerwehr S, Berry K, Carpenter N, Daumer C, Dignan P, Disteche C, Graham J, Hudgins L, Lewin S, McGillivray B, Miyasaki K, Ogasawara N, Pagon R, Pueschel S, Sack G, Say B, Schuffenhauer S, Soukup S, Yamanaka T (1994) Down syndrome phenotypes: the consequence of chromosomal imbalance. Proc Natl Acad Sci USA 91(11): 4997–5001.

Marino B, Vairo U, Corno A, Nava S, Guccione P, Calabrò R, Marcelletti C (1990a) Atrioventricular canal in Down syndrome. Am J Dis Child 144: 1120–2.

Marino B, Papa M, Guccione P, Corno A, Marasini M, Calabrò R (1990b) Ventricular septal defect in Down syndrome. Am J Dis Child 144: 544–5.

Mazzocco M, Arrigo P, Egeo A, Maffei M, Vergano A, Di Lisi R, Ghiotto F, Ciccone E, Cinti R, Ravazzolo R, Scartezzini P (2001) A novel human homologue of the SH3BGR gene encodes a small protein similar to glutaredoxin 1 of *Escherichia coli*. Biochem Biophys Res Commun 285: 540–5.

Mazzocco M, Maffei M, Egeo A, Vergano A, Di Lisi R, Ghiotto F, Scartezzini P (2002) The identification of a novel human homologue of the SH3BGR gene establishes a new family of highly conserved small protein related to Thioredoxin Superfamily. Gene 291: 233–9.

Ramos VC, Vidal-Taboada JM, Bergognon S, Egeo A, Fischer EMC, Scartezzini P, Oliva R (2002). Characterisation and expression analysis of the WDR9 gene, located in the Down syndrome critical region-2 of the human chromosome 21. Biochem Biophys Acta 1577: 377–83.

Reymond A, Marigo V, Yaylaoglu MB, Leoni A, Ucla C, Scamuffa N, Caccioppoli C, Dermitzakis ET, Lyle R, Banfi S, Eichele G, Antonarakis SE, Ballabio A (2002) Human chromosome 21 gene expression atlas in the mouse. Nature 420: 582–6.

Scartezzini P, Egeo A, Colella S, Fumagalli P, Arrigo P, Nizetic D, Taramelli R, Rasore-Quartino A (1997) Cloning a new human gene from chromosome 21q22.3 encoding a glutamic acid-rich protein expressed in heart and skeletal muscle. Hum Genet 99: 387–92.

Srivastava D, Olson EN (2000) A genetic blueprint for cardiac development. Nature 407: 221–6.

Vidal-Taboada JM, Bergonon S, Sanchez M, Lopez-Acedo C, Groet J, Nizetic D, Egeo A, Scartezzini P, Katsanis N, Fisher EMC, Delabar JM, Oliva R (1998a) A 342 kb high resolution physical restriction map and identification of transcribed sequences within the Down syndrome region-2. Biochem Biophys Res Commun 243: 572–8.

Vidal-Taboada JM, Sanz S, Egeo A, Scartezzini P, Oliva R (1998b) Identification and characterization of a new gene from human chromosome 21 between markers D21S343 and D21S268 encoding a leucine rich protein. Biochem Biophys Res Commun 250: 547–54.

Vidal-Taboada JM, Lu A, Pique M, Pons G, Gil J, Oliva R (2000) Down syndrome critical region gene 2: expression during mouse development and in human cell lines indicates a function related to cell proliferation. Biochem Biophys Res Commun 272: 156–63.

Chapter 4
Down syndrome and congenital heart disease

B. Marino, G. Assenza, F. Mileto, M. Digilio

Introduction

The diagnosis and treatment of congenital heart disease (CHD) is of primary importance in the general health care of people with Down syndrome (DS). CHD has a high prevalence in these subjects and cardiac care can prevent morbidity and mortality due to congestive heart failure and pulmonary vascular disease. Children with DS have particular anatomical and physiological cardiac problems and thus need specific management. Adults with DS also represent a new challenge from the cardiological point of view.

CHD and Down syndrome: a historical perspective

Although the first clinical description of DS has been ascribed to John Langdon Down in 1866 (Pueschel, 1996a), previous observation by Esquirol (1838) and Seguin (1846) had pointed out some features of DS before Down himself. John Down made the first clinical correlations between all the aspects of this syndrome, distinguishing them from other forms of mental handicap.

In the last decade of the nineteenth century, Garrod published many articles about the association between DS and CHD (Garrod, 1894, 1898). In the patient called Annie M., he noted a well marked cyanosis present from birth, clubbed fingers and toes, and he heard a systolic murmur all over the cardiac area. In other children with DS he pointed out many signs of CHD such as cardiac thrill, anomalous dullness of the cardiac area, anomalous position of apex beat out of the nipple line and intensity of the second tone being stronger than normal. Garrod went on to

39

discuss the prevalence of CHD in people with DS, reporting that there were many more cases of CHD in DS than in normal patients. Moreover Garrod speculated the adult patients with DS, in the asylum, did not have CHD because those with CHD died during infancy or early childhood (Pueschel, 1996a). For him, DS was the result of an 'inborn error of metabolism' (a term that he coined). In subsequent years, Shuttleworth mentioned that 'the heart is found incompletely finished not infrequently in children with this syndrome, the foramen ovale remaining patent, and defects involve also the interventricular septum' (Pueschel, 1996a).

To summarize, Garrod is the first physician who investigated and described CHD in DS; after him many investigators provided additional information, and now we have an explosion of knowledge in this field (Evans, 1950; Liu and Corlett, 1959; Berg et al., 1960; Rowe and Uchida, 1961; Warkany et al., 1966; Cullum and Lieban, 1969; Tandon and Edwards, 1973; Greenwood and Nadas, 1976; Laursen, 1976; Park et al., 1977; Clark, 1989; Marino, 1996).

Patterns of congenital heart disease in Down syndrome patients

CHD plays an important role in the natural history of DS. The prevalence of heart defects in DS is 40–50% compared with a 0.5–1% risk in infants with normal chromosomes. Why some children with DS have a cardiac defect and others have a normal heart is still a mystery. Not all the cardiac defects are equally represented in DS and numerous studies have confirmed that children with trisomy 21 present certain congenital heart defects and seem to be protected from others (de Biase et al., 1986; Ferencz et al., 1989; Marino et al., 1991; Ferencz et al., 1992; Marino and de Zorzi, 1993; Marino, 1989, 1990, 1992, 1996; Marino et al., 1990a, 1990b; Marino and Digilio, 2001).

The most common cardiac defect in DS is atrioventricular canal (AVC), also called atrioventricular septal defect. Atrioventricular canal represents about the 60% of cardiac malformations and occurs in about 20% of all children with DS. Also ventricular septal defect (VSD), tetralogy of Fallot (TOF) and atrial septal defect (ASD) can occur in patients with this aneuploidy. Other anomalies such as isolated pulmonary valve stenosis or atresia, aortic valve stenosis or atresia, and aortic coartation are quite rare. Some defects, regarding anomalies of segmental connection, such as left loop of the ventricles, atresia of atrioventricular valves, double-inlet left ventricle with two separate valves, and transposition of the great arteries, are virtually absent (Marino, 1996). For these types of malformation, trisomy 21 seems to represent a protective factor compared with the normal population.

In Chinese and Mexican children with DS there are some interesting differences in the prevalence and types of CHD. In these populations, the most common CHD is VSD; AVC is the second most prevalent (Sing Roxy et al., 1989; Vizcaino, 1993; Hijii et al., 1997). These data suggest that other genes and/or environmental factors can be involved in pathogenesis of various types of CHD (Marino, 1996).

Although DS is more common in males than in females, CHD in DS is more common in females (Pinto et al., 1990). However the role played by gender in the pathogenesis of this syndrome and of the cardiac defect is not known. Some studies have suggested that paternal genotype could have an influence on the presence of a cardiac defect.

It is interesting to note that in patients with mosaicism trisomy 21 there is a lower prevalence of CHD (30%) and the cardiac defects tend to be less severe (Marino and de Zorzi, 1993).

In the last 15 years, anatomical and clinical studies have shown that peculiar cardiac patterns are present in patients with this syndrome (Marino, 1989, 1990, 1992, 1996; Marino et al., 1990a, 1990b; Marino et al., 1991; Marino and de Zorzi, 1993; Marino and Digilio, 2001).

Atrioventricular canal

The complete form of AVC is the most frequent type of CHD associated with DS (Figure 4.1). About 70% of all children with a complete form of AVC have trisomy 21. The partial form is more prevalent in children without DS. Associated cardiac anomalies, and in particular left-sided obstructions, are significantly rarer in patients with AVC and DS than in

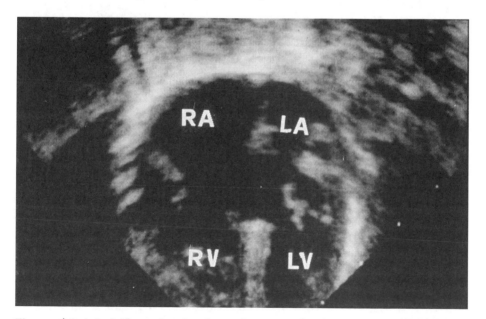

Figure 4.1 Apical 'four chambers' two-dimensional echocardiographic view in a patient with DS and complete AVC. RA= right atrium; LA= left atrium; RV= right ventricle; LV= left ventricle.

patients with AVC and normal chromosomes (de Biase et al., 1986; Marino et al., 1990a, 1990b; Marino, 1996). Children with DS show a 'simple' type of AVC: it is usually complete, and is rarely associated with other cardiac anomalies (if we exclude TOF). Particularly rare are left-sided anomalies, which are more frequent in patients with AVC but without DS. Genes located on different chromosomes could be responsible for AVC in patients without DS (Marino, 1996; Digilio et al., 1999).

Ventricular septal defect

In children with DS, a posterior perimembranous ventricular defect in the inlet segment of the ventricular septum is more frequent than in 'normal' patients. Muscular and subarterial ventricular defects are rare in this syndrome, and the most frequent associated cardiac anomaly is cleft of the mitral valve (Marino et al., 1990a, 1991) (Figure 4.2). In contrast, left ventricular outflow tract obstruction (LVOTO) is prevalent in children with VSD and without trisomy 21.

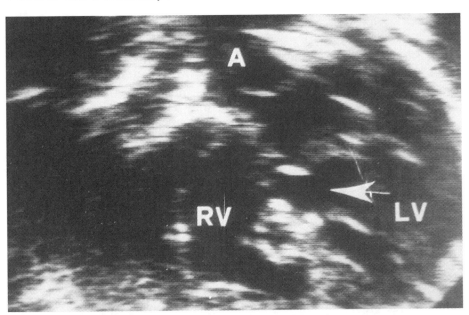

Figure 4.2 Subcostal 'long axis' two-dimensional echocardiographic view in a patient with DS and partial AVC. Note the cleft of the mitral valve (arrow). A= aorta.

Tetralogy of Fallot

Tetralogy of Fallot is the only conotruncal anomaly occurring in children with DS. In trisomy 21 patients, TOF is usually an isolated finding and usually in these patients the VSD is particularly large. The only additional cardiovascular anomaly is AVC, sometimes with hypoplastic right ventricle. Other cardiac defects, such as pulmonary atresia, absent pulmonary valve, discontinuity of pulmonary arteries, absent infundibular septum, sometimes associated with TOF in normal patients or in children with chromosome 22 deletion, are very rare in DS (Marino, 1996).

Atrial septal defect

The ASD ostium secundum type is a quite frequent cardiac malformation in children with DS. This cardiac defect can occur in isolation or associated with the other CHD such as AVC, TOF and VSD. In patients with ASD, the sinus venous type, the single atrium and the partial anomalous venous connection are extremely rare, while the presence of the valve flap of the 'foramen ovale' is frequent (Marino, 1996).

Conclusion

From an anatomical point of view, the patterns of congenital heart diseases in patients with DS are simpler than those observed in patients with normal chromosomes. Furthermore, cardiac malformations of subjects with trisomy 21 are less severe and more predictable. Therefore, surgical results in this group of patients can be similar and sometimes even better than those achieved in patients with the same heart defect who do not have chromosome anomalies.

Pulmonary disease

The main types of CHD in DS are associated with left-to-right shunt. Clinical and morphological studies support the idea that DS patients have a striking tendency to develop early and severe pulmonary vascular disease (Chi and Krovets, 1975; Clark et al., 1980; Loughlin et al., 1981; Frescura et al., 1987; Freedom, 1996).

The increased pulmonary blood flow can modify the stress–strain relationship in pulmonary arterioles and rapidly lead to irreversible damage to the pulmonary vascular bed. The pulmonary arterioles respond to chronic irritation by a staged response of intimal proliferation and medial hypertrophy.

The main difference between DS patients and those with a normal karyotype is the timing of these changes. In normal children, with the same types of CHD, pulmonary vascular changes become evident and irreversible in 2–3 years or more. In DS patients, there is a risk of a fixed vascular changes by 6–9 months (Frescura et al., 1987). We do not know exactly why DS patients have such an early form of pulmonary vascular disease; there are probably many mechanisms involved, and different aspects (including genetic ones) are now being considered.

Children with DS have often a chronic upper airway obstruction (Clark et al., 1980; Freedom, 1996). Structural abnormalities are often observed: midfacial hypoplasia with short nasal passages, small oral cavity, macroglossia, mandibular hypoplasia and narrowed hypopharynx. There are often airway anomalies: choanal stenosis and hypertrophy of tonsils and adenoids. Chest wall abnormalities like pectum excavatum and carinatum with a weak thoracic musculature can be present. The consequences of these defects can be an obstructive apnoea with hypoxaemia and hypercarbia. Moreover these infants may somewhat underventilate because of their hypotonia, and they can develop night-time hypercarbia and hypoxaemia (Soudon et al., 1975; Rowland et al., 1981). The vasoconstrictive chemical response of the pulmonary vascular bed, with an increased pressure, is the pathological conclusion (Frescura et al., 1987).

In DS, embryological failure of lung development has been suspected to occur. Cooney and Thurlbeck (1982) described such a defect as a gross diffuse and uniformly porous appearance of the cut surface of the lung, due to an enlargement of alveoli and alveolar ducts. From the histological point of view they introduced the 'radial alveolar count' as the average number of alveoli between terminal or respiratory bronchioles and the periphery of the acinus. In DS this number is reduced.

Another important cause of lung disease is recurrent pulmonary infection. The predisposition to infectious diseases in the respiratory tract is related to both structural and functional disorders and also to a genetic predisposition to immunodeficiency (Ugazio et al., 1978; Spina et al., 1981; Musiani et al., 1990). Pulmonary infections are one of the major causes of morbidity and mortality in DS. Sinus infection, through reduced mucociliary clearance, can be a starting point. Bacterial pneumonia (*Staphylococcus aureus* and *Haemophilus influenzae*) are often involved. Viral infection (RSV, parainfluenzal virus, adenoinfluenza virus) can be also present. Probably an indirect cause of pulmonary infection is the lung congestion due to the large intracardiac left-to-right shunt. Also aspiration and/or gastro-oesophageal reflux recurs due to an increased incidence of dysfunction, with *ab ingestis* pneumonia (Thiene et al., 1996).

Repeated respiratory infections of persons with DS result not only in increased morbidity and mortality but can also contribute to the early development of pulmonary hypertension.

Since the calculation of pulmonary vascular resistance, during cardiac catheterization, is not always accurate in DS, and diagnostic lung biopsy is an aggressive procedure and not always reliable, the best strategy to prevent pulmonary vascular disease is early echocardiographic diagnosis, aggressive management of pulmonary problems and early surgery based on echocardiography.

Access to cardiac care, clinical diagnosis and cardiac surgery

Since the majority of CHD in patients with DS need cardiac surgery in the first 6–12 months of life, early recognition of the cardiac defect is essential.

In the past, access to cardiac care was not always easy for children with DS. Late referral for diagnosis, preferential choice of medical *vs* surgical treatment and differences in health insurance, frequently characterized the medical approach to these patients (Bull et al., 1985). Nowadays there is general agreement that aggressive medical and surgical treatment must be offered to all infants with trisomy 21, without discrimination.

All infants with DS, including those without heart murmurs, must be examined by a paediatric cardiologist. An initial evaluation should be performed at birth, including a physical examination and an ECG. In those with anomalies on ECG or on physical examination, a complete echocardiographic study and chest radiography should be performed. It is very important to diagnose CHD in a DS patient before the baby is 4–6 months of age to permit planning for future care.

Some authors, including our group, suggest a large echocardiographic screening for all neonates with DS. Echocardiography has proved to be an essential tool for the diagnosis and surgical indication in all children with CHD and in particular in subjects with DS, as it avoids cardiac catheterization and unnecessary hospitalization (Tubman et al., 1991; di Carlo and Marino, 1996; Santoro et al., 1996).

One reason for the previous delay in referral has been the perception that DS babies are at increased risk for operative treatment; nowadays we know that this is not correct, and in western society the question of whether a child with mental handicap should be offered surgical treatment of a correctable CHD is no longer debated (Katlic et al., 1977; Kobel et al., 1982; Menahem and Mee, 1985; Sondheimer et al., 1985; Schneider et al., 1989; Vet and Ottenkamp, 1989; Morris et al., 1992; Rizzoli et al., 1992; di Carlo and Marino, 1994, 1996; Clark, 1996; di Carlo, 1996). It is the general philosophy today that cardiac surgery be offered to people with or without DS in the same manner.

In the past, the immediate mortality of complete repair of AVC, for example, has been higher in a DS group of patients compared with a non-trisomy 21 group. Nowadays, recent data relative to the experience acquired since the early 1980s in many centres throughout the world, represent a mortality rate of 10% or less (Katlic et al., 1977; Kobel et al., 1982; Schneider et al., 1989; di Carlo and Marino, 1994, 1996; Clark, 1996; di Carlo, 1996). An important observation is that, in spite of poorer pulmonary and infective conditions for children with DS, there is lower surgical mortality in comparison with other subjects without this aneuploidy. This phenomenon is usually attributed to the 'simpler' anatomy of the CHD in DS (Menahem and Mee, 1985; di Carlo and Marino, 1994, 1996; di Carlo, 1996; Formigari et al., 2004). The prevalence of reoperation because of left atrioventricular dysfunction is also lower in patients with DS (Williams et al., 1989; Marino, 1990).

Aggressive medical and surgical care increases the likelihood that these children will live longer than they would have in the era prior to surgical repair and decreases cumulative costs to families and society (Truesdell and Clark, 1991; Clark, 1996).

Post-operative results in these patients are quite good. The cardiac function in children and adolescents is adequate as well as the cardiorespiratory parameters and the results of the stress test (Russo et al., 1998; Pastore et al., 2000). Selected children with DS and without CHD, after a careful cardiorespiratory evaluation, can perform full physical activities and exercise including competitive sport (Fernhall et al., 1989; Russo et al., 1998; Pastore et al., 2000; Ulrich et al., 2001). In other subjects with minor cardiac anomalies or after surgical intervention, controlled recreational physical activities are indicated (Fernhall et al., 1989; Pitetti et al., 1992).

The adult Down syndrome patient: a new problem

Cardiologists have primarily focused their attention on CHD in children with DS. Nowadays, with the increased knowledge in this field, the adult Down syndrome patient has became less rare. Accordingly some recent investigations studied cardiac problems in adolescent and adults with DS (Goldhaber et al., 1986, 1987, 1988; Barnett et al., 1988; Pueschel, 1996b).

The cardiac status of a random group of DS patients was analysed and an elevated prevalence of mitral valve prolapse and aortic regurgitation was recognized (Goldhaber et al., 1986, 1987, 1988; Barnett et al., 1988; Pueschel, 1996b). Other research reported a higher prevalence of these cardiac defects in a group of patients with DS compared with subjects with other types of mental handicap. It is possible that both mitral valve prolapse and aortic regurgitation are due to a congenital laxity of connective tissue (Pueschel, 1996b). In fact we know that in trisomy 21 there is an increased prevalence of hip dislocation, patellar subluxation and atlantoaxial instability. Probably the same type of connective tissue anomalies are present also in cardiac valve structures (Pueschel, 1996b).

To prevent endocarditis, it is generally recommended that adults with DS and mitral valve prolapse or aortic regurgitation should be provided with antibiotic prophylaxis before dental procedures and before any form of surgical intervention (Pueschel, 1996b).

All adults with DS need a periodic cardiological examination to exclude and prevent the subtle cardiac anomalies that are not evident in childhood (Marino and Digilio, 2001).

In the near future, cardiologists could be involved in the study and treatment of ageing persons with DS affected by other types of degenerative heart disease such as atherosclerosis, arterial hypertension and coronary artery disease. Having to face these acquired clinical and research problems should be considered *per se* a great medical success.

References

Barnett ML, Friedman D, Kastner T (1988) The prevalence of mitral valve prolapse in patients with Down's syndrome: implications for dental management. Oral Surg Oral Med Oral Pathol 66: 445–7.

Berg JM, Crome L, France NE (1960) Congenital cardiac malformations in mongolism. Br Heart J 22: 331–46.

Bull C, Rigby M, Shinebourne EA (1985) Should management of complete atrioventricular canal defect be influenced by coexistent Down's syndrome? Lancet 1: 1147–9.

Chi TL, Krovets JL (1975) The pulmonary vascular bed in children with Down syndrome. J Pediatr 86: 533–8.

Clark EB (1989) Congenital cardiovascular defects in infants with Down syndrome. Pediatric Rev 11: 99–100.

Clark EB (1996) Acces to cardiac care for children with Down syndrome. In B Marino, SM Pueschel (eds) Heart Disease in Persons with Down Syndrome. Baltimore: Brookes, pp. 145–50.

Clark RW, Schimdt HS, Schuller DE (1980) Sleep-induced ventilatory dysfunction in Down's syndrome. Arch Inter Med 140: 45–50.

Cooney TP, Thurlbeck WM (1982) Pulmonary hypoplasia in Down's syndrome. N Engl J Med 307: 1170–3.

Cullum L, Lieban J (1969) The association of congenital heart disease with Down's syndrome (mongolism). Am J Med 24: 354–7.

de Biase L, di Ciommo V, Ballerini L, Bevilacqua M, Marcelletti C, Marino B (1986) Prevalence of left-sided obstructive lesions in patients with atrioventricular canal without Down's syndrome. J Thorac Cardiovasc Surg 91: 467–9.

di Carlo D (1996) Should coexisting Down syndrome affect the indication for surgery of congenital heart disease? In B Marino, SM Pueschel (eds) Heart Disease in Persons with Down Syndrome. Baltimore: Brookes, pp. 151–9.

di Carlo D, Marino B (1994) Atrioventricular canal with Down's syndrome or normal chromosomes: distinct prognosis with surgical management? J Thorac Cardiovasc Surg 107(5): 1368–9.

di Carlo D, Marino B (1996) Patient selection for repair of complete atrioventricular canal guided by echocardiography. J Am Coll Cardiol 26/2: 574.

Digilio MC, Marino B, Toscano A, Giannotti A, Dallapiccola B (1999) Atrioventricular canal defect without Down syndrome: a heterogeneous malformation. Am J Med Genet 85: 140–6.

Evans PR (1950) Cardiac anomalies in mongolism. Br Heart J 12: 258–62.

Ferencz C, Carmi R, Boughman JA (1992) Endocardial cushion defect: further studies of 'isolated' versus 'syndromic' occurrence. Am J Med Genet 43: 568–75.

Ferencz C, Neill CA, Boughman JA (1989) Congenital cardiovascular malformations with chromosome abnormalities: an epidemiologic study. J Pediatr 144: 79–86.

Fernhall B, Tymeson GT, Miller L, Burkett LN (1989) Cardiovascular fitness testing and fitness levels of adolescents and adults with mental retardation including Down syndrome. Educ Train Ment Retard 133–8.

Formigari R, di Donato RH, Gargiulo G, di Carlo D, Feltri C, Picchio FM, Marino B (2004) Better surgical prognosis for patients with complete atrioventricular canal and Down syndrome. Ann Thorac Surg (in press).

Freedom RM (1996) Hemodynamic evaluation in children with Down syndrome
    and congenital heart disease. In B Marino, SM Pueschel (eds) Heart Disease in
    Persons with Down Syndrome. Baltimore: Brookes, pp. 141–4.
Frescura C, Thiene G, Franceschini E, Talenti E, Mazzucco A (1987) Pulmonary
    vascular disease in infants with complete atrioventricular septal defects. Int J
    Cardiol 15: 91–100.
Garrod AE (1894) On the association of cardiac malformation with other con-
    genital defects. St Bart Hosp Rep 30: 53–61.
Garrod AE (1898) Congenital heart disease and the mongol type of idiocy. Br Med
    J 1: 1200–1.
Goldhaber SZ, Brown WD, Robertson N, Rubin IL, St. John Sutton NG (1988)
    Aortic regurgitation and mitral valve prolapse with Down's syndrome; a case-
    controlled study. J Ment Defic Res 32: 333–6.
Goldhaber SZ, Brown WD, St John Sutton NG (1987) High frequency of mitral
    valve prolapse and aortic regurgitation among asymptomatic adults with
    Down's syndrome. JAMA 258: 1793–5.
Goldhaber SZ, Rubin IL, Brown WD, Robertson N, Stubblefield F, Sloss LJ (1986)
    Valvular heart disease (aortic regurgitation and mitral valve prolapse) among
    institutionalized adults with Down's syndrome. Am J Cardiol 57: 278–81.
Greenwood RD, Nadas AS (1976) The clinical course of cardiac disease in Down's
    syndrome. Pediatrics 58: 893–7.
Hijii T, Fukishige J, Igarashi H, Takahashi N, Ueda K (1997) Life expectancy and
    social adaptation in individuals with Down syndrome with and without sur-
    gery for congenital heart disease. Clinical Pediatrics 6: 327–33.
Katlic MR, Clark EB, Neill CA, Haller JA (1977) Surgical management of congeni-
    tal heart disease in Down's syndrome. J Thorac Cardiovasc Surg 74: 204–9.
Kobel M, Creighton RE, Steward DJ (1982) Anaesthetic consideration in Down's
    syndrome: experience with 100 patients and review of the literature. Can
    Anaesth Soc J 29: 593–9.
Laursen HB (1976) Congenital heart disease in Down's syndrome. Br Heart J 38: 32–8.
Liu MC, Corlett K (1959) A study of congenital heart defects in mongolism. Arch
    Dis Child 12: 410–19.
Loughlin GM, Wynne JW, Victoria BE (1981) Sleep apnea as a possible cause of
    pulmonary hypertension in Down syndrome. J Pediatr 98: 435–7.
Marino B (1989) Left sided cardiac obstruction in patients with Down syndrome.
    J Pediatr 115: 834–5.
Marino B (1990) Valve insufficiency after atrioventricular septal defect repair: dif-
    ferences between patients with and without Down's syndrome? Ann Thorac
    Surg 50: 854.
Marino B (1992) Atrioventricular septal defect: anatomic characteristics in
    patients with and without Down's syndrome. Cardiol Young 2: 308–10.
Marino B (1996) Patterns of congenital heart disease and associated cardiac
    anomalies in children with Down syndrome. In B Marino, SM Pueschel (eds)
    Heart Disease in Persons with Down Syndrome. Brookes, pp. 133–40.
Marino B, Corno A, Guccione P, Marcelletti C (1991) Ventricular septal defect and
    Down's syndrome. Lancet 2: 245–6.
Marino B, de Zorzi A (1993) Congenital heart disease in trisomy 21 mosaicism. J
    Pediatr 122(3): 500–1.
Marino B, Digilio MC (2001) Health supervision for children with Down syn-
    drome. Pediatrics 108: 1384–5.

Marino B, Papa M, Guccione P, Corno A, Marasini M, Calabrò R (1990a) Ventricular septal defect in Down syndrome. Anatomic types and associated malformation. Am J Dis Child 144: 544–5.

Marino B, Vairo U, Corno A, Nava S, Guccione P, Calabrò R, Marcelletti C (1990b) Atrioventricular canal in Down syndrome: prevalence of associated cardiac malformations compared with patients without Down syndrome. Am J Dis Child 144: 1120–2.

Menahem S, Mee RBB (1985) Complete atrioventricular canal defect in presence of Down syndrome. Lancet 2: 834–5.

Morris CD, Magilke D, Reller M (1992) Down's syndrome affects results of surgical correction of complete atrioventricular canal. Pediatr Cardiol 13: 80–4.

Musiani P, Valitutti S, Castellino F, Larocca LM, Maggiano N, Piantelli M (1990) Intrathymic deficient expansion of T cell precursor in Down syndrome. Am J Med Genet, 7(suppl): 219–24.

Park SC, Mathews RA, Zuberbuhler JR, Rowe RD, Neches WH, Lenox CC (1977) Down syndrome with congenital heart malformation. Am J Dis Child 131: 29–33.

Pastore E, Marino B, Calzolari A, Digilio MC, Giannotti A, Turchetta A (2000) Clinical and cardiorespiratory assessment in children with Down syndrome without congenital heart disease. Arch Ped Adoles 154: 408–10.

Pinto FF, Nunes L, Ferraz F, Sanpayo F (1990) Down's syndrome: different distribution of congenital heart disease between the sexes. Int J Cardiol 27: 175–8.

Pitetti KH, Climstein M, Campbell KD, Barret PJ, Jackson JA (1992) The cardiovascular capacities of adults with Down syndrome: a comparative study. Med Sci Sports and Exerc 24: 13–19.

Pueschel SM (1996a) Historical perspective of heart disease in person with Down syndrome. In B Marino, SM Pueschel (eds) Heart Disease in Persons with Down Syndrome. Brookes, pp. 1–7.

Pueschel SM (1996b) Mitral valve prolapse and aortic regurgitation in adults with Down syndrome. In B Marino, SM Pueschel (eds) Heart Disease in Persons with Down Syndrome. Baltimore: Brookes, pp. 193–201.

Rizzoli G, Mazzucco A, Maizza F, Daliento L, Rubino M, Tursi V, Scalia D (1992) Does Down syndrome affect prognosis of surgically managed atrioventricular septal defects? J Thorac Cardiovasc Surg 104: 945–53.

Rowe RD, Uchida IA (1961) Cardiac malformation in mongolism. Am J Med 31: 726–35.

Rowland TW, Nodstrom LG, Bean MS, Burkhardt H (1981) Chronic upper airway obstruction and pulmonary hypertension in Down's syndrome. Am J Dis Child 135: 1050–2.

Russo MG, Pacileo G, Marino B, Pisacane C, Calabrò P, Ammirati A, Calabrò R (1998) Echocardiographic evaluation of left ventricular systolic function in the Down syndrome. Am J Cardiol 81: 1215–17.

Santoro G, Marino B, di Carlo D, Formigari R, Santoro G, Marcelletti C, Pasquini L (1996) Patient selection for repair of complete atrioventricular canal guided by echocardiography. Eur J Cardio-Thorac Surg 10: 439–42.

Schneider DS, Zahka KG, Clark EB, Neill CA (1989) Patterns of cardiac care in infants with Down syndrome. Am J Dis Child 143: 343–65.

Sing Roxy LN, Maurice LP, Chiu LK, Yung YC (1989) Congenital cardiovascular malformation in Chinese children with Down syndrome. Clin Med J 102/5: 382–6.

Sondheimer HM, Byrum CJ, Blackmann MS (1985) Unequal cardiac care for children with Down's syndrome. Am J Dis Child 139: 68–70.

Soudon P, Stijns M, Tremoroux-Wattiez M, Vliers A (1975) Precocity of pulmonary vascular obstruction in Down's syndrome. Eur J Cardiol 2/4: 473–6.

Spina CA, Smith D, Korn E, Fahey JL, Grossman HJ (1981) Altered cellular immune functions in patients with Down syndrome. Am J Dis Child 135: 251–5.

Tandon R, Edwards JE (1973) Cardiac malformations associated with Down's syndrome. Circulation 47: 1349–55.

Thiene G, Ventriglia F, Frescura C (1996) Heart and lung pathology in Down syndrome. In B Marino, SM Pueschel (eds) Heart Disease in Persons with Down Syndrome. Baltimore: Brookes, pp. 111–25.

Truesdell SC, Clark EB (1991) Health insurance status in a cohort of children and young adults with congenital cardiac diagnoses. Circulation 84: II-386.

Tubman TRJ, Shields MD, Craig BG, Mulholland HC, Nevin NC (1991) Congenital heart disease in Down's syndrome: two year prospective early screening study. Br Med J 302: 1425–7.

Ugazio AG, Lanzavecchia A, Jayakar S, Plebani A, Duse M, Bugio R (1978) Immunodeficiency in Down's syndrome. Acta Paediatr Scand 67: 705–8.

Ulrich DA, Ulrich BD, Angulo-Kinzler RM, Yun J (2001) Treadmill training of infants with Down syndrome: evidence based developmental outcomes. Pediatrics 108(5): 84.

Vet TW, Ottenkamp J (1989) Correction of atrioventricular septal defect: results influenced by Down syndrome? Am J Dis Child 143: 1361–5.

Vizcaino V (1993) Personal communication, Mexico City.

Warkany J, Passarge E, Smith LB (1966) Congenital malformations in autosomal trisomy syndromes. Am J Dis Child 112: 502–17.

Williams WH, Perrella AM, Plauth WH Jr, Hatcher CR Jr, Guyton RA (1989) Survival following repair of complete atrioventricular canal associated with Down's syndrome. In G Crupi, L Parezan, RH Anderson (eds) Perspectives in Pediatric Cardiology. Mount Kisco, NY: Futura Publishing, vol 2, pp. 131–4.

Chapter 5
Health status and disease in adults with Down syndrome

C. BACCICHETTI

Indroduction

There is evidence in ancient art of people with trisomy 21 being part of the human race for thousands of years but it was not until 1866 that Dr John Langdon Down first remarked on the facial similarities of a group of his mentally handicapped patients. Unfortunately, he used racial descriptors such as 'mongol' to describe their appearance, which led to a century of inaccurate and misleading terminology (Levitas and Reid, 2003). People who have Down syndrome (DS) and their advocates are understandably sensitive about the words used to describe this chromosomal condition. The identification of the chromosomal basis of DS in 1959 started a gradual process of acceptance of trisomy 21 as being a variation of normal; this has done a lot to remove some prejudice and end uninformed debate about the 'humanity' of people with DS. Down syndrome, the most frequently identified cause of mental handicap, has a prevalence of about 1 in 800 live births and stillbirths. Survival is lower in people with DS than in those without this disorder. In the past 50 years, survival beyond the first year of life has improved strikingly for DS, from below 50% to more than 90% (Young et al., 2002; Hermon et al., 2001).

Although the social integration of individuals with DS has been increasingly stressed in the last 10 years, very few studies have addressed this aspect.

The two-fold purpose of this investigation was to collect information regarding the occurence of disabilities and handicaps in an unselected population of DS patients living in the community in an area of northeast Italy, and develop a strategy that would prevent, where possible, the complications that make survival of these subjects demanding, both socially and personally. The family physician's holistic approach to patients forms the basic of good healthcare for adults with DS. The most

51

frequent causes of death in people with DS are congenital heart defects and respiratory infections (Young et al., 2002).

Patients with DS are likely to have a variety of illnesses, including thyroid disease, coeliac disease, diabetes, depression, obsessive-compulsive disorder, hearing loss, atlantoaxial subluxation and Alzheimer's disease. In addition to routine health screening, patients with DS should be screened for sleep apnoea, hypothyroidism, signs and symptoms of spinal cord compression and dementia.

Patients with DS may have an unusual presentation of an ordinary illness or condition, and behaviour changes or a loss of function may be the only indication of medical illness (Castro Lobera, 1993).

Materials, methods and results

A census of all subjects with DS living in the community was initiated in 1988 in northeast Italy (Baccichetti et al., 1990); this study reports data from the provinces of Belluno and Treviso and Pordenone. There are 1,285,000 inhabitants in this area, and we estimated that about 800 would have DS. The names of these individuals were obtained from a list, prepared by a medical commission, of subjects with mental deficit requiring some form of assistance. This list was checked with the entries in the Registry of Congenital Malformations of Northeast Italy, which has been operative since 1980, and the Italian Registry of Chromosomal Anomalies, which, since 1990, has collected information on all persons for whom the results of cytogenetic analysis are abnormal. In the district of Pordenone (125) and Belluno (104) a questionnaire was completed during a medical examination. For the district of Treviso a questionnaire was mailed in 1992 to each subject identified; the questionnaires concerned items on their medical history, cytogenetic analysis, social integration and relative living conditions, and the subjects were instructed to seek help from their attending physician in filling out the medical information. From the 540 questionnaires sent out, 355 replies were received.

During 2002, the parents' associations of Treviso reported a control sample of 128 DS patients and found that two were deceased and 30 were not previously 'captured'. Using capture–recapture estimation, we calculate that the number of persons with DS living in this community is 454 (Hook and Regal, 1995; Tilling, 2001).

Age distribution of subjects with DS living in Treviso and the change 10 years later are reported in Figure 5.1. Infant mortality has generally decreased in the past 20 years and a decrease in infant mortality in DS has also been noted. This is due to better medical treatment and increased parental involvement in the care for infants with DS. For adults, survival is also increased.

The number of individuals with DS over 50 years of age increased nearly three-fold. On the contrary, for children there is a decrease (31 vs. 20), due to the effect of prenatal diagnosis, but the total number of persons with DS is increased (427 vs. 454).

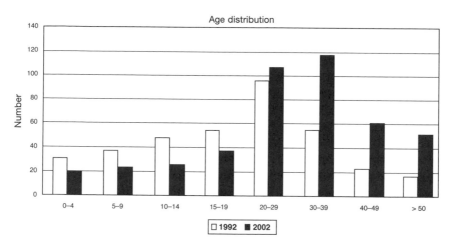

Figure 5.1 Age distribution of persons with Down syndrome living in Treviso (Italy).

Cytogenetic analysis

Only 44% of the surveyed subjects had undergone chromosome analysis. This finding, however, varies with age: analysis had been carried out in 70% of the subjects under 15 years of age, but in only 16% of those over this age. Considering the group as a whole, we found a single case of trisomy 21 from familial t (14:21) translocation; the other subjects either had free 21 trisomy, or *de novo* translocation. Among the patients with free 21 trisomy, there were two brothers, whose mother was 37 and 39 years of age at the time of their births, respectively, and two first cousins.

Associated pathologies

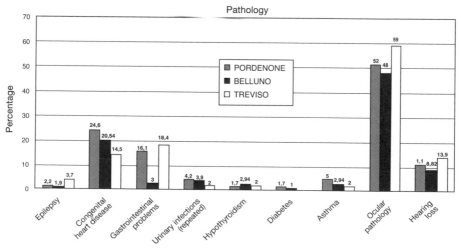

Figure 5.2 Distribution of associated pathologies in people with Down syndrome in three regions of northeast Italy.

Congenital heart disease

This was present in 54 subjects (17%), consisting of 26 females and 28 males. Heart surgery had been performed in 14 patients.

Deafness

Deafness was present in 11% of the subjects, and was mostly conduction type; in one case, deafness was sensorineural in type. Although middle ear problems appear to be the major cause of hearing impairment in individuals with DS, the accumulation of impacted cerumen in the outer ear canal is also a frequent problem.

Thyroid function

There is a growing body of literature that suggests a higher prevalence of thyroid dysfunction in individuals with DS in comparison to control populations for age and sex. All the patients were requested to have their thyroid status tested, and send the results; only 134 complied. Five patients, three males and two females, had overt hypothyroidism, and two were hyperthyroid. Nineteen subjects, 14 females and five males, had high TSH values, despite a normal range of thyroid hormone levels.

Epilepsy

This was reported in 21 patients giving a prevalence of 3%.

Social integration

Approximately 4% of the surveyed persons lived in an institution, mainly in a home for the aged. The others lived at home with the family. In 17 cases, both parents were dead, and six of these persons were institutionalized. Among the 12 subjects living in an institution, nine were older than 35 years. In addition, from Figure 5.3, it can be seen that about 40% of the subjects with DS were able to participate actively in society, even though only 1.7% could work without supervision.

Discussion

The aim of this study was to verify findings we had previously obtained from a small sample using a larger, unbiased sample (Baccichetti et al., 1990). In our earlier report, the incidence of congenital heart disease (CHD) was 13%; in this study, it was 17%. Since heart defects are reported to be present at birth in more than 40% of the children with DS (Rowe and Uchida, 1960), we can conclude that the mortality rate of subjects with CHD and DS is four times higher than in subjects without CHD.

Acute leukaemia has been documented to occur 10–20 times more in children with DS than in the non-DS population. We would expect to find DS subjects who survived leukaemia in our sample; the absence of these

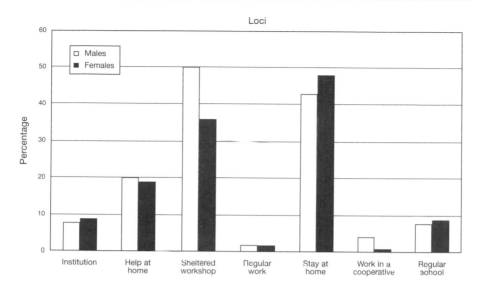

Figure 5.3 Social integration of a population of people with Down syndrome in northeast Italy.

people indicates that the mortality from leukaemia was very high. The results on thyroid status tests agreed with our previous findings in an out-patient sample (Rubello et al., 1995).

The incidence of epilepsy in subjects with DS has been described as increasing with age; in particular, a rate of 1.4% was reported in children (Tatsuno et al., 1984), while a figure of 12% was estimated in persons over 35 years of age (Veall, 1974). According to recent studies (Johannsen et al., 1996), the prevalence of epilepsy is 6.2% in an unselected population of children between 4 and 15 years of age, and 3.2% in an unselected population over 17 years of age. In our series of unselected DS subjects living in the community we found 21 patients with epilepsy, and the onset of this symptom in every case was before 35 years of age. Thus the prevalence of epilepsy was 3/100 (95% CI=1.2/100:4.9/100). In addition, it seems useful to stress that while epilepsy is certainly a more frequent event in DS subjects than in the general population, it does not reach the rate of 12% observed by others.

Moreover, as we consider it is important that not only the quantity but also the quality of life of subjects with DS should be enhanced, timely treatment of sensorineural handicaps is necessary to enable these individuals to be more useful to themselves as well as to the community. To this purpose, some complications, such as deafness and thyroid dysfunction, which present respectively in 11% and 7% of this population, should be prevented early; heart disease should receive prompt surgical attention at an appropriate age. We have not considered psychiatric disorders affecting one-third of DS adults because we need a better definition of psychiatric disorders. To our knowledge, other findings in non-selected populations of DS subjects living in the community are not available.

Plans for long-term living arrangements, estate planning and custody arrangements should be discussed with the parents or guardians. Because of improvements in healthcare and better education, and because more people with this condition are being raised at home, most adults with DS can expect to function well enough to live in a group home and hold a meaningful job.

Acknowledgements

The authors wish to thank Associazione Coordinamento Down, Associazione Italiana Persone Down Sezione di Belluno, A.N.F.A.A.S. di Treviso and Associazione Down Friuli Venezia Giulia.

Bibliography

Baccichetti C, Lenzini E, Pegoraro R (1990) DS in the Belluno district (Veneto Region, Northeast Italy): age distribution and morbidity. Am J Med Gen Suppl 7: 8–86.

Castro Lobera A (1993) The medical and social aspects of Down's syndrome. Aten Primaria 12(9): 604–6.

Comiskey CM, Barry JM (2001) A capture–recapture study of the prevalence and implications of opiate use in Dublin. Eur J Public Health 11(2): 198–200.

Goldberg-Stern H, Strawsburg RH, Patterson B, Hickey F, Bare M, Gadoth N, Dagrauw TJ (2001) Seizure frequency and characteristics in children with Down syndrome. Brain Dev 23(6): 375–8.

Hermon C, Alberman E, Beral V, Swerdlow AJ (2001) Mortality and cancer incidence in persons with Down's syndrome, their parents and siblings. Ann Hum Genet 65(2): 167–76.

Hook EB, Regal RR (1995) Capture–recapture estimation. Epidemiology 6(5): 569–70.

Johannsen P, Christensen JE, Goldstein H, Nielsen VK, Mai J (1996) Epilepsy in Down syndrome – prevalence in three age groups. Seizure 5(2): 121–5.

Levitas AS, Reid CS (2003) An angel with Down syndrome in a sixteenth century Flemish Nativity painting. Am J Med Genet 116A(4): 399–405.

Roizen NJ (2002) Medical care and monitoring for the adolescent with Down syndrome. Adolesc Med 13(2): 345–58

Roizen NJ, Wolters C, Nicol T, Blondis TA (1993) Hearing loss in children with Down syndrome. J Pediatr 123(1): S9–12.

Rowe RD, Uchida IH (1960) Congenital cardiac malformations in mongolism. Br Heart J 22: 331.

Rubello D, Pozzan GB, Casara D, Girelli ME, Boccato S, Rigon F, Baccichetti C, Piccolo M, Betterle C, Busnardo B (1995) Natural course of subclinical hypo-thyroidism in Down's syndrome: prospective study results and therapeutic considirations. J Endocrinol Invest 18(1): 35–40.

Tatsuno M, Hayashi M, Iwamoto H, Suzuki Y, Kuroki Y (1984) Epilepsy in child-hood DS. Brain & Develop 1: 37–44.

Tilling K (2001) Capture–recapture methods – useful or misleading? Int J Epidemiol 30(1): 12–14.

Veall RM (1974) The prevalence of epilepsy among mongols related to age. J Ment Def Res 18: 99–106.

Yang Q, Rasmussen SA, Friedman JM (2002) Mortality associated with Down's syn-drome in the USA from 1983 to 1997: a population-based study. Lancet 359: 1019–25.

Chapter 6
The endocrinology of adults with Down syndrome

C. ROMANO

Endocrinological involvement in Down syndrome (DS) refers mainly to four topics: thyroid disorders, growth, gonadal function and osteoporosis. The first two are addressed in other parts of the book, and will not be covered here.

Gonadal function

Gonadal function was studied in 1969 by Benda (1969), who found an increased incidence of abnormalities in sex development in subjects with DS. Several authors reported later on gonadal dysfunction shown by women with DS (Hojager et al., 1978; Hasen et al., 1980; Hsiang et al., 1987). Bellone et al. (1980) highlighted delayed puberty in both sexes with DS. Benda (1960) and Peters et al. (1975) underlined the ovarian abnormality, decreased total ovarian mass and decreased follicular growth in DS. With regard to menarche in DS, the first result from Bellone et al. (1980) of a delay has since been disputed by Goldstein (1988) and Scola and Pueschel (1992).

Ovulation and reproduction were first addressed by Tricomi et al. (1964), who observed a definite ovulatory pattern in 38.5% of its sample of women with DS, probable in 15.4%, possible in 15.4% and absent in the remaining 30.4%. Scola and Pueschel (1992) reported 88.5% of another sample of women with DS showing a biphasic basal body temperature curve, indicative of an ovulatory pattern. Rani et al. (1990) reported 31 documented pregnancies in 27 women with DS. Cento et al. (1996) matched 20 women with DS and 20 controls, reporting in the first group a significantly increased incidence of anovulatory cycles and defects in the luteal phase. Furthermore, ovulatory cycles showed a significant reduction in plasma levels of oestradiol and progesterone. The lesson that can be gathered from these results may be the following: a primary dysfunction in follicular maturation may be present in women with DS and can lead to anovulation or luteal function impairment.

It is important to increase our knowledge of the ovarian function of women with DS in order to be aware of potential reproductive problems: they can be sexually abused with resulting unwanted pregnancies.

The study of ovarian function in DS could be divided into the study of gonadotrophins, sex steroids and ovarian sensitivity to gonadotrophins. Conflicting results have been reported on the gonadotrophins. Hasen (1975) found aberrant function of the pituitary–gonadal axis, with plasma luteinizing hormone (LH) and follicle-stimulating hormone (FSH) significantly increased in women with DS. On the contrary, Bock (1974) reported normal function in the hypothalamic–pituitary–gonadal axis and normal FSH and LH plasma values in follicular and secretory phases. Cento et al. (1996) overlapped Bock's (1974) results regarding gonadotrophin plasma values, without any significant difference between women with DS and controls.

The development of ovaries in DS patients differs from the usual. Girls with DS show reduced total ovarian mass and number of small follicles, mainly after the age of 3 years (Benda 1960; Peters et al., 1975; Hojager et al., 1978; Cento et al., 1997). Their follicle growth is absent or retarded. Hypogonadism has been reported in DS (McCarthy and Rockette, 1986). Cento et al. (1996) compared the basal body temperature (BBT) curves and the endocrine patterns of 20 cycles in women with DS, regularly menstruating and at least 2 years since menarche, with age-matched healthy women with regular menses. Women with DS showed a significantly higher incidence of anovulatory cycles and, among the ovulatory cycles, 66% had a BBT curve representative of a short luteal phase. Plasma levels of oestradiol and progesterone were significantly decreased in ovulatory cycles of women with DS, advancing the consequent hypothesis that all the ovarian steps leading to ovulation and luteal function are impaired in women with DS.

The result of a subsequent study (Cento et al., 1997) of the same research team is also interesting. Ovarian sensitivity to FSH administration, expressed in terms of oestradiol production, was significantly blunted in normo-ovulating women with DS versus the controls. Plasma levels of growth hormone (GH) were decreased in the group with DS. Continuing their research path, Cento et al. (1998) proved that GH administration normalizes ovarian response to FSH in the early stages of a follicle's maturation in women with DS. These studies explain GH's role in ovarian function of women with DS. On the other hand, very recent studies (Frendo et al., 2000; Massin et al., 2001) have also demonstrated a prenatal origin of GH impairment in DS. These authors have shown that formation of syncytiotrophoblasts is abnormal in DS, since cytotrophoblasts aggregate in culture, but do not fuse or fuse poorly. This fact combines with the decreased production of human chorionic gonadotrophin (HCG) from the placenta and of pregnancy-specific hormones synthesized by syncytiotrophoblasts, such as human placental lactogen (HPL), placental growth hormone (PGH) and leptin.

The recent report by Kim et al. (2001) gives an example of the struggle to overcome the fertility impairment of DS. In this article a 30-year-old man, who is globozoospermic and mosaic for DS, fathered a healthy female neonate with a 46,XX karyotype, impregnating his wife through intracytoplasmic sperm injection (ICSI).

Osteoporosis

With regard to young adults with DS, an article (Sakadamis et al., 2002) evaluating bone mass and gonadal function has been just published. The results are important, mainly because they show that gonadal dysfunction and osteoporosis are coexistent in this sample. Particularly, while there is no statistical difference with the control group regarding FSH, testosterone, dehydroepiandrosterone sulphate (DHEA-S), serum calcium and phosphorus, and the calcium/creatinine urinary ratio, there is a statistically significant decrease of bone mineral density (BMD) and a statistically significant increase of LH, 17-hydroxy-progesterone (17-OH-P) and the hydroxyproline/creatinine urinary ratio. Such results highlight that reduced bone mass is present also in young adult males with DS and that hypogonadism, hypotonia, low muscular strength and stillness may be considered as promoting factors. A previous study (Angelopoulou et al., 2000) of the same research team proved that the strength of the femoral quadriceps predicts BMD significantly for people with DS. A practical and useful closing message is that an active lifestyle and increased physical exercise help to oppose osteoporosis in DS.

References

Angelopoulou N, Matziari C, Tsimaras V, Sakadamis A, Souftas V, Mandroukas K (2000) Bone mineral density and muscle strength in young men with mental retardation (with and without Down syndrome). Calcif Tissue Int 66: 176–80.

Bellone E, Tanganelli E, LaPlaca A et al. (1980) Menarca e fisiopatologia menstruale nella sindrome di Down. Minerva Ginecol 32: 579–88.

Benda CE (1960) The Child with Mongolism. New York: Grune & Stratton, p.120.

Benda CE (1969) Down's Syndrome. New York: Grune & Stratton, p. 98.

Bock JE (1974) The hypothalamic–pituitary–gonadal and adrenal cortical function in adult women with Down's syndrome. Acta Obstet Gynecol Scand 53: 69–72.

Cento RM, Ragusa L, Proto C, Alberti A, Fiore G, Colabucci F, Lanzone A (1997) Ovarian sensitivity to follicle stimulating hormone is blunted in normoovulatory women with Down's syndrome. Hum Reprod 12: 1709–13.

Cento RM, Ragusa L, Proto C, Alberti A, Fiore G, Soranna L, Colabucci F, Lanzone A (1998) Growth hormone administration normalizes the ovarian responsiveness to follicle-stimulating-hormone in the early stages of the follicular maturation in women with Down syndrome. J Endocrinol Invest 21: 342–7.

Cento RM, Ragusa L, Proto C, Alberti A, Romano C, Boemi G, Colabucci F, Lanzone A (1996) Basal body temperature curves and endocrine pattern of menstrual cycles in Down syndrome. Gynecol Endocrinol 10: 133–7.

Frendo JL, Vidaud M, Guibourdenche J, Luton D, Muller F, Bellet D, Giovagrandi Y, Tarrade A, Porquet D, Blot P, Evain-Brion D (2000) Defect of villous cytotrophoblast differentiation into syncytiotrophoblast in Down's syndrome. J Clin Endocrinol Metab 85: 3700–7.

Goldstein H (1988) Menarche, menstruation, sexual relations and contraception of adolescent females with Down syndrome. Eur J Obstet Gynecol Reprod Biol 27: 343–9.

Hasen J (1975) Aberrant pituitary–gonadal function in G-21 trisomy. Presented at the 57th Annual Meeting of the Endocrine Society, New York, p. 247.

Hasen J, Boyar RM, Shapiro LR (1980) Gonadal function in trisomy 21. Horm Res 12: 345–50.

Hojager B, Peters H, Byskov AG, Faber M (1978) Follicular development in ovaries of children with Down's syndrome. Acta Paediatr Scand 67: 637–43.

Hsiang YH, Berkovitz GD, Bland GL, Migeon CJ, Warren AC (1987) Gonadal function in patients with Down syndrome. Am J Med Genet 27: 449–58.

Kim ST, Cha YB, Park JM, Gye MC (2001) Successful pregnancy and delivery from frozen-thawed embryos after intracytoplasmic sperm injection using round-headed spermatozoa and assisted oocyte activation in a globozoospermic patient with mosaic Down syndrome. Fertil Steril 75: 445–7.

Massin A, Frendo JL, Guibourdenche J, Luton D, Giovangrandi Y, Muller F, Vidaud M, Evain-Brion D (2001) Defect of syncytiotrophoblast formation and human chorionic gonadotropin expression in Down's syndrome. Placenta 22 (Suppl A): S93–S97.

McCarthy JJ, Rockette HE (1986) Prediction of ovulation with basal body temperature. J Reprod Med 31: 742–7.

Peters H, Byskov AG, Himelstein-Braw R, Faber M (1975) Follicular growth: the basic event in the mouse and human ovary. J Reprod Fertil 45: 559–66.

Rani AS, Jyothi A, Reddy PP, Reddy OS (1990) Reproduction in Down's syndrome. Int J Gynecol Obstet 31: 81–6.

Sakadamis A, Angelopoulou N, Matziari C, Papameletiou V, Souftas V (2002) Bone mass, gonadal function and biochemical assessment in young men with trisomy 21. Eur J Obstet Gynecol Reprod Biol 100: 208–12.

Scola PS, Pueschel SM (1992) Menstrual cycles and basal body temperature curves in women with Down syndrome. Obstet Gynecol 79: 91–4.

Tricomi V, Valenti C, Hall JE (1964) Ovulatory patterns in Down's syndrome. Am J Obstet Gynecol 89: 651–6.

Chapter 7
Growth retardation in Down syndrome: thyroid disorders, coeliac disease and the effect of GH therapy

G. ANNERÉN, Å. MYRELID, J. GUSTAFSSON

Introduction

The growth pattern in Down syndrome (DS) differs markedly from that of normal children and short stature is a cardinal feature of DS. Growth retardation is not only due to the syndrome itself, but is also related to disorders such as coeliac disease and hypothyroidism. Data on DS-specific growth charts, autoimmune disorders, thyroid function, coeliac disease and a trial with growth hormone treatment will be covered in this chapter.

Growth pattern in individuals with Down syndrome, new Swedish growth charts

The growth pattern in DS is characterized by an impaired growth velocity from birth until adolescence, especially during the age interval of 6 months to 3 years and during puberty. Down syndrome-specific growth charts are important tools in medical follow-up of children with DS. There are several DS-specific growth charts available (Cronk et al, 1988; Piro et al., 1990; Cremers et al., 1996) The American growth charts for DS (Cronk et al., 1988) have been frequently used.

We have created Swedish growth charts based on a combination of longitudinal and cross-sectional data of 354 individuals with DS born between 1970 and 1997 (Myrelid et al., 2002). Mean birth lengths were 48 cm in both sexes. Mean birth weights were 3.0 kg for boys and 2.9 kg for girls. Head growth was impaired resulting in an SD for head circumference of –0.5 (Swedish standard, Karlberg et al., 1976) at birth decreasing to –2.0 at 4 years of age. This is similar to that reported for American children with DS (Palmer et al., 1992).

61

Final heights (161.5 cm for males, 147.5 cm for females) were reached at relatively young ages (16 and 15 years, respectively). Puberty was somewhat early and pubertal growth rate was decreased. The difference in height between the sexes was the same as that of healthy individuals. We have shown that there is a good correlation between final height and target height in children with DS (Arnell et al., 1996). Final height in DS individuals is about 18 cm below target height. In comparison with healthy boys, the males with DS had a mean birth length and a final height at 18 years of age corresponding to –1.5 SD and –2.5 SD, respectively. When our data for boys were compared with those of the DS growth charts created by Cronk and co-workers (1988) the final height corresponds to the 95th percentile of the American DS growth charts. The rather marked difference in final height between Swedish and American males with DS cannot be explained at present, but may be due to factors such as ethnic diversity and differences in size of the study groups. The difference in final mean height between males and females with DS in the present study was 14 cm, i.e. similar to that of healthy individuals. The girls with DS in the present study had a mean birth length of –1 SD and a mean final height, at the age of 18 years, of –2.5 SD according to the Swedish standard. The final height of the Swedish girls with DS was slightly greater than that of the American girls.

Obesity is a well known problem of adults with DS. In the present study, a body mass index (BMI) > 25 kg/m² at 18 years of age was observed in 31% of the males and 36% of the females. Our growth charts show that European DS boys are taller than corresponding American boys, whereas European DS girls, although being lighter, have a similar final height to corresponding American girls. If standard growth charts are used for DS children the development of associated diseases influencing linear growth may be overlooked.

Autoimmune disorders in Down syndrome

Individuals with DS are prone to develop autoimmune disease. The disorder autoimmune polyendocrine syndrome type I (APS I) is caused by a mutation in the AIRE gene on chromosome 21 (Nagamine et al., 1997). We have recently shown that about 15% (7/48) of patients with DS have elevated titres of autoantibodies which are common in APS I (to be published). The high prevalence of autoimmune disease, such as coeliac disease and hypothyroidism, in DS might be due to dysregulation of the AIRE gene.

Thyroid disorders in Down syndrome

Thyroid disease, mostly hypothyroidism, is common in DS. The prevalence of hypothyroidism in DS has been reported as 3–54% and thyroid autoantibodies have been found in 13–34% of DS individuals (Ivarsson et al., 1997). Congenital hypothyroidism has been reported to be about 30 times more common in newborns with DS compared to normal newborns (Fort et al., 1984).

One study has followed thyroid function during childhood and adolescence in DS in relation to sex, growth velocity and thyroid autoantibodies (Karlsson et al., 1998). Eighty-five individuals (42 males and 43 females) with DS, aged 1 to 25 years, were followed for up to 15 years. Height, weight, and serum levels of TSH and free T4 were recorded annually. Thyroid autoantibodies (thyroid peroxidase antibodies (TPO-ab) and thyroglobulin antibodies (Tg-ab)) were analysed when hypothyroidism was suspected. Hypothyroidism was found in 28/85 (32.9%) and hyperthyroidism in 2/85 (2.4%) of the subjects. No sex difference was observed. Of the hypothyroid subjects, 14/28 had developed the condition before the age of 8 years and only one of these displayed a detectable serum level of TPO-ab at diagnosis. Half (14/28) of the children with hypothyroidism acquired the disease after 8 years of age and of these 11/13 (84.6%) had elevated levels of one or both thyroid autoantibodies. There was a negative correlation between serum levels of free T4 and age ($r = 0.75$; $p < .001$). The mean level of TSH was elevated or in the upper normal range in all age groups. In the prepubertal (2–9 years of age) hypothyroid subjects, growth velocity was significantly lower the year before starting thyroxin therapy compared to the year after ($p < .05$) and also compared to that of sex- and age-matched euthyroid DS children ($p < .01$).

In conclusion, hypothyroidism develops in one-third of DS individuals before the age of 25 years. Autoimmune thyroid disease is uncommon in pre-school DS children, but occurs commonly after the age of 8 years. The cause of thyroid disorder in DS seems to be due a combination of thyroid gland hypoplasia and thyroid autoimmunity. Growth velocity was significantly improved in most children upon treatment with thyroxin.

Coeliac disease in Down syndrome

Coeliac disease is another autoimmune disorder reported to occur frequently in subjects with DS (George et al., 1996). In order to investigate the incidence of coeliac disease in children with DS and to find the best markers to detect the disease, a study was performed on 85 children with DS. We found that 5% of the children suffered from coeliac disease (Hansson et al., 1999). Elevated serum levels of antigliadin serum antibodies were commonly found (25%), and were shown to be a weak marker for coeliac disease. Determination of antiendomysium antibodies was a more useful screening test for the disease in DS.

Growth hormone (GH) secretion and the effect of GH therapy in children with Down syndrome

Endogenous growth hormone (GH) has a major influence on growth from the age of 6–9 months, through stimulation of the production of insulin-like growth factor I (IGF-I). Growth retardation in DS becomes pronounced during the period when GH starts to regulate growth. There is no obvious deficiency of GH in the serum of children with DS (Sara et al., 1983), although suboptimal endogenous GH production due to hypothalamic dysfunction has been demonstrated. Selective deficiency of IGF-I in serum has been observed in patients with DS older than 2 years (Sara et al., 1983). Subjects with DS have no deficiency of serum IGF-II (Annerén et al., 1984), and IGF receptors have been found to be present in brain cells from foetuses with trisomy 21 (Sara et al., 1984).

In a previous study we observed that children aged 3–6 years with DS who were short responded to short-term GH therapy with an increased growth velocity and normalization of the serum levels of IGF-I (Annerén et al., 1986). In order to find out if GH treatment of young children with DS could have an impact on mental development, 15 young children (average age at start 7.4 months) with DS were treated with growth hormone (GH) for 3 years (Annerén et al., 1999). The mean height of the children increased from −1.8 SD (Swedish standard) to −0.8 SD, whereas that of a control group fell from −1.7 to −2.2 SD during the same age period. After cessation of GH treatment the growth velocity declined. The growth of the head did not increase during the treatment and there was no effect on mental or gross motor function.

GH therapy given to children with Prader Willi syndrome, another syndrome with obesity as a cardinal feature (Gunay-Aygun et al., 1997), has been reported to influence lipid metabolism favourably (Lindgren et al., 1998). In an ongoing study we are investigating GH secretion as well as glucose production and lipolysis in adults with DS. There may be a similar mechanism in DS that might explain the obesity and other common problems (Annerén et al., 1996). In an ongoing study we are investigating GH secretion and metabolism in both adults and children with DS. However, GH therapy is still not recommended in children or adults with DS, except for those with a proven GH deficiency (Annerén et al., 2000).

Recommended medical programme for children with Down syndrome and growth retardation

Growth retardation in DS is sometimes due to treatable disorders. For this reason, the following medical investigations or measures are recommended in a child with DS and decreased growth velocity:

- Calculate target height from the heights of the parents
- Monitor growth on Down syndrome-specific growth charts
- Exclude hypothyroidism with serum tests of TSH and free T4. Repeat these tests annually during childhood and every third year in adulthood
- Exclude coeliac disease in case of symptoms
- If everything is normal analyse IGF-I in serum. If this is low exclude GH deficiency.

References

Annerén G, Engberg G, Sara VR (1984) The presence of normal levels of serum immunoreactive insulin-like growth factor 2 (IGF-2) in patients with Down's syndrome. Ups J Med Sci 89: 274–8.

Annerén G, Sara VR, Hall K, Tuvemo T (1986) Growth and somatomedin responses to growth hormone in Down's syndrome. Arch Dis Child 61: 48–52.

Annerén G, Bull MJ, Flórez J, Guyda HJ, Mortimer J, Pueschel SM (1996) Statement for parents on growth hormone treatment for children with Down syndrome. Down Syndrome Quarterly 1: 9.

Annerén G, Tuvemo T, Carlsson-Skwirut C, Lönnerholm T, Bang P, Sara VR, Gustafsson J (1999) Growth hormone treatment in young children with Down's syndrome: effects on growth and psychomotor development. Arch Dis Child 80: 334–8.

Annerén G, Tuvemo T, Gustafsson J (2000) Growth hormone therapy in young children with Down syndrome and clinical comparison between Down and Prader-Willi syndromes. Growth Horm IG Res Suppl B: 87–91.

Arnell H, Gustafsson J, Ivarsson SA, Annerén G (1996) Growth and pubertal development in Down syndrome. Acta Paediat 85: 1102–6.

Castells S, Torrado C, Bastian W, Wisniewski KE (1992) Growth hormone deficiency in Down's syndrome. J Intell Disabil Res 36: 29–43.

Cremers MJ, van der Tweel I, Boersma B, Wit JM, Zonderland M (1996) Growth curves of Dutch children with Down's syndrome. J Intell Disabil Res 40: 412–20.

Cronk C, Crocker AC, Pueschel SM, Shea AM, Zackai E, Pickens G, Reed RB (1988) Growth charts for children with Down syndrome: 1 month to 18 years of age. Pediatrics 81: 102–10.

Fort P, Lifshitz F, Bellisario R, Davis J, Lanes R, Pugliese M, Richman R, Post M, David R (1984) Abnormalities of thyroid function in infants with Down syndrome. J Pediatr 104: 545–9.

George EK, Mearin ML, Bouquet J, von Blomberg BM, Stapel SO, van Elburg RM, de Graaf EA, Hertzberg-ten Cate R, van Suijekom-Smith LW, Reeser HM, Oostdijk W (1996) High frequency of celiac disease in Down syndrome. J Pediatr 128: 555–7.

Gunay-Aygun M, Cassidy SB, Nicholls R (1997) Prader-Willi and other syndromes associated with obesity and mental retardation. Behav Genet 27(4): 307–24.

Hansson T, Dannaeus A, Annerén G, Sjöberg O, Klareskog L (1999) Celiac disease in relation to immunological serum markers, trace elements and HLA-DR and DQ antigens in Swedish children with Down syndrome. J Pediat Gastroent Nutr 29: 286–92.

Ivarsson S-A, Ericsson U-B, Gustafsson J, Forslund M, Vegfors P, Annerén G (1997) The impact of thyroid autoimmunity in children and adolescents with Down syndrome. Acta Paediat 86: 1065–7.

Karlberg P, Taranger J, Engström I Lichtenstein H, Lindström B, Svennberg-Redegren EM (1976) Physical growth from birth to 16 years and longitudinal outcome of the study during the same period. Acta Paediat Scand Suppl 258: 7–76.

Karlsson B, Gustafsson J, Hedow G, Ivarsson SA, Annerén G (1998) Thyroid function in children and adolescents with Down syndrome in relation to age, sex, growth velocity and thyroid antibodies. Arch Dis Childhood 79: 242–5.

Lindgren AC, Hagenäs L, Müller J, Blichfeldt S, Rosenborg M, Brismar T, Ritsen M (1998) Growth hormone treatment of children with Prader-Willi syndrome affects linear growth and body composition favourably. Acta Paediat 87: 28–31.

Myrelid Å, Gustafsson J, Ollars B, Annerén G (2002) Growth charts for Down's syndrome from birth to 18 years of age. Arch Dis Child 87: 97–103.

Nagamine K, Peterson P, Scott HS, Kudoh J, Minoshima S, Heino M, Krohn KJ, Lalioti MD, Mullis PE, Antonarakis SE, Kawasaki K, Asakawa S, Ito F, Shimizu N (1997) Positional cloning of the APECED gene. Nat Genet 17: 393–8.

Palmer C, Cronk C, Pueschel SM, Wisniewski KE, Laxova R, Crocker AC, Pauli RM (1992) Head circumference of children with Down syndrome (0–36 months). Am J Med Genet 42: 61–7.

Piro E, Pennino C, Cammarata M, Corsello G, Grenci A, Lo Giudio C, Morabito M, Piccione M, Giuffre L (1990) Growth charts of Down's syndrome in Sicily: evaluation of 382 children 0–14 years of age. Am J Med Genet Suppl 7: 66–70.

Sara VR, Gustavson K-H, Annerén G, Hall K, Wetterberg L (1983) Somatomedins in Down's syndrome. Biol Psychiat 18: 803–11.

Sara VR, Sjögren B, Annerén G, Gustavson K-H, Forsman A, Hall K, Wahlström J, Wetterberg L (1984) The precence of normal receptors for somatomedin and insulin in foetuses with Down's syndrome. Biol Psychiatr 19: 591–8.

Chapter 8
The audiological diagnosis in subjects with Down syndrome

A. Mura, M. Medicina

A major incidence of hearing deficit in subjects with Down syndrome compared with the normal population has been described by many authors, although great controversy exists, with results varying from 8% (McIntire et al., 1965) to 78% (Balkany et al., 1979). The results of deafness, even if the impairment is slight, on the psychophysical development in Down subjects can be important because these people usually need special rehabilitation and major stimulation of learning.

An early diagnosis of deafness is therefore very important, as are hearing checks over a long period of time. Diagnosis is difficult in very young Down patients, as it is in normal children; it may also be difficult in older people due to lack of cooperation.

There are many techniques used in the diagnosis of deafness of Down subjects, both subjective (standard tonal audiometry, pure-tone play audiometry) and objective (impedance tests, auditory brainstem response examination, otoacoustic emissions).

Pure-tone air and bone conduction threshold permits a rapid evaluation of hearing deficit. It is only possible in cooperative subjects, under suitable conditions. A summary of the literature is as follows:

- Fulton and Lloyd (1968) found normal auditory function in 58% of subjects; of the remaining people 55% showed conductive deafness, 22% mixed and 23% neurosensorial impairment
- Medicina et al. (1986) reported normal hearing function in 67.3% of subjects
- Paludetti et al. (1982) detected the audiometric threshold, ranging between 15 and 40 dB HL, in 33% of cases
- Brooks et al. (1972) reported normal hearing in 23% of Down subjects on the basis of pure-tone and impedance audiometry

- Hildmann et al. (2002) conducted a study of 102 subjects (32 were younger than 2 years) which showed an incidence of 88% conductive deafness, 7% mixed and 5% neurosensorial

We should also take into consideration the fact that the average hearing level of DS children with normal hearing function seemed lower than that of a normal group control (Dahle and McCollister, 1986).

Types of deafness

Conductive deafness

There is agreement in the literature that when deafness is present, it is of the conductive type in most cases (60–70%). Impedance tests show the presence of pathology of the middle ear with great accuracy. This is a very common condition in Down subjects, mostly due to middle ear otitis with effusion, which lasts longer than in normal children of the same age (Schwartz and Schwartz, 1978).

Conductive deafness is caused by anatomical and functional alterations of the oronasopharynx, for example a constricted nasopharynx, an acute angle of insertion of the Eustachian tube in the nasopharynx, macroglossia, a more superficial position of the palatine tonsils, hypotonia of muscles of the palate and the middle ear (Strome, 1981). Congenital alterations of the ossicular chain, including the stapes, are also important in the aetiology of conductive deafness (Fulton and Lloyd, 1968; Schwartz and Schwartz, 1978; Balkany et al., 1979).

Neurosensorial impairment

The incidence of neurosensorial hearing loss is lower. In some cases it can be due to anomalies of the inner ear in the cochlear turns (Igarashi et al., 1977); in other cases the appearance of a neurosensorial component in the early phase compared to normal subjects is due to histological alteration similar to presbiacusis of the temporal bone of Down subjects (Krmpotic-Nemanic, 1970).

Anatomofunctional alterations of the central nervous system have been described, consisting of a minor cerebellum and brainstem weight change and abnormal myelinization and speed of nervous conduction (Crome et al., 1967; Scott et al., 1983).

Auditory testing techniques

The main audiological problem of Down subjects is detecting the possible deafness and establishing the type and the level of hearing loss.

Otomicroscopy

Otomicroscopy is very important because often the external auditory meatus is stenotic or obstructed by cerumen and a view of the tympanic membrane can be difficult. The diagnostic strategy, as in a normal subject, varies according to the age and level of cooperation of the subject.

Play and tonal audiometry

Play and tonal audiometry are generally difficult to do and produce controversal results (Figure 8.1). A functional audiological diagnosis can be made by applying objective methods, which include impedance tests, otoacoustic emissions and brainstem audiometry. These techniques may be used in combination in many cases.

Impedance audiometry

Impedance audiometry (tympanometry and acoustic reflex) (Figure 8.2) allows a diagnosis of middle ear pathology, either inflammatory or not, which contributes to deafness and can be treated with pharmacological

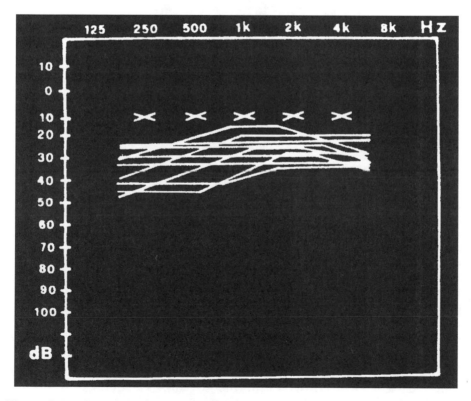

Figure 8.1 Pure-tone audiometry results in Down's syndrome showing a prevalence of conductive hearing loss (Paludetti et al., 1982).

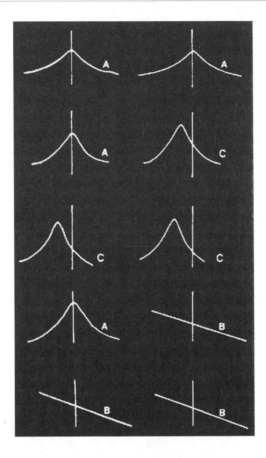

Figure 8.2 Different types of tympanograms with the type A indicating normal condition and the types B and C suggesting pathological middle ear function (Paludetti et al., 1982).

therapy or surgery, to avoid the disease becoming chronic. Tympanometry, moreover, permits an evaluation of the tubaric functionality and the stapedial reflex; if this is present, it can be used to obtain the auditory threshold.

Auditory brainstem responses

Analysis of auditory brainstem responses (ABR) is an objective, non-invasive technique, which provides information about the cochlear function and the auditory pathway in the brain. Many discordant anomalies have been described in ABR of Down subjects in relation to waves and interpeak intervals latency and amplitude (Straumanis et al., 1973; Folsom et al., 1983; Kaga and Marsh, 1986; Kakigi and Kuroda, 1992) (Figure 8.3 a, b and c). However this method allows an evaluation of auditory threshold by determining the level of the wave V at progressively decreasing intensity.

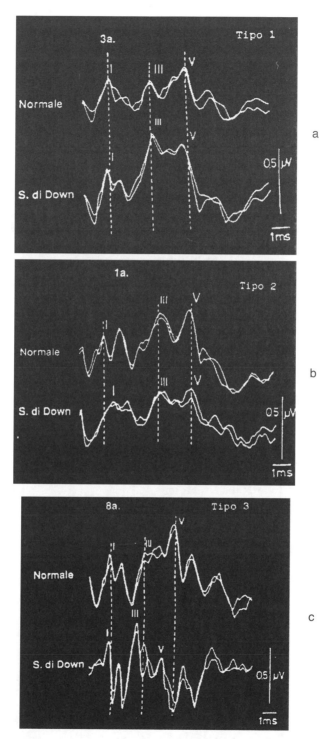

Figure 8.3 a, b and c Brainstem acoustic responses (ABR) in Down syndrome and in normal subjects. Note the great inter-individual variability of waves and interpeak-intervals latency (Kaga and Marsh, 1986).

Other techniques

The acoustic otoemission to clicks stimulus (TEOAE) and products of acoustic distortion (DPOAE) have become important in recent years in the early diagnosis of deafness; these are used as a method at the first stage of a child's audiological screening (Molini et al., 1997). These tests have important characteristics of objectivity, non-invasiveness, sensitivity and

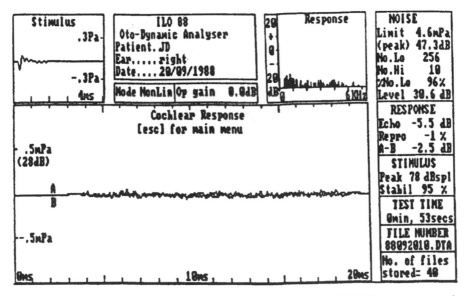

Figure 8.4 Absence of transient evoked otoacoustic emission (TEOAE) in a Down subject with conductive hearing loss.

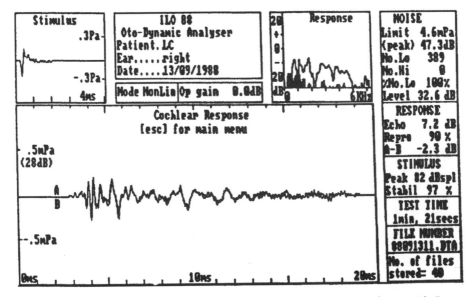

Figure 8.5 Transient evoked otoacoustic emissions (TEOAE) in a subject with Down syndrome, classified as having normal hearing.

low cost. DPOAE is a sensitive indicator of the inner ear function. It is known, however, that the presence of middle ear disorders limits their use in audiological diagnosis (Figures 8.4 and 8.5).

It is generally agreed that where middle ear disorders are present, the cochlea functions normally in DS (Salata et al., 1998). The reported alterations of the amplitude of DPOAE in adult Down subjects with normal function of the middle ear could be the result of anomalies of the inner ear connected with age (Hassmann et al., 1998).

Conclusions

In audiological screening during the first days of life or in successive months, both impedance tests and DPOAE should be used and repeated as a follow-up. This is also the case where normal results were obtained at the first examination. To evaluate hearing threshold, we prefer the ABR technique.

The early diagnosis of deafness in Down subjects is extremely important; correct medical therapy can then be started or rehabilitation with an acoustic prothesis can reduce the damage caused by a hearing deficit. If untreated, deafness can dramatically exacerbate the deficits typical of DS.

References

Balkany J, Downs M, Jafek B, Krajicek M (1979) Hearing loss in Down's syndrome. A treatable handicap more common than generally recognized. Clin Ped 18: 116–18.

Brooks D, Wooley H, Kanijlal G (1972) Hearing loss and middle ear disorders in patients with Down's syndrome. J Ment Defic Res 16: 21–9.

Crome L, Cowie W, Slater E (1966) A statistical note on cerebellar and brainstem weight in mongolism. J Ment Defic Res 10: 69–72.

Dahle A, McCollister F (1986) Hearing and otologic disorders in children with Down syndrome. Am J Ment Defic 90: 636–42.

Folsom R, Widen J, Wilson W (1983) Auditory brainstem responses in infants with Down's syndrome. Arch Otolarygol Head Neck Surg 109: 607–10.

Fulton R, Lloyd L (1968) Hearing impairment in a population of children with Down's syndrome. Am J Ment Defic 73: 298–302.

Hassmann E, Skotnicka B, Midro A, Musiatowicz M (1998) Distortion products otoacustic emissions in diagnosis of hearing loss in Down syndrome. Intern Journ Ped Otorhinolaryngol 45: 199–206.

Hildmann A, Hildmann H, Kesser A (2002) Hearing disorders in children with Down's syndrome. Laryngo-Rhino-Otol 81: 3–7.

Igarashi M, Takahashi M, Alford B, Johnson P (1977) Inner ear morphology in Down's syndrome. Acta Otolaryngol 83: 175–85.

Kaga K, Marsh R (1986) Auditory brainstem responses in young children with Down's syndrome. Int J Pediat Otolaryngol 11: 29–38.

Kakigi R, Kuroda Y (1992) Brainstem auditory potentials in adults with Down's Syndrome. EEG and Clin Neurophysiol 84: 293–5.

Krmpotic-Nemanic J (1970) Down's syndrome and presbycusis. Lancet 2: 670–1.

McIntire M, Menolascino F, Wiley J (1965) Mongolism – some clinical aspects. Am J Ment Defic 69: 780–94.

Medicina MC, Mura A, Felicioli F, Moretti A (1987) Indagini audiologiche nella sindrome di Down. Riv ORL Audiol Foniat 7(3): 275–9.

Molini E, Ricci G, Alunni N, Simoncelli C, Brunelli B (1997) Risultati e considerazioni a proposito di uno screening audiologico neonatale basato sull'impiego delle otoemissioni acustiche evocate transienti. Acta Otorhinilaringol Ital 17: 1–8.

Paludetti G, Lungarotti S, Ottaviani F, Rosignoli M, Tassini A (1982) Reperti audiologici nei bambini Down. Riv ORL Audiol Foniat 4: 429–34.

Salata J, Jacobson J, Strasnick B (1998) Distortion product otoacoustic emissions hearing screening in high risk newborns. Otolaryngol Head Neck Surg 118: 37–43.

Schwartz D, Schwartz R (1978) Acoustic impedance and otoscopic findings in young children with Down's syndrome. Arch Otolaryngol 104: 652–6.

Scott B, Becker L, Petit T (1983) Neurobiology of Down's syndrome. Prog Neurobiol 21: 199–237.

Straumanis J, Shagass C, Overton D (1973) Auditory evoked responses in young adults with Down's syndrome and idiopathic mental retardation. Biol Psychiatr 6: 75–9.

Strome M (1981) Down's syndrome: a modern otorhinolaryngological perspective. Laryngoscope, 91: 1581–94.

Chapter 9
Surgical treatment of occipitoatlantoaxial instability in Down syndrome

D. Fabris Monterumici, C. Baccichetti, P. Drigo

Although the earliest report of atlantoaxial subluxation dates back some 4,500–5,000 years when the Edwin Smith Papyrus described a displacement of a person's cervical vertebra (Power d'Arcy, 1933), atlantoaxial instability in Down syndrome (DS) was first reported by Spitzer et al. in 1961.

In 1984, the Committee on Sports Medicine of the American Academy of Pediatrics published a statement on the remarkably high incidence of atlantoaxial instability among individuals with DS. On the assumption that this instability, demonstrable through a specified series of lateral radiographs of the neck, constituted a predisposition to cervical spine dislocation with subsequent spinal cord compression, it recommended screening procedures that should be followed before individuals with DS engage in strenuous activities. It also recommended that children with asymptomatic atlantoaxial instability should not participate in any sporting activity that could potentially injure the neck.

Because the implementation of these recommendations could deprive individuals with DS of activities that are emotionally and physically beneficial and because of the rarity of reported cervical dislocations associated with injury, several epidemiological studies have been published on the prevalence of atlantoaxial instability in people with DS and the frequency of this disorder is reported to be between 9 and 40%. The discrepancy between the results is due mainly to variation in methodology and the lack of a definition for atlantoaxial instability.

Tredwell et al. (1990) measured the atlanto–occipital relationship as the distance between the anterior margin of the condyles at the base of the skull and the sharp contour of the anterior aspect of the concave joint of the atlas.

Gabriel et al. (1990) showed the translational anterior–posterior motion on each side for flexion and extension.

Karol et al. (1996) compared the reproducibility of three techniques used to measure translation between the occiput and C1 in children with DS. Intraobserver and interobserver variability were computed to determine if there is a reliable way to measure occiput–C1 instability. They concluded that measurement of atlanto–occipital translation by any of these methods is not reproducible. On the other hand Ferguson et al. (1997) examined 84 patients with DS and had flexion–extension lateral radiographs of the C1–C2 articulation for the purpose of dividing the group into subluxators (more than or equal to 4 mm atlanto–dens interval and 2 mm translation) and non-subluxators (those who did not meet these criteria). Neurological examinations and chart review were carried out on all patients to ascertain those with a positive neurological finding and concluded that positive neurological findings and an abnormal atlanto–dens interval are not related. In 1995, the Committee on Sports Medicine and Fitness of the American Academy of Pediatrics published a position paper on atlantoaxial instability in children with DS in which the previous statement on the same subject published in 1984 was retracted. The Committee concluded that 'lateral plain radiographs of the cervical spine are of potential but unproved value in detecting patients at risk of developing spinal cord injury during sports participation'. The Committee suggested that clinical evaluation, attending to complaints and physical signs of spinal cord injury, rather than radiological evaluation provided a more reliable way of detecting individual risk of serious injury during athletic competition.

Selby et al. (1991) studied 135 children with DS for clinical signs and symptoms that might predict atlantoaxial subluxation and failed to identify any reliable clinical predictor.

Indications for treatment

Over the last 10 years there have been great discussions about the indication criteria (clinical and/or radiological) for surgery. As far as clinical criteria are concerned, surgery is mandatory, in our opinion, when neurological impairment is seen. If a patient has only radiographic evidence of occipitoaxial hypermotility without any neurological signs, this does not represent an imperative indication for surgery, owing to the difficulties and the possible complications related to surgery. In these cases, a periodic radiographic study is the only control that must be carried out (every 6 months or yearly).

It is important, however, that in cases where there is radiographic evidence of severe atlantoaxial instability even without neurological impairment, the surgical option must be carefully evaluated; in these cases, it is essential to carry out sequential, regular radiographic checks.

One must consider that in these cases, there may be a 'neurological' deterioration; this deterioration can only be stopped, but not definitely corrected, by surgery.

Symptomatic atlantoaxial subluxation is reported to be present in 1% of children and adults with DS. These persons exhibit a variety of symptoms compatible with spinal cord injury, including brisk deep tendon reflexes (64%), extensor plantar responses (52%), muscle weakness (52%), gait abnormalities (43%), difficulties in walking (40%), ankle clonus (40%), and quadri- or hemiplegia (52%). Furthermore, about one-third displayed local symptoms such as neck pain and torticollis with limited neck mobility and head tilt. It is of note that 17% of symptomatic patients reported in the literature had sustained an injury to the cervical spine, which either had caused atlantoaxial subluxation leading to neurological symptoms or was a contributing factor augmenting the pre-existing symptoms.

Surgical technique

The anterior and/or posterior decompression techniques, postulated by some authors (Taggrad et al., 2000), do not seem to guarantee better results (double surgical approach; anterior transoral surgery) than stabilization techniques. The reducibility, or alternatively the stiffness, of the occipito–atlantoaxial dislocation may suggest different surgical strategies, but an obstinate intraoperative attempt to obtain a reduction is potentially extremely dangerous and must be avoided. An occipitocervical fusion, carried out with large iliac chips, carved from both sides of the ilium, combines the principles for good biological stability and is able to guarantee maintenance of the reduction over time. Healing of the fusion is better when the corticocancellous bone grafts are fixed to the C2 neural arch by means of a loop driven through two holes made in the grafts (Figures 9.1 and 9.2), whereas the occipital bone and the C1 and C2 posterior arches are well decorticated.

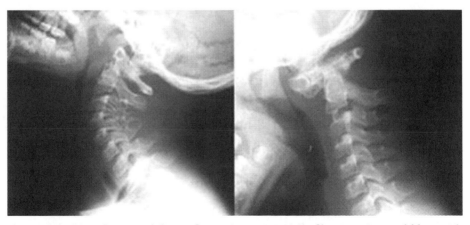

Figure 9.1 C1 and C2 instability in flexion/extension X-ray films in a 5-year-old boy with Down syndrome and neurological impairment.

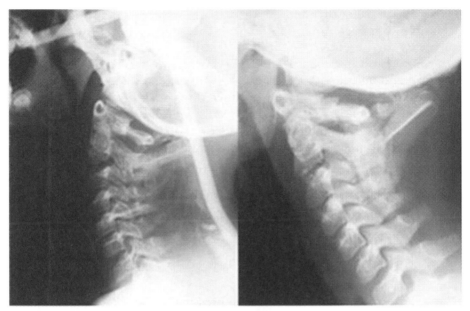

Figure 9.2 Posterior occipitocervical fusion with iliac bone graft, and reduction maintained until fusion healed with halo-vest device.

The use of internal fixation devices (plates and screws) cannot be advocated on a routine basis, owing to the young age of these patients (and the thinness of the occiput). This technique may be used when a pseudoarthrosis of a previous fusion occurs (and this is not rare in Down patients) (Figures 9.3, 9.4 and 9.5).

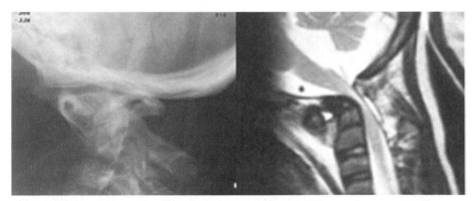

Figure 9.3 Severe neurological impairment in a 6-year-old boy with Down syndrome and an almost complete C1/C2 dislocation.

Postoperative treatment

In order to obtain a solid fusion it is essential to avoid any motion between the bone segments. Absolute immobilization is therefore necessary, and this can be only guaranteed by a trans-skeletal fixation. In our

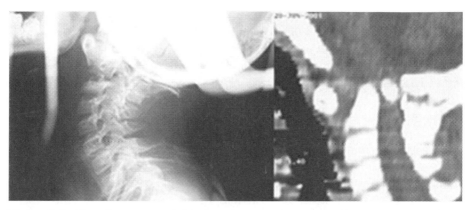

Figure 9.4 (Case from Figure 9.3.) Occipitocervical posterior fusion was carried out and despite strong post-op immobilization in halo-vest device for 3 months, a pseudo-arthrosis was seen after halo vest removal.

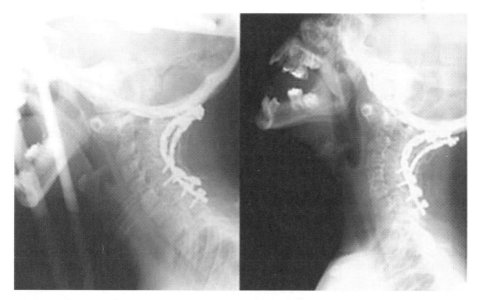

Figure 9.5 (Case from Figure 9.3.) New surgical approach: repair was carried out, the pseudoarthrosis was repaired and an internal fixation put in place, with a fair result and a solid fusion at follow-up.

experience the halo-vest device is the ideal means of fixation. Following this method in four patients, we were able to see an improvement of the preoperative tetraperesis without any complications in three cases; stabilization of the neurological status occurred in the fourth case.

Conclusion

As far as we know, in our district, since 1992, only six DS paediatric patients have undergone surgery because of severe neurological impairment. In this area there are over 2,500 subjects with DS of which 1,000 are children. Frost et al. (1999) presented a case of a 49-year-old DS patient whose triplegia, subacute progressive respiratory failure and death could be attributed to severe spinal canal stenosis. Bosma et al. (1999) reported five patients with a mean age at diagnosis of 42 years, with severe symptoms due to cervical spondylarthritic myelopathy. In conclusion we think that while mental handicap, skull and brain anomalies, and the development of Alzheimer-type neuropathological changes in patients older than 40 years are well recognized by neurologists and neuropathologists, the various cervical spine abnormalities that can occur are less appreciated. Progressive walking difficulties, bladder dysfunction and pathological reflexes may be attributed to Alzheimer disease or atlantoaxial subluxation in adults with DS, and radiography should be considered for this population in order to rule out the latter. Early diagnosis may prevent irreversible neurological deficits.

Bibliography

American Academy of Pediatrics Committee on Sport Medicine and Fitness (1995) Atlantoaxial instability in Down syndrome. Pediatrics 96: 151–4.

Bosma GP, van Buchem MA, Voormolen JH, van Biezen FC, Brouwer OF (1999) Cervical spondylarthrotic myelopathy with early onset in Down's syndrome: five cases and a review of the literature. J Intellect Disabil Res 43: 283–8.

Ferguson RL, Putney ME, Allen BL Jr (1997) Comparison of neurologic deficits with atlanto–dens intervals in patients with Down syndrome. J Spinal Disord 10(3): 246–52.

Frost M, Huffer WE, Sze CI, Badesch D, Cajade-Law AG, Kleinschmidt-DeMasters BK (1999) Cervical spine abnormalities in Down syndrome. Clin Neuropathol 18(5): 250–9.

Gabriel KR, Mason DE, Carango P (1990) Occipito–atlantal translation in Down syndrome. Spine 15: 977–1002.

Karol LA, Sheffield EG, Crawford K, Moody MK, Browne RH (1996) Reproducibility in the measurement of atlanto–occipital instability in children with Down syndrome. Spine 21: 2463–7.

Power D'Arcy L (1933) Some early surgical cases: The Edwin Smith Papyrus. Brit J Surgery 21:1–6.

Powell JF, Woodcock T, Luscombe FE (1990) Atlanto–axial subluxation in Down's syndrome. Anaesthesia 45(12): 1049–51.

Pueschel SM, Herndon JH, Gelch MM, Senft KE, Scola FH, Goldberg M (1984) Symptomatic atlantoaxial subluxation in persons with Down syndrome. J Pediatr Orthop 4: 682–8.

Selby KA, Newton RW, Gupta S, Hunt L (1991) Clinical predictors and radiological reliability in atlantoaxial subluxation in Down's syndrome. Arch Dis Child 66(7): 876–8.

Spitzer R, Rabinowiich JY, Wybar KC (1961) A study of abnormalities of the skull, teeth and lenses in mongolism. Can Med Assoc J 87: 567–72.

Taggrad DA et al. (2000) Treatment of Down syndrome-associated craniovertebral abnormalities. J Neurosurg (Spine 2) 93: 205–13.

Tredwell SJ, Newman DE, Lockitch G (1990) Instability of the upper cervical spine in Down syndrome. J Pediatr Orthop 10(5): 602–6.

Chapter 10
Down syndrome and coeliac disease

M. Bonamico, P. Mariani, M. Ferri, M. Carbone, R. Nenna

Coeliac disease

Coeliac disease (CD) is an autoimmune gastrointestinal disorder characterized by flat intestinal mucosa with hyperplasia of crypts and abnormal surface epithelium, due to a permanent intolerance to gluten contained in wheat, barley and rye.

Pathogenesis and clinical signs

The pathogenesis of CD is believed to involve interaction between genetic and environmental factors. In particular, a significant part of the genetic susceptibility to CD seems associated with products of the major histocompatibility complex (MHC), encoded within the Class II region on chromosome 6. In fact, in a group of Italian paediatric patients we have reported (Mazzilli et al., 1992) that 92% of CD patients carried the high-risk DQ2 α/β dimer, while most of the dimer negative patients were typed as DR4, DQ8.

The clinical presentation of CD may be as:

- A classic form, characterized, usually at weaning, by chronic diarrhoea, growth failure, vomiting and/or abdominal pain
- An atypical form, with extraintestinal symptoms, such as short stature, anaemia, osteoporosis, dental enamel defects, neurological manifestations, etc.
- A silent form, identified in a high number of asymptomatic subjects, among first-degree relatives of CD patients, blood donors, or in the general population during screening programmes performed using serological tests

Diagnosis of coeliac disease

Due to the variety of uncharacteristic symptoms, sensitive and specific screening tests are developed as an aid in detecting subjects in which intestinal biopsy should be performed. The first antibodies to be detected during the 1980s were the antigliadin antibodies (AGA) IgA and IgG, assayed by an enzyme-linked immuno sorbent assay (ELISA) method; these are particularly sensitive in children, but without a good specificity. Antiendomysium antibodies (AEA), detected by an indirect immunofluorescent method, are specific, but require cryostatic sections of monkey oesophagus and are observer-dependent. More recently, anti-tissue transglutaminase (tTG) antibodies, particularly using a human recombinant antigen and a radioimmunoassay, have proved to be very sensitive as a screening method for CD patients (Bao et al., 1999; Bazzicalupi et al., 1999; Bonamico et al., 2001). The screening procedures have allowed CD to be identified over a wide Italian population; the results demonstrate a high frequency of the disease (1:180) (Catassi et al., 1996).

The diagnosis of CD requires the detection of the typical villous atrophy with crypt hyperplasia on small intestine mucosa samples, obtained by peroral capsule or during upper endoscopy, on free diet. On a gluten-free diet, symptoms and serum AGA and AEA, if these antibodies were present at the time of the diagnosis, must subside. According to the new criteria established in the 1990s (Walker-Smith et al., 1990) by the European Society for Paediatric Gastroenterology, Hepatology and Nutrition (ESPGHAN), additional biopsies are required if there are doubts about the initial diagnosis and the adequacy of the clinical response to a gluten-free diet, particularly in children aged 2 years or less at presentation.

CD may become symptomatic at different ages, not only at the paediatric stage, as the period from gluten consumption to intestinal damage and the onset of symptoms may vary significantly from one subject to another. In adults, and even in the elderly, CD can show a classic presentation with digestive symptoms (chronic diarrhoea, weight loss and malnutrition), or atypical presentation with extraintestinal manifestations (anaemia, repeated abortions) or it can be silent. Compared to the disease in children, CD in adults has a higher mortality rate than expected and is associated with different complications, such as hyposplenism, which are infrequent in children.

Various diseases are associated with CD, both in children and in adults: herpetiform dermatitis, insulin-dependent diabetes, autoimmune thyropathy, active chronic hepatitis, alveolitis, alopecia and chromosomal disorders (Down syndrome and Turner syndrome).

Coeliac disease and Down syndrome

In 1975, Bentley reported the case of a 14-year-old boy with DS and CD, affected by a retinoblastoma. Other case reports of the association of these two conditions have been described in the literature in subsequent years (Nowak et al., 1983; Ruch et al., 1985; Santer et al., 1991). More recently efforts have been made to evaluate the prevalence of DS in CD patients (Amil Dias and Walker-Smith, 1990; Granditsch and Rossipal, 1990) and the prevalence of CD in DS subjects (Storm, 1990; Zubillaga et al., 1993; Castro et al., 1993; Jansson and Johansson, 1995; Failla et al., 1996; Gale et al., 1997; Carlsson et al., 1998; Hansson et al., 1999; Pueshel et al., 1999; Csizmadia et al., 2000; Zachor et al., 2000; Carnicer et al., 2001; Mackey et al., 2001; Bonamico et al., 2001; Agardh et al., 2002). These studies, concerning children more frequently than adults, have led to the conclusion that CD is significantly more frequent in DS patients than in the general population. In fact, in selecting studies on large populations, we were able to evaluate the results of 15 papers published over the period 1990–2002 (Table 10.1); according to these studies the prevalence of CD in DS ranges from 2.5% to 20.3%. The largest series has been collected by a multicentre study concerning 1202 Italian DS subjects (Bonamico et al., 2001) (1110 children and 92 adults; 609 males and 593 females) submitted to serological screening using both AGA and AEA. In this study it was possible to identify 55 biopsy-proved CD patients, obtaining a prevalence of CD in DS patients

Table 10.1 Numbers and percentages of Down syndrome patients (children and adults) IgA, AGA and AEA positive and with partial/total intestinal villous atrophy.

Authors	Patients N	AGA IgA pos N (%)	AEA pos N (%)	Partial/total villous atrophy N (%)
(Storm, 1990	78	8 (10.2)	n.d.	2 (2.5)
(Zubillaga et al., 1993	70	9 (12.8)	n.d.	3 (4.2)
(Castro et al., 1993	155	41 (26.4)	n.d.	7 (4.5)
(Jansson and Johansson, 1995	54	22 (40.7)	n.d.	9 (20.3)
•Failla et al., 1996	57	6 (10.5)	n.d.	6 (12.2)
° Gale et al., 1997	55	21 (43.6)	n.d.	2 (3.6)
(Carlsson et al., 1998	43	16 (37.2)	7 (16.3)	8 (18.6)
(Hansson et al., 1999	76	28 (36.8)	5 (6.6)	3 (3.9)
•Pueschel et al., 1999	105	12 (11.4)	5 (4.8)	4 (3.8)
(Csizmadia et al., 2000	137	n.d.	15 (10.9)	11 (8.0)
•Zachor et al., 2000	75	8 (10.7)	10 (13.3)	5 (6.7)
•Carnicer et al., 2001	284	17 (5.9)	14 (4.9)	18 (6.3)
•Mackey et al., 2001	93	36 (37.6)	5 (5.4)	3 (3.2)
•Bonamico et al., 2001	1,202	259 (21.5)	65 (5.4)	55 (4.6)
•Agardh et al., 2002	48	15 (31.2)	7 (14.6)	8 (16.6)

n.d.= not done; (children only; • both children and adults; ° adults only of 4.6%, which far exceeds the prevalence of CD in the general Italian population (0.55%). Therefore, we can assume that this association is not by chance.

Over the last two decades the same issues concerning the diagnosis of CD in the general population have arisen in screening for CD in DS patients, with some particular characteristics. In fact it is clear that invasive procedures in DS patients, already subject to many diagnostic procedures and to a long follow-up (e.g. cardiac follow-up), should be avoided, unless strictly necessary. In addition, sometimes parents of antibody-positive children and adults did not give permission for intestinal biopsy to be performed, particularly in asymptomatic cases.

The 55 DS subjects with CD in the multicentre study (Bonamico et al., 2001), compared with two other groups of DS subjects without CD, showed lower height and weight and a statistically significant increase of some symptoms, such as diarrhoea, vomiting, anorexia and constipation and more frequently low levels of serum iron and calcium, while sometimes aminotransferases increased. The possible transient increase of such enzymes has already been observed in CD patients (Bonamico et al., 1986; Volta et al., 1998).

It is worth noting that in this study, 69% of coeliac DS persons showed the classic presentation of the disease, with gastrointestinal symptoms, 11% had the atypical form (short stature and/or anaemia), while the remaining 20% were clinically silent. Therefore it can be seen that only one patient out of five showed a silent form, in contrast with the general population, where seven out of eight subjects are asymptomatic (Catassi et al., 1996). We can presume that some cases of patients with CD and DS may not be diagnosed, especially if they involve symptoms of various organ systems or involve minor symptoms, such as growth failure or constipation, which may be overlooked by a doctor.

Recently, in a multicentre study, we reported a high prevalence of CD in another chromosomal disorder, Turner syndrome (Bonamico et al., in press); in these patients the ratio between symptomatic and silent forms (2.7:1) was reversed with respect to those in the general population. We could hypothesize that, whereas in CD patients without these chromosomal syndromes mechanisms of compensation may be present, so that for a long time enteropathy may exist without symptoms, in DS patients and in Turner syndrome girls these mechanisms are less able to overcome the overt clinical manifestation of CD. Alternatively, in both syndromes an increase of autoimmune pathologies, such as insulin-dependent diabetes and thyroiditis, have been detected, and CD is also considered an autoimmune disease. We can conclude that in DS and TS subjects a careful clinical evaluation, considering the possibility of CD, may be very useful, in addition to serological screening, in order to select subjects for intestinal biopsy.

Often the anamnesis, physical examination and nutritional status indices do not allow DS subjects to be selected for intestinal biopsy; these patients are screened for CD using specific antibodies. Nevertheless, the first widely used antibodies, the AGA, which allowed the non-causal association between DS and CD to be recognized, proved unsuitable in DS subjects. In fact, from an analysis of the 14 papers (Table 10.1), AGA were detected in percentages ranging from 10.2% to 43.6% in DS patients, whereas the percentages of biopsy proved CD were far lower, from 2.5% to 20.3%. The possibility of finding positive IgA AGA in patients with a normal mucosa may be the result of elevated immunoglobulin levels in patients with DS, compared with the total population (Burgio et al., 1975), particularly for food antigens (Reichelt et al., 1994), or to a permeability defect (Ferrante et al., 1991), which allows gliadin fragments to pass through the intestinal mucosa with subsequent production of antibodies.

Since the end of the 1990s, AEA determination has become widespread in screening CD patients both in the general population and in DS persons (Carlsson et al., 1998; Hansson et al., 1999; Pueshel et al., 1999; Csizmadia et al., 2000; Zachor et al., 2000; Carnicer et al., 2001; Mackey et al., 2001; Bonamico et al., 2001; Agardh et al., 2002); AEA have proved to have high senstivity and specificity, except for children aged less than 2 years, in which they could be negative (Burgin-Wolff et al., 1991). In the above mentioned studies, these antibodies have been detected over the whole Down population considered, obtaining a prevalence ranging from 4.8% to 13.3%.

The determination of anti-tTG antibodies, the more recent assay, represents a reliable marker for CD. It is worth noting that tTG is an enzyme that plays a key pathogenetic role in CD, as it activates the autoimmune process responsible for the disease, through the modification of the gliadine peptides (Dieterich et al., 1998). Up to now, these antibodies in DS patients have only been assayed in two studies (Csizmadia et al., 2000; Agardh et al., 2002); using a recombinant human antigen, these autoantibodies seem to be as useful as AEA in screening for CD in DS subjects (Agardh et al., 2002).

The absence of a full correspondence of the serological markers and the intestinal damage (villous atrophy with crypt hyperplasia) diagnostic for CD, led to a search for genetic markers in DS subjects, as performed on first-degree relatives of CD patients, in order to select a high risk population for follow-up. The HLA class II typing (Zubillaga et al., 1993; Castro et al., 1993) and more recently the HLA DQ-A1 and DQ-B1 typing (Hansson et al., 1999; Csizmadia et al., 2000; Agardh et al., 2002) showed that in DS subjects the gene distribution of susceptibility for CD is comparable with the gene distribution of the whole CD population. As HLA represents only 30% of the CD genetic risk (Petronzelli et al., 1997), indicating the contribution by other, non-HLA genes, several attempts have been made in recent years to detect other genes that predispose CD. However, no non-HLA loci have been conclusively identified, despite a number of studies using genome-wide or candidate gene approaches. Particularly, a British study on 21 families with multiple cases of CD, none of whom had DS, was carried out. Using typing information of six microsatellite markers across chromosome 21 to test linkage, no support was provided for genetic linkage of CD to this chromosome (Morris et al., 2000). It is, however, most likely that other genes in addition to the HLA loci contribute to the susceptibility. The discrepancies between the different studies and the difficulties in detecting novel genes suggest few individual effects in non-HLA loci on the development of the disease, or alternatively, a large degree of genetic heterogeneity as to which loci contribute in individual patients (Mazzilli et al., in press).

The role of genetic factors in CD indicates that a serological follow-up should be performed for all patients with the genetic predisposition, particularly for DS persons. In fact, recently Cszimadia et al. (2000) demonstrated that some DS patients genetically at risk, and previously AEA negative, became positive later, and that intestinal biopsy showed villous atrophy. Conversely, Agardh et al. (2002) suggest screening HLA-DQB1*02 and anti-tTG autoantibodies together in silent CD, while in patients with gastrointestinal symptoms or malabsorption, anti-tTG autoantibodies could be combined with AGA to detect other forms of enteropathies or CD.

It is well known that, over the last few decades, the average life expectancy of DS patients has increased, as it has in the general population. This is due to a wider knowledge of some medical specialities, such as cardiosurgery, which is responsible for the mortality decrease in the first years of life. Much of the improvement is related to the detection and the treatment of diseases affecting adolescents and adults, such as thyroid pathologies. Finally, a substantial contribution has come from an improvement in psychosocial welfare promoted by paediatricians, infant neuropsychiatrists and general physicians (early detection of psychomotor retardation, programmes stimulating cognitive functions, integration in schools and thereafter in working life). Notwithstanding that, various diseases are more frequent in DS adults than in the general population, such as thyroid disorders, gonadic disfunction and osteoporosis. A higher mortality rate in DS patients is due to neoplastic diseases, particularly related to the blood-forming organs. About 30–40% of DS patients over 50 years of age are affected by some disabling osteoarticular pathologies, such as atlanto–axial and atlanto–occipital instability. Ocular and ear diseases affect 30–40% and 60–90%, respectively, of DS patients over 50 years of age. Finally, nearly all DS patients over 40 are affected by a neurological disease which is Alzheimer-like, with a faster and more premature loss of cognitive functions than the general population.

Only a small series of DS adults have been screened for CD. Nevertheless it is evident that even a late diagnosis could improve the quality of life of these disadvantaged persons. In fact, with a gluten-free diet, some signs and symptoms wrongly considered minor in DS patients could subside; in addition, the increase of autoimmune pathologies and neoplasia, which are the harmful complications of both diseases, could probably be prevented.

References

Agardh D, Nilsson A, Carlsson A, Kockum I, Lernmark Å, Ivarsson SA (2002) Tissue transglutaminase autoantibodies and human leucocyte antigen in Down's syndrome patients with coeliac disease. Acta Paediatr 91: 34–8.

Amil Dias J, Walker-Smith J (1990) Down's syndrome and celiac disease. J Pediatr Gastroenterol Nutr 10: 41–3.

Bao F, Yu L, Babu S, Wang T, Hoffenberg EJ, Rewers M, Eisenbarth GS (1999) One third of HLA DQ2 homozygous patients with type 1 diabetes express celiac disease associated transglutaminase autoantibodies. J Autoimmun 13: 143–8.

Bazzicaluppi E, Lampasona V, Barera G, Venerando A, Bianchi C, Chiumello G, Bonifacio E, Bosi E (1999) Comparison of tissue transglutaminase-specific antibody assays with established antibody measurements for coeliac disease. J Autoimmun 12: 51–6.

Bentley D (1975) A case of Down's syndrome complicated by retinoblastoma and celiac disease. Pediatrics 56: 131–3.

Bonamico M, Mariani P, Danesi HM, Crisogianni M, Failla P, Gemme G, Rasore Quartino A, Giannotti A, Castro M, Balli F, Lecora M, Andria G, Guariso G, Gabrielli O, Catassi C, Lazzari R, Ansaldi Balocco N, De Virgiliis S, Culasso F, Romano C (2001) Prevalence and clinical picture of celiac disease in Italian Down syndrome patients: a multicenter study. J Pediatr Gastroenterol Nutr 33: 139–43.

Bonamico M, Pasquino AM, Mariani P, Danesi HM, Culasso F, Mazzanti L, Petri A, Bona G, Sigep and ISGTS (2002) Prevalence and clinical picture of celiac disease in Turner Syndrome. J Clin Endocrinol Metab 87: 5495–8.

Bonamico M, Pitzalis G, Culasso F, Vania A, Monti S, Benedetti C, Mariani P, Signoretti A (1986) Il danno epatico nella malattia celiaca del bambino. Minerva Pediatr 38: 959–62.

Bonamico M, Tiberti C, Picarelli A, Mariani P, Rossi D, Cipolletta E, Greco M, Di Tola M, Sabbatella L, Carabba B, Magliocca FM, Strisciuglio P, Di Mario U (2001) Radioimmunoassay to detect antitransglutaminase autoantibodies is the most sensitive and specific screening method for celiac disease. Am J Gastroenterol 96: 1536–40.

Burgin-Wolff A, Gaze H, Hadziselimovic F, Huber H, Lentze MJ, Nussle D, Reymond-Berthet C (1991) Antigliadin and antiendomysium antibody determination for coeliac disease. Arch Dis Child 66: 941–7.

Burgio GR, Ugazio AG, Nespoli L, Marcioni AF, Bottelli AM, Pasquali F (1975) Derangements of immunoglobulin levels, phytohemagglutinin responsiveness and T and B cell markers in Down's syndrome at different ages. Eur J Immunol 5: 600–3.

Carlsson A, Axelsson I, Borulf S, Bredberg A, Forslund M, Lindberg B, Sjöberg K, Ivarsson SA (1998) Prevalence of IgA-antigliadin antibodies and IgA-antiendomysium antibodies related to celiac disease in children with Down's syndrome. Pediatrics 101: 272–5.

Carnicer J, Farre C, Varea V, Vilar P, Moreno J, Artigas J (2001) Prevalence of celiac disease in Down's Syndrome. Eur J Gastroenterol Hepatol 13: 263–7.

Castro M, Crinò A, Papadatou B, Purpura M, Giannotti A, Ferretti F, Colistro F, Mottola L, Digilio MC, Lucidi V, Borrelli P (1993) Down's syndrome and celiac disease: the prevalence of high IgA-antigliadin antibodies and HLA-DR and DQ antigens in trisomy 21. J Pediatr Gastroenterol Nutr 16: 265–8.

Catassi C, Fabiani E, Ratsch IM, Coppa GV, Giorgi PL, Pierdomenico R, Alessandrini S, Iwanejko G, Domenici R, Mei E, Miano A, Marani M, Bottaro G, Spina M, Dotti M, Montanelli A, Barbato M, Viola F, Lazzari R, Vallini M, Guariso G, Plebani M, Cataldo F, Traverso G, Ughi C, Chiaravalloti G, Baldassarre M, Scarcella P, Bascietto F, Ceglie L, Valenti A, Paolucci P, Caradonna M, Bravi E, Ventura A (1996) The coeliac iceberg in Italy. A multicentre antigliadin antibodies screening for coeliac disease in school-age subjects. Acta Paediatr Suppl 412: 29–35.

Csizmadia CG, Mearin ML, Oren A, Krombout A, Crusius JBA, von Blomberg BME, Peña AS, Wiggers MNL, Vandenbroucke JP (2000) Accuracy and cost-effectiveness of a new strategy to screen for celiac disease in children with Down syndrome. J Pediatr 137: 756–61.

Dieterich W, Laag E, Schopper H, Volta U, Ferguson A, Gillett H, Riecken EO, Shuppan D (1998) Autoantibodies to tissue transglutaminase as predictors of celiac disease. Gastroenterology 115: 1317–21.

Failla P, Ruberto C, Pagano MC, Lombardo M, Bottaro G, Perichon B, Krisnamoorthy R, Romano C, Ragusa A (1996) Coeliac disease in Down's syndrome with HLA serological and molecular studies. J Pediatr Gastroenterol Nutr 23: 303–6.

Ferrante E, Bonamico M, Mariani P, Cherubini C, Triglione P, Lionetti P, Ballati G (1991) High serum antigliadin antibodies in children with Down syndrome and in a subject with 18q-syndrome. Eur J Epidemiol 7: 732.

Gale L, Wimalaratna H, Brotodiharjo A, Duggan JM (1997) Down's syndrome is strongly associated with coeliac disease. Gut 40: 492–6.

Granditsch G, Rossipal E (1990) Down's syndrome and celiac disease. J Pediatr Gastroenterol Nutr 11: 279.

Hansson T, Annerén G, Sjoberg O, Klareskog L, Dannaeus A (1999) Celiac disease in relation to immunologic serum markers, trace elements and HLA-DR and DQ antigens in Swedish children with Down syndrome. J Pediatr Gastroenterol Nutr 29: 286–92.

Jansson U, Johansson C (1995) Down syndrome and celiac disease. J Pediatr Gastroenterol Nutr 443–5.

Mackey J, Treem WR, Worley G, Boney A, Hart P, Kishnani PS (2001) Frequency of celiac disease in individuals with Down syndrome in the United States. Clinical Pediatrics May: 249–52.

Mazzilli MC, Ferrante P, Mariani P, Martone F, Triglione P, Bonamico M (1992) A study of Italian pediatric celiac disease patients confirms that the primary HLA association is to the DQ (alpha1*0501, beta 1*0201) heterodimer. Human Immunology 33: 133–9.

Mazzilli MC, Lie BA, Mora B, Bonamico M, Thorsby E (2002) Contribution of genetics to the understanding of coeliac disease. Proceedings of the 10th International Symposium on coeliac disease. Paris, 2–5 June 2002, in press.

Morris MA, Yiannakou JY, King AL, Brett PM, Biagi F, Vaughan R, Curtis D, Ciclitira PJ (2000) Coeliac disease and Down syndrome: associations not due to genetic linkage on chromosome 21. Scand J Gastroenterol 35: 177–8.

Nowak TV, Ghisham FK, Schulze-Delrieu K (1983) Celiac sprue in Down's syndrome: considerations on a pathogenic link. Am J Gastroenterol 78: 280–3.

Petronzelli F, Bonamico M, Ferrante P, Grillo R, Mora B, Mariani P, Apollonio I, Gemme G, Mazzilli MC (1997) Genetic contribution of HLA region to the familial clustering of coeliac disease. Ann Hum Genet 61: 307–17.

Pueshel SM, Romano C, Failla P, Barone C, Pettinato R, Castellano Chiodo A, Plumari DL (1999) A prevalence study of celiac disease in persons with Down syndrome residing in the United States of America. Acta Paediatr 88: 953–6.

Reichelt KL, Lindback T, Scott H (1994) Increased levels of antibodies to food proteins in Down syndrome. Acta Paediatr Japonica 36: 489–92.

Ruch W, Schurmann K, Gordon P, Burgin-Wolff A, Girard J (1985) Coexistent coeliac disease, Graves' disease and diabetes mellitus type I in a patient with Down syndrome. Eur J Pediatr 144: 89–90.

Santer R, Sievers E, Oldigs HD (1991) Celiac disease in Down's syndrome. J Pediatr Gastroenterol Nutr 13: 121.

Storm W (1990) Prevalence and diagnostic significance of gliadin antibodies in children with Down syndrome. Eur J Pediatr 149: 833–4.

Volta U, De Franceschi L, Lari F, Molinaro N, Zoli M, Bianchi FB (1998) Coeliac disease hidden by cryptogenic hypertransaminasaemia. Lancet 352: 26–9.

Walker-Smith JA, Guandalini S, Schmitz J, Shmerling DH, Visakorpi JK (1990) Revised criteria for diagnosis of coeliac disease. Arch Dis Child 65: 909–11.

Zachor DA, Mroczek-Musulman E, Brown P (2000) Prevalence of celiac disease in Down syndrome in the United States. J Pediatr Gastroenterol Nutr 31: 275–9.

Zubillaga P, Vitoria JC, Arrieta A, Echaniz P, Garcia-Masdevall MD (1993) Down's syndrome and coeliac disease. J Pediatr Gastroenterol Nutr 16: 168–70.

Chapter 11
Neurophysiology of ageing in Down syndrome

R. FERRI, S. MIANO

Nervous excitability and epilepsy in Down syndrome

Down syndrome (DS) is characterized by a peculiar increase in excitability of different nervous system structures; we have studied such an increase by means of different neurophysiological approaches, mostly during development. From the clinical point of view, the report of a significantly increased prevalence of early-onset epilepsy (EOE) in DS (Romano et al., 1990; Goldberg-Stern et al., 2001) is an indirect confirmation of the increase in nervous excitability. In particular, no relationship has been found between type of epilepsy, age at onset, and eventual presence or absence of known aetiology. The cause of the onset of epilepsy is thought to be correlated with a decrease in the number of inhibitory interneurons at the cortical level, abnormalities in cortical layer structure, persistence of foetal dendritic arborization and alteration of the neuronal membrane permeability to potassium which would induce a decrease of the threshold for the activation of epileptiform abnormalities (Goldberg-Stern et al., 2001).

Studies aimed at evaluating specifically neurophysiological processes of ageing in DS are scarce; however, we know that life expectancy of these individuals is approaching that of the general population, because of the increased level and quality of healthcare in modern society. The most important cause of death in DS is dependent on the presence of congenital heart abnormalities; with progressing age, the incidence of leukaemia increases together with that of thyroid and immune dysfunctions and, probably, early ageing processes (van Buggenhout et al., 1999).

For these reasons, it is important to start research on the neurophysiological aspects of individuals with DS during adulthood and/or ageing. In recent years, some investigations have been carried out on the epidemiology of central nervous system pathology in DS, such as epilepsy and dementia. In particular, late-onset epilepsy (LOE) seems to show an age-related increase in DS because it is present in 75–85% of DS subjects who show signs of Alzheimer's disease (AD) after 50 years of age, and can be found in association with myoclonus and a history of traumatic brain injury (van Allen et al., 1999; Tyrrell et al., 2001; Tsiouris et al., 2002).

In 1990, Evenhius reported an eight-fold increase in the frequency of epilepsy and myoclonus in subjects with DS and dementia compared to non-demented age-matched DS subjects; the same author considered epilepsy to be an initial sign of the dementia process and his findings were later confirmed by Pueschel et al. (1995) who reported a particular increase in the incidence of epilepsy during the third decade of life. DS males are likely to present LOE at a younger age than females (22 years vs. 51 years) (Puri et al., 2001). Thus, in DS, epilepsy shows a bimodal distribution of age at onset, with a peak during development and another during adulthood (Puri et al., 2001).

Interestingly, three patients with DS who developed progressive myoclonic epilepsy during adulthood (after 50 years of age), after the onset of dementia, were reported in the literature (Li et al., 1995; Moller et al., 2001). They showed some similarities with myoclonic epilepsy in some forms of familial Alzheimer's disease and with Unverricht-Lundborg progressive myoclonic epilepsy, which are determined by mutations of chromosome 21 (Lalioti et al., 1997; Saunders, 2001). The same reports are also interesting because they show that abnormalities in nervous excitability of DS are age-related, being more evident with increasing age; these abnormalities need a better neurophysiological characterization.

Some of the studies we have carried out in the past, however, contain important indications on age-related changes in nervous excitability in DS and might constitute the starting point for future research.

Brainstem auditory evoked potentials in Down syndrome

Brainstem auditory evoked potentials (BAEPs) are recorded during the first few milliseconds following auditory stimulation and are generated at the level of peripheral and central brainstem auditory pathways. They represent a very reliable tool for the evaluation of the auditory function and can also be recorded with an uncooperative subject, even during sedation or sleep. They can be used for the assessment of the hearing threshold in subjects who do not cooperate at tone audiometry. Typically, BAEPs are characterized by five main peaks and the interval between the first and the fifth peak reflects the central brainstem conduction time, which shows significant prolongation in various diseases influencing central nervous transmission. In our first study on BAEPs (Gigli et al., 1984), we reported that children with DS show a peculiar alteration, characterized by a shortening in central conduction time. This is not detectable in other pathological conditions. This finding has been repeatedly confirmed in the literature both in infants (Folsom et al., 1983) and adults (Kakigi and Kuroda, 1992; Squires et al., 1980, 1982).

In our report (Gigli et al., 1984) we were able to exclude the possibility that the shortening in brainstem conduction time was due to physical reasons such as short stature and, consequently, short brainstem; in agreement with other authors, we hypothesized that DS subjects show a disturbance in excitability at the level of the brainstem, probably related to a decrease in inhibitory mechanisms.

Some years later, we recorded BAEPs in a much larger group of patients (Ferri et al., 1995a) and were able to describe the effects of age on them during a period ranging from 1.5 to 45 years. With this study, we confirmed the previous findings and were also able to demonstrate that, unlike normal controls, DS subjects show even shorter BAEP latencies with increasing age. Obviously, we suggested that the deficit in inhibitory mechanisms responsible for the shortening of the BAEP latencies in DS, already present in early life, seems to undergo an age-related worsening during adulthood.

Middle-latency somatosensory evoked potentials in Down syndrome

Middle-latency somatosensory evoked potentials (MLSEPs) are recorded between 15 and 100 milliseconds following stimulation of a peripheral nerve. In particular, MLSEPs recorded after stimulation of the median nerve at the wrist represent the sequential activation of different structures and regions located within the parietal and frontal lobes, mostly contralateral to the stimulated side. These potentials can be obtained reliably in subjects who offer only partial cooperation as they are not asked to do particular tasks. MLSEPs are able to demonstrate changes in cortical excitability over the activated areas in detail; this is the case especially if they are recorded by means of several electrodes on the scalp, because this allows the construction of topographic scalp colour maps.

In our first study (Ferri et al., 1994), we recorded MLSEPs in DS subjects aged 7.75–27.42 years. In these subjects we were able to demonstrate that, in addition to the increased subcortical nervous excitability reported above (BAEPs), an increased cortical nervous excitability over the parietal and frontal lobes can be detected. In the same investigation, we could also demonstrate a significant difference between DS subjects and normal controls, not only in terms of amplitude of the potentials, but also in terms of morphology and topographic scalp distribution. It is important to underline that the comparison was carried out with both age-matched normal controls and normal elderly subjects, who also show an increase in amplitude of some components of MLSEPs. MLSEPs of DS individuals were clearly different in morphology and showed higher amplitudes than those of normal elderly subjects.

The consequent conclusion of our investigation was that the clear-cut changes in cortical excitability/inhibition in DS were peculiar to this condition and not correlated with the presence of eventual early brain ageing processes.

This conclusion was further confirmed and reinforced by our subsequent work (Ferri et al., 1996a) in which we included DS subjects with a wider age range (6.4–34.4 years); this allowed us to analyse age-related changes in MLSEP parameters which were not interpretable in terms of early brain ageing processes. Finally, it is important to note that the morphological and topographical features of MLSEPs in DS subjects are very different from those of patients affected by AD (pathological brain ageing) (Ferri et al., 1996b).

Sleep neurophysiology in Down syndrome

Similarly to other groups of subjects with mental handicap, DS individuals show some characteristic sleep neurophysiological features:

- Significant decrease in the percentage of REM sleep (more evident in subjects with severe mental handicap)
- Marked increase in REM sleep latency
- Significant reduction in number and frequency of rapid eye movements during REM sleep (Colognola et al., 1988)

In the past, we repeatedly evaluated the effects of the administration of an organic compound, butoctamide hydrogen succinate (BAHS), on sleep patterns of DS subjects (Yanagisawa and Yoshikawa, 1973). This compound is normally found in the cerebrospinal fluid, and causes an increase in the amount of REM sleep. Administration of BAHS has clarified the mechanisms responsible for the decrease of this sleep stage (Gigli et al., 1985a, 1985b; Grubar et al., 1984, 1986). These studies confirmed the importance of sleep in the memory and learning capabilities of these subjects, from the neurophysiological point of view.

On this basis, we then focused our attention on the correlation between sleep abnormalities and growth hormone secretion in DS (Ferri et al., 1995b). We found that in these subjects, the amplitude of nocturnal hormone secretion peaks is greatly reduced and that the pulsatility of such a secretion is in poor synchrony with slow-wave sleep, contrary to that observed in normal controls. Thus, the production of growth hormone in DS, if studied during sleep and with the contemporaneous monitoring of sleep stages, shows significant abnormalities.

This study prompted us to consider that many patients with DS are affected by obstructive sleep apnoea (OSA) (Marcus et al., 1991). It is known that the secretion of growth hormone is decreased in children with disturbed sleep respiratory patterns, probably because of sleep fragmentation; it is also known that the effective treatment of OSA can determine not only the re-establishment of normal growth hormone production (Grunstein et al., 1992; Matsumoto et al., 1985) but also the consequent correction of the tendency of these children to be of short stature (Brouillette et al., 1982; Goldstein et al., 1987).

There are several reports in the literature describing the presence of OSA in subjects with DS (Southall et al., 1987; Marcus et al., 1991; Stebbens et al., 1991). In order to evaluate the eventual consequences of the central nervous dysfunction described above on nocturnal breathing in DS, we selected a group of subjects without evident risk factors for OSA and studied their sleep respiratory patterns (Ferri et al., 1997). Surprisingly, we were able to demonstrate the presence of a significant number of central apnoea and peripheral blood oxygen desaturation episodes. Central apnoea episodes were very often preceded by sighs, were most frequent during sleep stage 1 and REM. The episodes were often organized in long sequences constituting pseudoperiodic respiration. Sleep structure was not significantly modified by the presence of central apnoea and by oxygen desaturation.

In this study, we hypothesized that the increase in number of central apnoea episodes during sleep might be correlated with the presence of hyperresponsive central respiratory control mechanisms, located at the level of the brainstem. We had already indicated the brainstem as a structure in which abnormal excitability/inhibition was evident (see above, Gigli et al., 1984). Similarly to the characteristic abnormality of BAEPs which becomes more evident with increasing age (Ferri et al., 1995a), the frequency of central sleep apnoea was also found to be significantly correlated with age in our DS subjects: it was higher in adults than in children in the age range between 8.6 and 32.2 years (Ferri et al., 1997).

Finally, in order to confirm once more the role of a possible brainstem dysfunction in the aetiopathogenesis of central sleep apnoea, we also evaluated the heart rate variability during sleep in a group of DS subjects (Ferri et al., 1998) and were able to confirm the original hypothesis.

Conclusions

The data briefly described above mostly consider subjects with ages ranging from childhood to adulthood; further insights are needed in order to understand the neurophysiological characteristics of DS elderly subjects better. However, some conclusions can be drawn.

The increase in excitability (or decrease in inhibition) involving several structures of the central nervous system of DS subjects seems to cause different clinical consequences, such as central apnoea and seizures, which seem to worsen with age.

Subjects with DS show neurophysiological abnormalities which seem to be unique and peculiar and cannot be explained by the presence of other pathological processes, such as early brain ageing.

These abnormalities are characterized by diffuse changes in excitability of the central nervous system; excitability seems to be increased. This might be a consequence of decreased inhibitory mechanisms subserved by different neurotransmitters.

Neurotransmitter abnormalities in DS might be understood by means of the analysis of genes involved in the determinism of DS. The gene thought to be one of the most important molecular factors involved in DS, designated as DSCR1, is located in the region 21q22.1–q22.2 (Fuentes et al., 1995). The DSCR1 transcript is expressed at the highest levels in foetal brain and adult heart and at lower levels in various other tissues; Fuentes et al. (2000) demonstrated that DSCR1 protein is overexpressed in the brain of Down syndrome foetuses, and interacts physically and functionally with calcineurin A. DSCR1 belongs to a family of evolutionarily conserved proteins and its overexpression inhibits calcineurin-dependent gene transcription. Fuentes et al. (2000) also hypothesized that members of this family of human proteins are endogenous regulators of calcineurin-mediated signalling pathways and may be involved in many physiological processes. Kingsbury and Cunningham (2000) showed that DSCR1 inhibits calcineurin function. These authors proposed that increased expression of DSCR1 in trisomy-21 individuals may contribute to the neurological, cardiac or immunological defects of DS. Calcineurin regulates NMDA receptor activity; NMDA receptors are glutamate-sensitive ion channel receptors that mediate excitatory synaptic transmission and are widely implicated in synaptic plasticity and integration of synaptic activity in the CNS (Rycroft and Gibb, 2002). This might be one of the mechanisms at the basis of the abnormal central nervous excitability in DS; however, we must be aware that more than one neurotransmitter system might be involved.

References

Broulliette RT, Fernbach SK, Hunt CE (1982) Obstructive sleep apnea in infants and children. J Pediatrics 100: 31–40.

Colognola RM, Musumeci SA, Ferri R, Grubar JC, Bergonzi P, Gigli GL (1988) REM sleep and mental retardation (MR): Comparison among three groups with homogeneous karyotype. In WP Koella, F Obal, H Schulz, P Visser (eds) Sleep '86. Stuttgart: Gustav Fischer Verlag, pp. 370–2.

Evenhuis HM (1990) The natural history of dementia in Down's syndrome. Arch Neurol 47: 263–7.

Ferri R, Curzi-Dascalova L, del Gracco S, Elia M, Musumeci SA, Pettinato S (1998) Heart rate variability and apnea during sleep in Down's syndrome. J Sleep Res 7: 282–7.

Ferri R, Curzi-Dascalova L, del Gracco S, Elia M, Musumeci SA, Stefanini MC (1997) Respiratory patterns during sleep in Down's syndrome: importance of central apnoeas. J Sleep Res 6: 134–41.

Ferri R, del Gracco S, Elia M, Musumeci SA, Scuderi C, Bergonzi P (1994) Bit-mapped somatosensory evoked potentials in Down's syndrome individuals. Neurophysiologie Clinique 24: 357–66.

Ferri R, del Gracco S, Elia M, Musumeci SA, Spada R, Stefanini MC (1996b) Scalp topographic mapping of middle-latency somatosensory evoked potentials in normal aging and dementia. Neurophysiologie Clinique 26: 311–19.

Ferri R, del Gracco S, Elia M, Musumeci SA, Stefanini MC (1995a) Age, sex and mental retardation related changes of brainstem auditory evoked potentials in Down's syndrome. It J Neur Sci 16: 377–83.

Ferri R, del Gracco S, Elia M, Musumeci SA, Stefanini MC (1996a) Age- and height-dependent changes of amplitude and latency of somatosensory evoked potentials in children with Down's syndrome and young adult controls. Neurophysiologie Clinique 26: 321–7.

Ferri R, Ragusa L, Alberti A, Elia M, Musumeci SA, del Gracco S, Romano C, Stefanini MC (1995b) Growth hormone and sleep in Down syndrome. Dev Brain Dysfunction 9: 114–20.

Folsom RC, Widen JE, Wilson WR (1983) Auditory brain-stem responses in infants with Down's syndrome. Arch Otolaryngol 109: 607–10.

Fuentes JJ, Genesca L, Kingsbury TJ, Cunningham KW, Perez-Riba M, Estivill X, de la Luna S (2000) DSCR1, overexpressed in Down syndrome, is an inhibitor of calcineurin-mediated signaling pathways. Hum Mol Genet 9: 1681–90.

Fuentes JJ, Pritchard MA, Planas AM, Bosch A, Ferrer I, Estivill X (1995) A new human gene from the Down syndrome critical region encodes a proline-rich protein highly expressed in fetal brain and heart. Hum Mol Genet 4: 1935–44.

Gigli GL, Bergonzi P, Grubar JC, Colognola RM, Amata MT, Pollicina C, Musumeci SA, Ferri R (1985b) Effects of intensive learning sessions on nocturnal sleep in Down's syndrome (DS) children. Comparison with the effects of an experimental drug (BAHS). In WP Koella, E Ruther, H Schulz (eds) Sleep '84. Gustav Fischer Verlag: Stuttgart, pp. 361–3.

Gigli GL, Ferri R, Musumeci SA, Tomassetti P, Bergonzi P (1984) Brainstem auditory evoked responses in children with Down's syndrome. In JM Berg (ed.) Perspectives in Progress in Mental Retardation. Vol. II. Biomedical Aspects. University Park Press: Baltimore, pp. 277–86.

Gigli GL, Grubar JC, Colognola RM, Amata MT, Pollicina C, Ferri R, Musumeci SA, Bergonzi P (1985a) Butoctamide hydogen succinate and intensive learning sessions: effects on night sleep of Down's syndrome patients. Sleep 10: 563–9.

Goldberg-Stern H, Strawsburg RH, Patterson B, Hickey F, Bare M, Gadoth N, Degrauw TJ (2001) Seizure frequency and characteristics in children with Down syndrome. Brain Dev 23: 375–8.

Goldstein JC, Wu RHK, Thorpy MJ, Shprintzen RJ, Marion RE, Saenger P (1987) Reversibility of deficient sleep entrained growth hormone secretion in a boy with achondroplasia and obstructive sleep apnea. Acta Endocrinologica (Copenh) 116: 95–101.

Grubar JC, Gigli GL, Colognola RM, Ferri R, Musumeci SA, Bergonzi P (1984) Effects of butoctamide (BAHS) on nocturnal sleep of Down's syndrome children. Comparison with the effects of an experimental drug. In WP Koella, E Ruther, H Schulz (eds) Sleep '84. Stuttgart: Gustav Fischer Verlag, pp. 420–2.

Grubar JC, Gigli GL, Colognola RM, Ferri R, Musumeci SA, Bergonzi P (1986) Sleep patterns of Down's syndrome children: effects of BAHS administration. Psychopharmachology 90: 119–22.

Grunstein R, Stewart D, Sullivan C (1992) Endocrine and metabolic disturbances in obstructive sleep apnea. In S Smirne, M Franceschi, L Ferini-Strambi,

M Zucconi (eds) Sleep, Hormones and Immunological System. Milano: Masson, pp. 111–22.

Kakigi R, Kuroda M (1992) Brain-stem auditory evoked potentials in adults with Down's syndrome. Electroencephalogr Clin Neurophysiol 84: 293–5.

Kingsbury TJ, Cunnigham KW (2000) A conserved family of calcineurin regulators. Genes Dev 14: 1595–604.

Lalioti MD, Mirotsou M, Buresi C, Peitsch MC, Rossier C, Ouazzani R, Baldy-Moulinier M, Bottani A, Malafosse A, Antonarakis SE (1997) Identification of mutations in cystatin B, the gene responsible for the Unverricht-Lundborg type of progressive myoclonus epilepsy (EPM1). Am J Hum Genet 60: 342–51.

Li LM, O'Donoghue MF, Sander JW (1995) Myoclonic epilepsy of late onset in trisomy 21. Arq Neuropsiquiatr 53: 792–4.

Marcus CL, Keens TG, Bautista DB, von Pechmann WS, Davidson Ward SL (1991) Obstructive sleep apnea in children with Down syndrome. Pediatrics 88: 132–9.

Matsumoto AM, Sandblom RE, Schoene RB, Lee KA, Giblin EC, Pierson DJ, Bremner WJ (1985) Testosterone replacement in hypogonadal males: effects on obstructive sleep apnea, respiratory drives and sleep. Clin Endocrinol (Oxf) 22: 713–21.

Moller JC, Hamer HM, Oertel WH, Rosenow F (2001) Late-onset myoclonic epilepsy in Down's syndrome (LOMEDS). Seizure 10: 303–6.

Pueschel SM, Anneren G, Durlach R, Flores J, Sustrova M, Verma IC (1995) Guidelines for optimal medical care of persons with Down syndrome. International League of Societies for Persons with Mental Handicap (ILSMH). Acta Paediatr 84: 823–7.

Puri BK, Ho KW, Singh I (2001) Age of seizure onset in adults with Down's syndrome. Int J Clin Pract 55: 442–4.

Romano C, Tiné A, Fazio G, Rizzo R, Colognola RM, Sorge G, Bergonzi P, Pavone L (1990) Seizures in patients with trisomy 21. Am J Med Genet 7(Suppl): 298–300.

Rycroft BK, Gibb AJ (2002) Direct effects of calmodulin on NMDA receptor single-channel gating in rat hippocampal granule cells. J Neurosci 22: 8860–8.

Saunders AM (2001) Gene identification in Alzheimer's disease. Pharmacogenomics 2: 239–49.

Southall DP, Stebbens VA, Mirza R, Lang MH, Croft CB, Shinebourne EA (1987) Upper airway obstruction with hypoxaemia and sleep disruption in Down syndrome. Dev Med Child Neurol 29: 734–42.

Squires N, Aine C, Buchwald J, Norman R, Galbraith G (1980) Auditory brain stem response abnormalities in severely and profoundly retarded adults. Electroenceph Clin Neurophys 50: 172–85.

Squires N, Buchwald J, Liley F, Strecker J (1982) Brainstem auditory evoked potential abnormalities in retarded adults. In J Courjon, F Mauguière, M Revol (eds) Clinical Application of Evoked Potentials in Neurology. New York: Raven Press, pp. 233–40.

Stebbens VA, Dennis J, Samuels MP, Croft CB, Southhall DP (1991) Sleep related upper airway obstruction in a cohort with Down's syndrome. Arch Dis Childhood 6: 1333–8.

Tsiouris JA, Patti PJ, Tipu O, Raguthu S (2002) Adverse effects of phenytoin given for late-onset seizures in adults with Down syndrome. Neurology 59: 779–80.

Tyrrell J, Cosgrave M, McCarron M, McPherson J, Calvert J, Kelly A, McLaughlin M, Gill M, Lawlor BA (2001) Dementia in people with Down's syndrome. Int J Geriatr Psychiatry 16: 1168–74.

van Allen MI, Fung J, Jurenka SB (1999) Health care concerns and guidelines for adults with Down syndrome. Am J Med Genet 89: 100–10.

van Buggenhout GJ, Trommelen JC, Schoenmaker A, De Bal C, Verbeek JJ, Smeets DF, Ropers HH, Devriendt K, Hamel BC, Fryns JP (1999) Down syndrome in a population of elderly mentally retarded patients: genetic-diagnostic survey and implications for medical care. Am J Med Genet 85: 376–84.

Yanagisawa I, Yoshikawa H (1973) A bromine compound isolated from human cerebrospinal fluid and synthesis-related compounds. Acta Biochem Biophys 329: 283–94.

Chapter 12
Down syndrome and Alzheimer's disease

K.E. WISNIEWSKI, E. KIDA, G. ALBERTINI

Introduction

Individuals with Down syndrome (DS) all have varying degrees of mental handicap (MH); only a few have learning disabilities (Wisniewski et al., 1988; Capone, 2001; Jenkins and Velinov, 2001). Also, individuals with DS have developmental delays (speech and motor) and are prone to infection, endocrinopathy, malignancies, visual/auditory problems and seizures and some also develop AD earlier than the general population (Wisniewski et al., 1978, 1979a, 1979b, 1985b, 1992, 1996; Stafstrom et al., 1991).

Recently, when the entire DNA sequence of the human genome was completed, it was estimated that 50–65% of the 30,000 genes of the human genome expressed in the brain may contribute to normal development. Chromosome 21 is the smallest human autosome, containing about 418 genes (www.ncbi.nlm.nih.gov). In trisomy 21, an individual has an extra copy of chromosome 21, creating a 'gene dose effect', leading to a 50% increase in messenger RNA (mRNA), transcription products, and its gene products (proteins) that may lead to functional overexpression in all cells or tissues (Peterson et al., 1994; Rosenberg, 1997; Antonarakis, 1998; Hattori et al., 2000; Capone, 2001). This increase contributes to the pathogenesis and phenotype (clinical symptoms and brain abnormalities) of DS (Wisniewski and Schmidt-Sidor, 1989; Wisniewski 1990; Wisniewski et al., 1984, 1997; Korenberg et al., 1990; Schmidt-Sidor et al., 1990; Wisniewski and Kida, 1994). Also, overexpression of some genes and their gene products on chromosome 21 (e.g., amyloid precursor protein (APP)) and/or products of genes localized to other chromosomes may cause earlier signs of AD in DS, including dementia and brain abnormalities (shrinkage of the brain, neuronal loss), senile plaques, neurofibrillary tangles and synaptic abnormalities (Wisniewski et al., 1985a, 1985b, 1987; Neve et al., 1988; Rosen et al., 1993; Kida et al., 1995a, 1995b).

Proteolytic cleavage of APP generates a peptide with 40–42 amino acid residues, amyloid-β (Aβ), the major component of senile plaques and vascular Aβ in AD. Indeed, most individuals with DS develop AD neuropathology after 30–40 years of age, around 20–30 years earlier than the general population (Wisniewski et al., 1979a, 1985a, 1985b, 1987; Wisniewski and Hill, 1985). Some people with DS develop diffuse Aβ deposits in the brain parenchyma as early as their first decade of life. Recent data suggest that extracellular deposition of Aβ deposits in DS brain is preceded by intracellular accumulation of Aβ in neurons and astrocytes, followed by neuritic plaques, neurofibrillary tangles and neuronal loss. The latter, another neuropathological feature of the AD brain, is distinctly more severe in some brain areas (fronto-temporal cortex) in DS than AD (Wisniewski et al., 1985b). Further study is needed to determine whether neuronal loss is caused by amyloid cascade or reflects the consequences of overexpression of other genes located in the DS critical region (DSCR), e.g., chaperone proteins, SOD1, S100-calcium binding protein, β subunit, or genes located on other chromosomes, which also show altered expression in DS (Capone, 2001).

Recent data suggest that the clinical features of DS are multifactorial and that the gene-dosage hypothesis may simplify the complex pathogenetic events underlying DS phenotypes. Thus, it appears that altered coordinated expression and interactions among numerous proteins may also be associated with AD pathology in DS. The clinicopathological and biochemical aspects and treatment of AD in DS will be discussed.

Clinical studies

Premature ageing and dementia among people with DS has been recognized since a report by Fraser and Mitchell in 1876. Until recently, however, accelerated ageing among this population was not considered to be an important issue affecting major programme development, because typically, the majority of people with DS were not expected to live past adolescence or young adulthood (Thase et al., 1982, 1984).

Presently, extensive data indicate that people with DS are more likely to show declines in cognitive functioning after 50 years of age, but this is still earlier than adults with MH of other aetiologies (Wisniewski et al., 1978; Thase et al., 1982, 1984; Devenny et al., 1993, 1996; Zigman et al., 1996). These declines have been attributed to the presence of AD neuropathology in virtually all cases older than 30 years of age (Wisniewski et al., 1985b; Wisniewski and Schmidt-Sidor, 1989).

A 6-year longitudinal study comparing 91 adults (31–63 years of age) with DS and mild or moderate MH to 64 adults (31–76 years of age) with other forms of MH (taking yearly measures of mental status, short- and long-term memory, speeded psychomotor function and visuospatial organization) suggests that adults with DS with mild or moderate MH may be at lower risk for dementia during their fourth and fifth decades of life than previous studies have suggested (Devenny et al., 1993, 1996).

Neuropathological studies

The presence of AD-type pathology in the brains of almost all people with DS 30 years of age and older has been the cornerstone for the widely held view that people with DS will develop AD at a much younger age than non-DS individuals (Malamud, 1972; Wisniewski et al., 1978, 1985a, 1985b, 1992; Rabe et al., 1990). Because of this relationship between DS and AD, it has been widely assumed that knowledge about almost any aspect of one of these conditions will illuminate the other (Mann et al., 1985, 1987a, 1987b, 1990; Mann, 1989; Wisniewski, 1990). The brain abnormalities (cortical, synaptic dysgenesis, neuronal loss and microencephaly) are associated with impairment of central nervous system maturation, differentiation and function that is observed at various stages of life. Usually, the brain weight of individuals with DS is lower than that of controls (Figure 12.1).

AD-type pathology is characterized by two major neuropathological features: amyloid (senile) plaques and neurofibrillary tangles (NFTs). NFTs

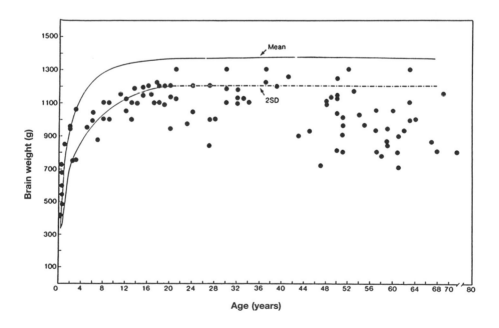

Figure 12.1 Brain weights at death in 100 patients with Down syndrome.

comprise paired helical filaments (PHFs), abnormal cytoplasmic fibres that result from the hyperphosphorylation of the microtubule-associated protein tau (Wisniewski et al., 1985a, 1985b; Wisniewski and Hill, 1985; Mann, 1989; Flament et al., 1990; Selkoe, 1999). Senile plaques are primarily composed of Aβ, which is proteolytically generated from the β-amyloid precursor protein (βAPP) (Selkoe, 1999). The βAPP gene is encoded on chromosome 21 (Robakis et al., 1987). DS subjects have three copies of chromosome 21, and, thus an additional copy of the βAPP gene, leading to increased production of Aβ very early in life and the development of Alzheimer-type neuropathology in young and middle-aged subjects (Mann, 1989; Rumble et al., 1989). The development of amyloid deposits was described in teenage DS subjects by silver staining techniques (Wisniewski et al., 1985a, 1985b). Subsequently, sensitive antibodies to Aβ42 were used to detect abundant diffuse Aβ42 plaques (thioflavin S-negative) as early as 12 years in DS subjects (Lemere et al., 1996). Typically, by around 30–40 years of age, and infrequently in younger subjects, a subset of plaques in DS brains shows fibrillar Aβ, i.e. thioflavin-positive amyloid. The number of such fibrillar plaques increases with age (Lemere et al., 1996). Many of these plaques are associated with local gliosis and neuronal changes such as NFTs. The presence of senile plaques (plaques containing Aβ fibrils associated with neuritic changes), NFTs and clinically progressive dementia with behavioural changes (Lai and Williams, 1989) in DS subjects all suggest that DS brains can provide a powerful model for studying the temporal development of AD-type neuropathology (Wisniewski et al., 1985a, 1985b; Tagliavini et al., 1989).

In AD brains, compacted Aβ plaques are often associated with such inflammatory markers as activated microglia, reactive astrocytes and complement proteins, including C1q, C3, C9, C3d and C4d (McGeer and McGeer, 1992). The complement cascade comprises a series of enzymatic steps that play a role in the immune response (Kuby, 1998). C1q, C3 and C9 are three proteins involved in the beginning, middle and end, respectively, of the classical complement cascade. Whereas the classical complement pathway is more commonly activated by the binding of C1q to the Fc portion of an immunoglobulin, aggregated Aβ but not monomeric Aβ (Snyder et al., 1994) has been reported to activate the classical complement cascade by directly binding to C1q *in vitro* (Velazquez et al., 1997). Synthetic preaggregated Aβ42 peptides were observed to bind C1q much more effectively than Aβ40 peptides, and the binding site of the Aβ42 peptides was localized to the C1q A chain collagen-like region, residues 14–26 (Jiang et al., 1994). Binding of Aβ to C1q has been shown to enhance Aβ aggregation because of the complementary spacing in the structures of the two proteins (Webster et al., 1995). Moreover, *in situ* evidence for the activation of the classical complement pathway has been observed in AD brain (Afagh et al., 1996; Yasojima et al., 1999). This cascade marks cells for attack by macrophages and causes the release of various proteins to serve as anaphylotoxins that further stimulate the immune response. The cascade ends in the assembly of two molecules of preassembled C5b, 6, 7 with two molecules of C8 and subsequently, 12–18 molecules of C9 to form the membrane attack complex (MAC), C5b–9, which creates a leaky pore in the plasma membrane and leads to lysis of target cells (McGeer et al., 1989a). C4d and C3d constitute by-products of degradation of C4b and C3b on the cell surface and indicate complement activation; immunoreactivity (IR) for each has been observed in senile plaques, dystrophic neurites and NFTs in AD (McGeer et al., 1989b). The presence of C4d is indicative of activation of the classical pathway, whereas C3d is indicative of either the classical or alternative complement pathways (Ayakima et al., 1991). C5b–9 IR has been detected in dystrophic neurites in senile plaques (but not in association with extracellular amyloid) and in NFTs in AD (McGeer et al., 1989a, 1989b). Apolipoprotein J (apo J), an inhibitor of the membrane attack complex, has been shown to colocalize with senile plaques in AD and DS cerebral cortex (Kida et al., 1995a). Furthermore, apo J has been observed to form a complex with soluble Aβ in cerebrospinal fluid (Ghiso et al., 1993).

Activation of the alternative complement pathway by Aβ peptides has also been described (Bradt et al., 1998). Stoltzner et al. (2000) studied 24 DS cases for the temporal appearance of several complement proteins (Clq, C3, C4d, and C5b–9) as well as the complement inhibitor, apo J, in DS brains, and related this process to other AD neuropathological changes (Aβ42 deposits, dystrophic neurites, reactive astrocytes and activated microglia). Thus, markers of AD neuropathology and the activation, progression and completion of the classical complement cascade were analysed looking at the IR of PHF tau, Aβ42, classical complement proteins (Clq and C3), markers indicating activation of complement (C4d and C5b–9), the complement inhibitor, apo J, in a temporal series of 24 DS brains of increasing ages, from 12 to 73 years, and compared to the classical changes of AD. Aβ42-labelled diffuse plaques were first detected in a 12-year-old DS subject and were not labelled by any of the complement antibodies. Colocalization of Aβ42 with Clq, C3, C4d, and/or apo J was first detected in compacted plaques in the brain of a 15-year-old DS patient with features of mature AD pathology, such as reactive astrocytes, activated microglia, dystrophic neurites and a few NFTs. Our data suggest that in AD and DS, the classical complement cascade is activated after compaction of Aβ42 deposits and, in some instances, can progress to the local neuronal expression of the MAC as a response to Aβ plaque maturation (Stoltzner et al., 2000).

In another immunohistochemical study of intraneuronal Aβ accumulation in DS brains (temporal cortex) of 70 cases aged 3–73 years, for the Aβ-terminal, Aβ40 C-terminus and Aβ42 C-terminus and N-terminal antibodies did not detect intracellular Aβ (Mori et al., 2002). Aβ40 antibodies did not detect significant intracellular Aβ, but older cases showed Aβ40 IR in mature plaques. In contrast, Aβ42 antibodies revealed clear-cut intraneuronal IR in very young DS patients, but this IR declined as extracellular Aβ plaques gradually accumulated and matured (Figure 12.2a–d). No inflammatory changes were associated with intraneuronal Aβ. We also studied the temporal development of gliosis and NFT formation, revealing that in DS temporal cortex, inflammation and NFT follow Aβ deposition. We conclude that Aβ42 accumulates intracellularly prior to extracellular Aβ deposition in DS and that subsequent maturation of extracellular Aβ deposits elicits inflammatory responses and precedes NFTs (Mori et al., 2002).

Presynaptic markers for cholinergic, noradrenergic and serotonergic markers are all reduced in the brains of aged individuals with DS. These

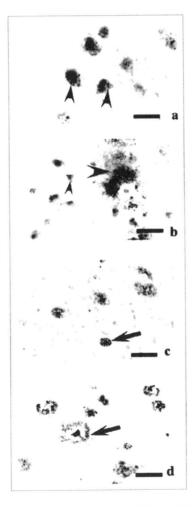

Figure 12.2a. Intense cytoplasmic neuronal staining of DS, 3–4 years old (arrowheads); **b.** Temporal cortex of DS, 17 years old, had both diffuse plaques (large arrowhead) and neuronal staining (small arrowhead); **c.** Fully matured plaques (arrow) were present as early as 29 years. **d.** At 62 years, mature, cored plaques were present (arrow), but intraneuronal Ab42 was nearly absent. Magnification bar = **a** 10 μm, **b** and **d** 50 μm, **c** 20 μm.

neurochemical changes seem to be caused by degeneration and cell loss of the cortical projection neurons arising from the nucleus basalis of Meynert (cholinergic), locus ceruleus (noradrenergic) and dorsal raphae nuclei (serotonergic). Pharmacological interventions, designed to enhance cholinergic neurotransmission in the brain, appear to hold some promise for enhancing communication and adaptive behaviour in young adults with DS (Kishnani et al., 1999).

It was also documented that in DS brains there was a defective repair of oxidative mtDNA damage in fibroblasts was comparable to that in controls (Druzhyna et al., 1998). Several proteins necessary for nucleotide excision-repair have also been studied in brains from adults with DS or AD compared with control subjects (Hemon et al., 1998). The expression of excision-repair-cross-complementing proteins 80 and 89 was consistently higher in frontal and temporal cortex samples from DS subjects and in all brain regions studied from AD subjects. Such findings are consistent with increased oxidative DNA damage *in vivo* and suggest that chronic oxidative injury constitutes a risk factor for subsequent neuronal death in aged individuals with DS (Buscigilo and Yankner, 1995; Slater et al., 1995).

The gene that encodes the cholesterol-carrying apolipoprotein E (*APOE*) and that maps to chromosome 19 has three allelic forms (Mahey, 1988). In the general population, *APOE E3* is the most common allele (0.78), followed by *APOE E4* (0.14) and *APOE E2* (0.07). Accordingly, three different homozygous or heterozygous genotypes are possible, resulting in six distinct phenotypes. Certain phenotypes have been linked to increased risk for developing both late-onset, familial and sporadic forms of AD (Saunders et al., 1993). Gene dose for *APOE E4* is correlated with both increased risk and earlier onset of AD, whereas the *APOE E2* gene dose appears to confer some protective effect (Corder et al., 1994). To determine whether this relationship holds true in DS, several studies have examined *APOE* allele frequency in adults with and without clinical symptoms of dementia (Wisniewski et al., 1995; Schupf et al., 1996; Prasher et al., 1997).

Treatment

The high risk of developing AD-type dementia in individuals with DS makes it clear that a neuroprotection strategy offers the best hope for palliation or prevention (Oken and McGeer, 1995). Current clinical research strategies are focused on the use of antioxidants, anti-inflammatory agents, neurotrophic factors or hormone replacement (Peskind, 1998). Recent epidemiological studies and clinical trials have been encouraging regarding possible benefits derived from using indomethacin (a nonsteroidal anti-inflammatory drug) (Stewart et al., 1997), oestrogen (Bender, 1997) and the antioxidants selegiline (monoamine oxidase inhibitor) and β-tocopherol (vitamin E) (Sano et al., 1997). Novel compounds designed to improve the clearance and/or to prevent the deposition of the neurotoxic Aβ peptide are also on the horizon. Also, treatment with Aβ vaccinations in transgenic mice is promising for amelioration of AD pathology in individuals with DS, but more research must be done. Clinical trials of Aβ vaccinations in subjects with AD are already under way (McLaurin et al., 2002).

References

Afagh A, Cummings BJ, Cribbs DH, Cotman CW, Tenner AJ (1996) Localization and cell association of Clq in Alzheimer's disease brain. Exp Neurol 138: 22–32.

Antonarakis S (1998) 10 years of genomics, chromosome 21, and DS. Genomics 51: 1–16.

Ayakima H, Yamada T, Kawamata T, McGeer PL (1991) Association of amyloid P component with complement proteins in neurologically diseased brain tissue. Brain Res 548: 349–52.

Bender K (1997) Evidence of estrogen benefit in dementia and cognition. Psychiatr Times 14(suppl): 20–22.

Bradt BM, Kolb WP, Cooper NR (1998) Complement-dependent pro-inflammatory properties of the Alzheimer's disease β-peptide. J Exp Med 188: 431–8.

Buscigilo J, Yankner B (1995) Apoptosis and increased generation of reactive oxygen species in Down's syndrome neurons in vitro. Nature 378: 776–9.

Capone GT (2001) Down syndrome: advances in molecular biology and the neurosciences. J Dev Behav Pediatr 22(1): 40–59.

Corder EH, Saunders AM, Risch NJ, Strittmatter WJ, Schmechel DE, Gaskell PC, Rimmler JB, Locke PA, Conneally PM, Schmader KE, Small GW, Roses AD, Haines JL, Pericak-Vance MA (1994) Protective effect of apolipoprotein E type 2 allele for late onset Alzheimer disease. Nat Genet 7: 180–4.

Devenny DA, Silverman WP, Hill AL, Jenkins E, Sersen EA, Wisniewski KE (1996) Normal aging in adults with Down's syndrome: a longitudinal study. JIDR 40(3): 208–21.

Devenny DA, Wisniewski KE, Silverman WP (1993) Dementia of the Alzheimer's type among high-functioning adults with Down's syndrome: individual profiles of performance. In B Corain, K Iqbal, M Nicolini, B Winblad, HM Wisniewski, P Zatta (eds) Alzheimer's Disease: Advances in Clinical and Basic Research. New York: John Wiley & Sons, pp. 47–53.

Druzhyna N, Nair RG, LeDoux SP, Wilson GL (1998) Defective repair of oxidative damage in mitochondrial DNA in Down's syndrome. Mutat Res 409(2): 81–9.

Flament A, Delacourte A, Mann DM (1990) Phosphorylation of tau proteins: a major event during the process of neurofibrillary degeneration. A comparative study between Alzheimer's disease and Down's syndrome. Brain Res 516(1): 15–19.

Fraser J, Mitchell A (1876) Kalmuc idiocy: report of a case with autopsy with notes on 62 cases. J Ment Sci 22: 161.

Ghiso J, Matsubara E, Koudinov A, Choi-Miura NH, Tomita M, Wisniewski T, Frangione B (1993) The cerebrospinal-fluid soluble form of Alzheimer's amyloid β is complexed to SP-40, 40 (apolipoprotein J) an inhibitor of the complement membrane-attack complex. Biochem J 293: 27–30.

Hattori M, Fujiyama A, Taylor TD, Watanabe H, Yada T, Park HS, Toyoda A, Ishii K, Totoki Y, Choi DK, Groner Y, Soeda E, Ohki M, Takagi T, Sakaki Y, Taudien S, Blechschmidt K, Polley A, Menzel U, Delabar J, Kumpf K, Lehmann R, Patterson D, Reichwald K, Rump A, Schillhabel M, Schudy A, Zimmermann W, Rosenthal A, Kudoh J, Schibuya K, Kawasaki K, Asakawa S, Shintani A, Sasaki T, Nagamine K, Mitsuyama S, Antonarakis SE, Minoshima S, Shimizu N, Nordsiek G, Hornischer K, Brant P, Scharfe M, Schon O, Desario A, Reichelt J, Kauer G, Blocker H, Ramser J, Beck A, Klages S, Hennig S, Riesselmann L, Dagand E, Haaf T, Wehrmeyer S, Borsym K, Gardincr K, Nizctic D, Francis F, Lchrach H, Reinhardt R, Yaspo ML (2000) The DNA sequence of human chromosome 21. Nature 405(6784): 311–19.

Hemon M, Cairns N, Egly JM, Fery A, Labudova O, Lubec G (1998) Expression of DNA excision-repair-cross-complementing proteins p80 and p89 in brain of patients with Down syndrome and Alzheimer's disease. Neurosci Lett 251(1): 45–8.

Jenkins EC, Velinov MT (2001) Down syndrome and the human genome. DS Quart 6(4): 1–12.

Jiang H, Burdick D, Glabe CG, Cotman CW, Tenner AJ (1994) β-amyloid activates complement by binding to a specific region of the collagen-like domain of the Clq A chain. J Immunol 152: 5050–9.

Kida E, Choi-Miura N-H, Wisniewski KE (1995a) Deposition of apolipoproteins E and J in senile plaques is topographically determined in both Alzheimer's disease and Down's syndrome brain. Brain Res 685: 211–16.

Kida E, Wisniewski KE, Wisniewski HM (1995b) Early amyloid-deposits show different immunoreactivity to the amino- and carboxy-terminal regions of ß-peptide in Alzheimer's disease and Down's syndrome brain. Neurosci Lett 193: 105–8.

Kishnani P, Sullivan J, Walter B, Spiridigliozzi GA, Doraiswamy PM, Krisman KR (1999) Cholinergic therapy for Down's syndrome. Lancet 353: 1064–5.

Korenberg JR, Kawashima H, Pulst SM, Allen L, Magenis E, Epstein CJ (1990) Down syndrome: toward a molecular definition of the phenotype. Am J Med Genet Suppl 7: 91–7.

Kuby J (1998) The Complement System. In Immunology. New York: WH Freeman & Co, pp. 335–55.

Lai F, Williams RS (1989) A prospective study of Alzheimer's disease in Down syndrome. Arch Neurol 46: 849–53.

Lemere CA, Blustzjan JK, Yamaguchi H, Wisniewski T, Saido TC, Selkoe DJ (1996) Sequence of deposition of heterogeneous amyloid β-peptides and Apo E in Down syndrome: implications for initial events in amyloid plaque formation. Neurobiol Dis 3: 16–32.

Mahey R (1988) Apolipoprotein E: cholesterol transport protein with expanding role in cell biology. Science 240: 622–30.

Malamud N (1972) Neuropathology of organic brain syndromes associated with aging. In CM Gaitz (ed.) Aging and the Brain. New York: Plenum, p. 63.

Mann DMA (1989) Cerebral amyloidosis, aging and Alzheimer's disease: a contribution from studies on Down's syndrome. Neurobiol Aging 10: 397–9.

Mann DMA, Royston MC, Ravindra CR (1990) Some morphometric observations on the brains of patients with Down's syndrome: their relationship to age and dementia. J Neurol Sci 99: 153–64.

Mann DMA, Yates PO, Marcyniuk B (1984) Alzheimer's presenile dementia, senile dementia of Alzheimer type and Down's syndrome in middle age form an age related continuum of pathological changes. Neuropathol Appl Neurobiol 10: 185–207.

Mann DMA, Yates PO, Marcyniuk B (1987b) Dopaminergic neurotransmitter systems in Alzheimer's disease and in Down's syndrome at middle age. J Neurol Neurosurg Psychiatry 50: 341–4.

Mann DMA, Yates PO, Marcyniuk B, Ravindra CR (1985) Pathological evidence for neurotransmitter deficits in Down's syndrome of middle age. J Ment Defic Res 29: 125–35.

Mann DMA, Yates PO, Marcyniuk B, Ravindra CR (1987a) Loss of neurons from cortical and sub-cortical areas in Down's syndrome patients at middle age. Quantitative comparisons with younger Down's patients and patients with Alzheimer's disease. J Neurol Sci 80: 79–89.

McGeer PL, Akiyama H, Itagaki S, McGeer EG (1989a) Activation of the classical complement pathway in brain tissue of Alzheimer patients. Neurosci Lett 107: 341–6.

McGeer PL, Akiyama H, Itagaki S, McGeer EG (1989b) Immune system response in Alzheimer's disease. Can J Neurol Sci 16: 516–27.

McGeer PL, McGeer EG (1992) Complement proteins and complement inhibitors in Alzheimer's disease. Res Immunol 143: 621–4.

McLaurin JA, Cecal R, Kierstead ME, Phinney AL, Manea M, French JE, Lambermon MH, Darabie AA, Brown ME, Janus C, Chishti MA, Horne P, Westaway D, Fraser PE, Mount HT, Przybylski M, St George-Hyslop P (2002) Therapeutically effective antibodies against amyloid-beta peptide target amyloid-beta residues 4–10 and inhibit cytotoxicity and fibrillogenesis. Nat Med 8(11): 1263–9.

Mori C, Spooner ET, Wisniewski KE, Wisniewski TM, Yamaguchi H, Saido TC, Tolan DR, Selkoe DJ, Lemere CA (2002) Intraneuronal Aβ42 accumulation in Down syndrome brain. Amyloid: J Protein Folding Disord 9: 88–102.

Neve R, Finch E, Dawes E (1988) Expression of the Alzheimer's amyloid precursor gene transcripts in the human brain. Neuron 1: 669–77.

Oken R, McGeer P (1995) Down's syndrome: prophylaxis and therapy for the frequently comorbid Alzheimer's disease. Med Hypotheses 44: 233–4.

Oliver C, Holland AJ (1986) Down's syndrome & Alzheimer's disease. Psych Med 16: 307–22.

Peskind E (1998) Pharmacologic approaches to cognitive deficits in Alzheimer's disease. J Clin Psychiatry 59(Suppl 9): 22–7.

Peterson A, Patil N, Robbins C, Wang L, Cox DR, Myers RM (1994) A transcript map of the Down syndrome critical region on chromosome 21. Hum Mol Genet 3(10): 1735–42.

Prasher VP, Chowdhury TA, Rowe BR, Bain SC (1997) ApoE genotype and Alzheimer's disease in adults with Down syndrome: meta-analysis. Am J Ment Retard 102(2): 103–10.

Rabe A, Wisniewski KE, Schupf N, Wisniewski, HM (1990) Relationship of Down syndrome to Alzheimer disease. In SI Deutsch, A Weizman, R Weizman (eds) Application of Basic Neuroscience to Child Psychiatry. New York: Plenum Publishing Corp, pp. 325–40.

Robakis NK, Wisniewski HM, Jenkins EC, Devine-Gage EA, Houck GE, Yao XL, Ramakrishna N, Wolfe G, Silverman WP, Brown WT (1987) Chromosome 21q21 sublocalisation of gene encoding beta-amyloid peptide in cerebral vessels and neuritic (senile) plaques of people with Alzheimer disease and Down syndrome. Lancet 1: 384–5.

Rosen DR, Siddique T, Patterson D, Figlewicz DA, Sapp P, Hentati A, Donaldson D, Goto J, O'Regan JP, Deng HX (1993) Mutations in Cu/Zn superoxide dismutase gene are associated with familial amyotrophic lateral sclerosis. Nature 362(6415): 59–62.

Rosenberg R (1997) Molecular neurogenetics: genome is settling the issue. JAMA 278: 1282–3.

Rumble B, Retallack R, Hilbich C, Simms G, Multhaup G, Martins R, Hockey A, Montgomery P, Beyreuther K, Masters CL (1989) Amyloid A4 protein, and its precursor in Down's syndrome and Alzheimer's disease. N Engl J Med 320: 1446–52.

Sano M, Ernesto C, Thomas RG, Klauber MR, Schafer K, Grundman M, Woodbury P, Growdon J, Cotman CW, Pfeiffer E, Schneider LS, Thal LJ (1997) A controlled trial of selegiline, alpha-tocopherol, or both as treatment for Alzheimer's disease. The Alzheimer's Disease Cooperative Study. N Engl J Med 336(17): 1216–22.

Saunders AM, Strittmatter WJ, Schmechel D, George-Hyslop PH, Pericak-Vance MA, Joo SH, Rosi BL, Gusella JF, Crapper-MacLachlan DR, Alberts MJ (1993) Association of apolipoprotein E allele epsilon 4 with late-onset familial and sporadic Alzheimer's disease. Neurology 43(8): 1467–72.

Schmidt-Sidor B, Wisniewski KE, Shepard TH, Sersen EA (1990) Brain growth in Down syndrome subjects ages: 15 to 22 weeks of gestational age and birth to 60 months. Clin Neuropathol 9: 181–90.

Schupf N, Kapell D, Lee JH, Zigman W, Canto B, Tycko B, Mayeux R (1996) Onset of dementia is associated with apolipoprotein E epsilon4 in Down's syndrome. Ann Neurol 40(5): 799–801.

Selkoe DJ (1999) Translating cell biology into therapeutic advances in Alzheimer's disease. Nature 399: A23–A31.

Slater A, Nobel C, Orrenius S (1995) The role of intracellular oxidants in apoptosis. Biochim Biophys Acta 1271: 59–62.

Snyder SW, Wang GT, Barrett L, Ladror US, Casuto D, Lee CM, Krafft GA, Holzman RB, Holzman TF (1994) Complement C1q does not bind monomeric β-amyloid. Exp Neurol 128: 136–42.

Stafstrom CE, Patxot OF, Gilmore HE, Wisniewski KE (1991) Seizures in children with Down syndrome: etiologies, characteristics, and outcome. Dev Med Child Neurol 33: 191–200.

Stewart WF, Kawas C, Corrada M, Metter EJ (1997) Risk of Alzheimer's disease and duration of NSAID use. Neurology 48(3): 626–32.

Stoltzner SE, Grenfell TJ, Mori C, Wisniewski KE, Wisniewski TM, Selkoe DJ, Lemere CA (2000) Temporal accrual of complement proteins in amyloid plaques in Down's syndrome with Alzheimer's disease. Am J Path 156(2): 489–99.

Tagliavini F, Giaccone G, Linoli G, Frangione B, Bugiani O (1989) Cerebral extracellular preamyloid deposits in Alzheimer's disease, Down syndrome and nondemented elderly individuals. Prog Clin Biol Res 317: 1001–5.

Thase ME, Liss L, Smeltzer D, Maloon J (1982) Clinical evaluation of dementia in Down's syndrome: a preliminary report. J Ment Defic Res 26: 239–44.

Thase ME, Tigner R, Smeltzer DJ, Liss L (1984) Age-related neuropsychological deficits in Down's syndrome. Biol Psychiatry 19: 571–85.

Velazquez P, Cribbs D, Poulos T, Tenner A (1997) Aspartate residue 7 in amyloid β-protein is critical for classical complement pathway activation: implications for Alzheimer's disease pathogenesis. Nature Med 3: 77–9.

Webster S, Glabe C, Rogers J (1995) Multivalent binding of complement protein Clq to the amyloid β-peptide promotes the nucleation phase of Aβ aggregation. Biochem Biophys Res Commun 217: 869–75.

Wisniewski KE (1990) Down syndrome children often have brain with maturation delay; retardation of growth and cortical dysgenesis. Am J Med Genet 37: 274–81.

Wisniewski KE, Cobill JM, Wilcox CB, Caspary EA, Williams DG, Wisniewski HM (1979a) T lymphocytes in patients with Down's syndrome. Biol Psychiatry 14: 463–71.

Wisniewski KE, Dalton AJ, Crapper McLachlan DR, Wen GY, Wisniewski HM (1985a) Alzheimer disease in Down syndrome: clinicopathological studies. Neurology 35: 957–61.

Wisniewski KE, Hill AL (1985) Clinical aspects of dementia in mental retardation and developmental disabilities. In M Janicki, HM Wisniewski (eds) Aging and Developmental Disabilities: Issues and Approaches. Baltimore: Brookes Pub Co, pp. 195–210.

Wisniewski KE, Hill L, Wisniewski HM (1992) Aging and Alzheimer's disease in people with Down syndrome. In I Lott, E McCoy (eds) Down Syndrome: Advances in Medical Care. New York: Wiley-Liss Division, pp. 167–83.

Wisniewski KE, Howe J, Williams D, Gwyn D, Wisniewski HM (1978) Precocious aging and dementia in patients with Down's syndrome. Biol Psychiatry 13: 619–27.

Wisniewski KE, Jervis GA, Moretz RC, Wisniewski HM (1979b) Alzheimer neurofibrillary tangles in disease other than senile and presenile dementia. Ann Neurol 5: 288–94.

Wisniewski KE, Kida E (1994) Abnormal neurogenesis and synaptogenesis in Down syndrome brain. Dev Brain Dysfunct 7: 289–301.

Wisniewski KE, Kida E, Kuchna I, Wierzba-Bobrowicz T, Dambska M (1997) Regulators of neuronal survival (Bcl-2, Bax, c-Jun) in prenatal and postnatal human frontal and temporal lobes in normal and Down syndrome brain. IPSEN Found. In AM Galaburda and Y Christen (eds) Research Perspectives in the Neurosciences. Paris: Springer-Verlag, pp. 179–95.

Wisniewski KE, Laure-Kamionowska M, Wisniewski HM (1984) Evidence of arrest of neurogenesis and synaptogenesis in brains of patients with Down syndrome. N Engl J Med 311: 1187–8.

Wisniewski KE, Miezejeski CM, Hill AL (1988) Neurological and psychological status of individuals with Down syndrome. In L Nadel (ed.) The Psychobiology of Down Syndrome. Cambridge, MA: The MIT Press, pp. 316–43.

Wisniewski T, Morelli L, Wegiel J, Levy E, Wisniewski HM, Frangione B (1995) The influence of apolipoprotein E isotypes on Alzheimer's disease pathology in 40 cases of Down's syndrome. Ann Neurol 37(1): 136–8.

Wisniewski KE, Rabe A, Wisniewski HM (1987) Pathological similarities between Alzheimer's disease and Down's syndrome: is there a genetic link? Integr Psychiatry 5: 159–70.

Wisniewski KE, Schmidt-Sidor B (1989) Postnatal delay of myelin formation in brains from some Down syndrome infants and children. Clin Neuropathol 8: 55–62.

Wisniewski KE, Wisniewski HM (1983) Age-associated changes in Down's syndrome. In B Reisberg (ed.) Textbook of Alzheimer's Disease. New York: New York Free Press, pp. 319–26.

Wisniewski KE, Wisniewski HM, Wen GY (1985b) Occurrence of neuropathological changes and dementia of Alzheimer's disease in Down's syndrome. Ann Neurol 17: 278–82.

Wisniewski KE, Zimmerli E, Mlodzik B, Devenny DA, Wisniewski HM (1996) Invecchiamento e malattia di Alzheimer negli adulti con sindrome di Down con ritardo mentale lieve o moderato. (Accelerated aging and Alzheimer disease in mild/moderate mentally retarded Down syndrome individuals.) In G Albertini, G Biondi (eds) Disabilita Dello Sviluppo Ed Inbecchiamento. Italy: Omega Edizioni, pp. 47–59.

Yasojima K, Schwab C, McGeer EG, McGeer PL (1999) Up-regulated production and activation of the complement system in Alzheimer's disease brain. Am J Pathol 154: 927–36.

Zigman W, Schupf N, Sersen E, Silverman W (1996) Prevalence of dementia in adults with and without Down syndrome. Am J Men Retard 100: 403–12.

Chapter 13
Pharmacological therapies in Down syndrome: facts and fancy

A. RASORE-QUARTINO

Introduction

The possibility of actively treating children with Down syndrome (DS) is a reality today. We must keep in mind, however, that genetic influences of the extra chromosome are already operating *in utero*, causing physical and neurological defects that are present at birth. Moreover, such influences go on throughout the whole life; many defects appearing late in life are the result of continuous genetic action expressing itself on the evolving organism.

The question is: how can we interfere with these processes and which therapies can we avail ourselves of, in order to counterbalance the ongoing disabilities?

Different methodological approaches exist that are aimed at the prevention and treatment of symptoms and their consequences or that are possibly aimed even at the 'normalization' of the syndrome itself. Such studies can start from the phenotypic anomalies, from chemical research, even from basic research or from the study of the genes located on chromosome 21 (Epstein, 1999). All these methods have their importance and each of them has given very interesting and positive results.

Accurate knowledge of the different diseases or complications that are most frequently associated with DS has led to the elaboration of preventive and therapeutic strategies which have contributed to the prolongation of life and to the amelioration of its quality. Similarly, the social modifications that have taken place in the last 20–30 years in western Europe and in the United States in relation to the inclusion of people with DS (inclusion in the family, in school and in work) have contributed to these improvements. Changing expectations with regard to the actual possibilities of treatments have been important.

Both the most significant pharmacological therapies, which can actually modify specific diseases affecting DS, and non-conventional treatments are discussed below.

Thyroid disorders

Since the first descriptions of DS and for almost a century, hypothyroidism was considered a constant feature of the syndrome. Only when laboratory tests for thyroid function became commonly available, was it pointed out that most people with DS were actually euthyroid. It was also demonstrated that a higher incidence of thyroid disorders, mainly hypothyroidism, is characteristic of DS. According to the literature, congenital hypothyroidism in DS varies from 0.7% to 10%, while in non-trisomic newborns it varies from 0.015% to 0.020%. Figures for acquired hypothyroidism are also variable (from 13% to 54% in DS, versus 0.8% to 1.1% in the normal population) (Fort et al., 1984).

Two forms of hypothyroidism can be distinguished. The most frequent one, so-called compensated hypothyroidism, shows only a variable increase of serum thyroid stimulating hormone (TSH), while serum levels of thyroid hormones (T3 and T4) are within normal limits: this can be assumed to be a temporary phase preceding a possible condition of hypofunction. Increased TSH represents a central response to the reduction of functional thyroid tissue, often on an immunological basis and is followed by a progressive decrease of T3 and T4 values. Although this is commonly the course of the disease, in DS TSH levels often fluctuate without any modification of thyroid function. These transient thyroid dysfunctions are possibly related to inappropriate secretion of TSH or to reduced sensitivity to TSH itself. A neuroregulatory disorder is also a possible cause. Some authors found significantly lower IQs in persons with DS and elevated TSH (Pueschel and Pezzullo, 1985). In DS hypothyroidism can also be the consequence of an autoimmune disorder. In this case, serum levels of antithyroid antibodies (antithyroglobulin and antiperoxidase antibodies) are constantly elevated.

The second form of hypothyroidism is clinically expressed, manifesting when hormone deficiency develops and showing reduced T3 and T4 levels. In DS most symptoms may not be recognized or can even be mistaken for the features of the syndrome itself, including lethargy, dullness, increased fatigability, loss of attention, slowing of motor activity and intellectual functioning, coarsness of voice, dry and rough skin, tendency to gain weight, etc., mainly in adolescents and adults (Pueschel and Pueschel, 1992). Periodic checks of thyroid function are therefore mandatory. Since untreated hypothyroidism can interfere with normal neuronal function, causing decreased intellectual abilities, appropriate substitutive therapy is strongly recommended.

About one third of subjects with constant TSH elevation and the presence of antithyroid antibodies sooner or later develop a clinical form of hypothyroidism. Some authors therefore think that early treatment can have a protective effect and either prevent or at least postpone the appearance of symptoms.

The results of personal investigations confirm that persons with DS are at increased risk of developing hypothyroidism at any age. One person out of 12, during his/her life, has either compensated or clinically apparent hypothyroidism (Rasore-Quartino and Cominetti, 1994).

Coeliac disease

Coeliac disease is a genetic and immunological disorder in which ingestion of wheat gliadin and related proteins (rye, barley) triggers an immunological response and injury to the small intestine.

Severe, albeit infrequent, forms exist, mainly in small children, that are characterized clinically by prominent abdomen, bulky diarrhoea, poor growth and hypovitaminosis. More frequent forms show only one or two symptoms (anaemia, growth deficiency etc.), but most affected persons are completely asymptomatic (the so-called silent form of coeliac disease) representing about 80% of the total. Long-term complications include: stunted growth, nutritional deficiencies, deficiency of liposoluble vitamins (A, D, E, K), sideropenia, anaemia, delayed onset of puberty, neurological disease, osteoporosis, other autoimmune disorders and intestinal lymphomas. The prevalence in the general population is around 0.5%.

Screening for coeliac disease is done through the determination of antiendomysium (EMA) IgA and antigliadin (AGA) IgA antibodies, the latter being less specific. IgA transglutaminase antibodies are also useful. Positive subjects undergo peroral intestinal biopsy (by Watson capsule or by paediatric or adult endoscopes).

The mainstay of treatment for coeliac disease is the gluten-free diet, i.e. the abolition of any gluten-containing food from the diet. Of course this diet requires a strong commitment and constant surveillance.

The discussion as to whether oats are tolerated or not, has been going on for over 20 years. It has been shown that oat products do not have toxic effects in affected adults. Even in children, according to a very recent publication (Hoffenberg et al., 2000), oats are harmless. These studies, although very important, are not conclusive, mainly because they do not give any evidence of long-term safety. Moreover, most manufacturers do not guarantee their oat products to be free of gluten. For these reasons, it is wise to keep oats off the diet of coeliac disease affected persons, especially children.

In 1975, Bentley described a boy with DS and coeliac disease. Since then, other reports of the association of these two conditions have appeared in the literature (Amil Dias and Walker-Smith, 1990). Epidemiological studies have led to the conclusion that coeliac disease is significantly more frequent in patients with DS than in the general population. In one recent and extensive epidemiological study (Bonamico et al., 2001), 1202 persons with DS of different ages were examined: the prevalence of coeliac disease was 5.4%, the silent form representing only 20% of the total. This is different from the data collected from the general population, where the ratio between symptomatic and silent forms is 1:8. In DS this ratio is reversed to 4:1 since 80% of the patients with DS show a symptomatic form of disease. One can hypothesize that, whereas in coeliac patients without DS, mechanisms of compensation may be present, so that entheropathy can exist for a long time without symptoms, in patients with DS these mechanisms are less able to overcome the overt clinical manifestations of coeliac disease. It is common knowledge that in DS a long period of time elapses from the onset of symptoms to the diagnosis. This could be caused by a misinterpretation of the symptoms in people with DS.

The screening of coeliac disease in DS, as well as dietary treatment is therefore necessary, otherwise there is a risk of severe complications (Bonamico et al., 1996).

Blood disorders and malignancies

In trisomic newborns, inefficient regulation of myelopoiesis is usual, its cause being either delayed maturation or a deficiency of committed stem cells (Weinstein, 1978). A generalized cellular dysfunction is substantiated by the presence of various haematological abnormalities: polycythaemia, thrombocytopenia, thrombocytosis, higher or lower leukocyte count. These abnormalities are time-limited and are the consequence of defective control in the production of haemopoietic cells in one or more cell lines (Miller and Cosgriff, 1983). The extreme aspect of defective haemopoiesis is leukaemia. In DS the risk of developing leukaemia is 10–20 times higher than in normal children (Rosner and Lee, 1972); 25% of all leukaemias are evident at birth; 15% of congenital leukaemias develop in newborns with DS. The ratio of acute lymphocytic leukaemia to acute non-lymphocytic leukaemia is similar in both populations, except for the first 2 years of life.

The response to treatment, prognosis and other characteristics are similar. The abnormal sensitivity to methotrexate found in children with DS has been correlated to the prolonged clearance of the drug in these persons (Garré et al., 1987).

In 17% of DS infants, a form of acute, transitory leukaemia, mainly of the myeloid type, can develop. Its clinical and haematological features are undistinguishable from those of the common acute leukaemia, except for the spontaneous and complete remission. The differential diagnosis is usually very difficult and severe problems can arise for therapeutical decisions (Cominetti et al., 1985). Acute transitory leukaemia possibly represents a myelodysplastic phase preceding an overt form of megakaryoblastic leukaemia, with thrombocytopenia, lasting from several months to a few years. In DS megakaryoblastic leukaemia has a 500-fold higher than expected incidence, with its peak under 4 years of age (Creutzig et al., 1996).

The association between DS and leukaemia decreases with age and is not apparent after 40 years. In recent, extended population surveys, malignant neoplasms other than leukaemia are less frequent in DS than expected, with the exception of testicular cancer, ovarian cancer and retinoblastomas, which were seen more often than expected, but not significantly so (Hasle et al., 2000; Yang et al., 2002).

Growth deficiency

Linear growth retardation is characteristic of DS. Stature is generally stabilized at minus 2–3 standard deviations on normal growth charts. The mechanisms responsible for short stature are not yet completely explained. Defective growth hormone (GH) secretion has been hypothesized as a cause of short stature in DS (Castells et al., 1992). Most authors have confirmed a normal GH secretion. A great deal of interest was focused on the role of somatomedins/insulin-like growth factors (IGF), as these peptides are essential not only for body growth, but also for the development and the maintenance of the nervous system. In children with DS, IGF-I is low or clearly pathological, with values similar to those found in hypopituitarism. However, a decreased IGF concentration does not seem to be accompanied by an impaired GH responsiveness to secretogogues (Barreca et al., 1994). These results appear to exclude the notion that short stature and reduced IGF-I concentrations in DS are due to an alteration of GH secretion or of the GH receptor and point out the occurence of a GH molecular anomaly in some of these patients (Barreca et al., 1994).

GH treatment has been proposed in children with DS and impaired growth, irrespective of GH and IGF-I levels. Interesting results have been obtained, with acceleration of growth velocity (Annerèn et al., 1993). Nevertheless, at present, the role of that therapy is still controversial due to the lack of long-term experience and the possible complications (hypertension, hyperglycaemia).

Nutritional problems

Nutritional problems in DS, although not strictly correlated with drugs, have been followed with particular interest, for at least three reasons: the tendency to obesity, possible food intolerance or allergy and the administration of vitamin or mineral supplements.

The whole problem is complicated by a number of variables, both genetic and environmental. The latter have acquired special relevance, contributing to the prolongation of life expectancy in the general population. In DS, significant prolongation of life is seen, along with the reduction of the life in institutions, the progressive inclusion in the society and the constant improvement of medical care.

Obesity

Obesity was a common problem for people with DS. At present, it is less frequent, but is more common in adults than children with DS. In a controlled study, body composition of children with DS did not significantly differ from controls. Energy intake was lower in subjects with DS and several micronutrients were consumed at less than 80% of the recommended dietary allowances (Luke et al., 1996). To avoid an inadequate intake of vitamins and minerals, it is suggested that treatment or prevention of obesity combines a balanced diet, without unnecessary energy restriction, vitamin and mineral supplementation and increased physical activity.

Studies on nutrition are biased by heterogeneity of age, environment and alimentary habits; these vary from one region to another.

Vitamins and minerals

Specific vitamin and mineral deficiencies have been described, but studies are often contradictory. Discordant results have been obtained studying serum concentrations of some vitamins (thiamine, niacin, ascorbic acid, vit A, beta-carotene) (Storm, 1990).

Low serum blood levels of calcium and copper have been described in subjects living in institutions (Barlow et al., 1981). Selenium, whose antioxidative activity is well known, has reduced levels in people with DS, as does vitamin E (Jackson et al., 1988).

Franceschi et al. (1988) published interesting studies on zinc serum values and their relationships with thymic hormone and immunological functions. Serum zinc concentrations in DS were low, similar to those found in normal ageing persons. A corresponding reduction of thymic hormone and immunological functions was detected. In persons with reduced zinc values, reduced thyroid activity was described. In hypozincaemic patients, higher TSH levels were found, that were significantly reduced after zinc supplementation (Bucci et al., 1999). Zinc supplementation increases thymic hormone levels and enhances immunological defences. Other investigations have shown normal zinc values in persons of different ages with DS.

It must be pointed out that vitamins are organic compounds which, in very small quantities, are indispensable for the normal metabolism in man. When they are employed in high doses, they do not act as vitamins any more, but as drugs. There is a real risk of damage, especially in children. It has been known for a long time that liposoluble vitamins can be toxic, if taken in excess. Recent studies have shown that high doses of hydrosoluble vitamins can be toxic too. They can also interfere with the action of other vitamins or of drugs. The same can be said of the minerals that are necessary for normal metabolism.

As highlighted below, excessive doses of vitamins and minerals can be harmful:

- High dose vitamin A is toxic both for children (increased endocranial pressure, stunted growth) and adults (decreased appetite, dry and itching skin, loss of hair, bone pain). Hydrosoluble preparations are six times more toxic than liposoluble ones. If taken in pregnancy, vitamin A increases the risk of spontaneous abortion and of foetal malformations (ear anomalies, cleft palate, congenital heart disease and central nervous system malformations)
- High dose vitamin D is very frequently toxic, but individual sensitivity is very variable. Main symptoms of toxicity are nausea, anorexia, weight loss, headache, muscular weakness, poliuria, hypercalcaemia with calcifications, bone pain, hypertension and sometimes nephrocalcinosis leading to renal failure
- Vitamin E is largely used as an antioxidant. Symptoms of excessive intake are quite vague, going from muscular weakness to headache, nausea, vomiting, weariness. Excessive vitamin E can interfere with the metabolism of vitamin K, leading to haemorragic diathesis. It can also act as an antagonist of vitamin A, causing visual defects
- High dose vitamin C can cause the formation of urinary stones and cause diarrhoea. It interferes with the metabolism of vitamin B12, causing anaemia. In glucose-6-phosphate-dehydrogenase deficient subjects, it can cause haemolytic crises; in diabetics it can interfere with glucose dosage
- Excessive vitamin B6 has toxic effects on the nervous system, causing nerve degeneration
- Nicotinic acid, used without success in the treatment of schizophrenia, infantile psychoses and mental disorders, can cause, if taken in excess, the release of histamine, and provoke severe skin redness, itching and haematological disorders. Very high doses are hepatotoxic and can cause hyperuricaemia and acute gout arthritis; they can aggravate peptic ulcer or asthma and moreover cause abdominal colics, nausea and diarrhoea
- Calcium can cause constipation and alteration of renal function
- Iron can increase the risk of heart damage (haemosiderosis)
- Zinc is said to enhance the immune response, but excessive doses interfere with the metabolism of iron and copper
- Selenium at high doses is harmful, causing hair and nail loss

During the 1970s, the first advocates of megadoses of vitamins for the treatment of behaviour and learning disorders in children made their appearance. For DS, Turkel (1975) proposed the so-called 'U therapy', a complex of many substances (vitamins, minerals, enzymes, hormones and drugs) to be administered many times a day (up to 30–35 pills!) and capable of improving mental abilities of such children.

In 1981 Harrel et al. claimed that a trial with megadoses of vitamins and minerals had shown a critical improvement of intellectual, educational and linguistic abilities of a group of children with mental disabilities, among whom were some children with DS.

Several controlled studies performed in the following years failed to show any increased intelligence in the observed populations of children with DS (Weathers, 1983; Smith et al., 1984).

In a controlled study with high dosage multivitamin and mineral supplements, this treatment was associated with decreased developmental progress and various side effects (Bidder et al., 1989). More recently, a systematic review of controlled trials of dietary supplements and of drugs, identifying 373 randomized participants, provided no positive evidence that any combination of drugs, vitamins and minerals could enhance either cognitive function or psychomotor development in persons with DS, although some minor effect could not be completely excluded at this point (Salman, 2002). Such regimens should be reserved only for large well designed trials. Parents of children with DS should be actively discouraged from giving these 'miracle drugs' to their children.

Nevertheless new preparations of this type in pseudoscientific associations are publicized every day, with high costs and an absence of any positive results!

It is necessary to say that a correct supplementation of vitamins and minerals can have beneficial effects on the health status of children and adults with DS, but it is also necessary to warn parents and caregivers against enthusiasm about the miracles of unconventional therapies that, on the contrary, cause only bitter disappointments and health risks.

Unconventional therapies for DS

Among the well known unconventional therapies for DS, the application of sicca cell therapy (foetal tissue of sheep, goats and rabbits in Germany and foetal tissue in eastern Europe) was popularized from 1970 to 1980. The injection of foreign protein into any human carries the potential for allergic or toxic reactions.

Treatment with 5-hydroxytryptophan, a precursor of the neuroregulatory amine serotonin (5-hydroxytryptamine) whose blood levels in DS are reduced, increased the risk of convulsions.

Dimethil-sulfoxide (a solvent extracted from lignin found in wood pulps) was also useless (Giuffré, 1983; Pueschel and Pueschel, 1992).

Based on anecdotal experiences, a new treatment has recently been advocated to improve cognitive functions of children with DS. It is Piracetam, a cyclic derivative of gamma-amino-butyric acid (GABA), a component of psychoactive nootropic drugs. Concern about the uncontrolled administration of Piracetam to children with DS was expressed by Holmes (1999) and the American College of Human Genetics, pointing out the necessity of controlled studies on the efficacy of the treatment before giving it to children with DS. In the only controlled study published to date (Lobaugh et al., 2001), the drug did not significantly improve cognitive performances over placebo use, but was associated with CNS stimulatory effects in seven children out of 18: aggressiveness (four), agitation or irritability (two), sexual arousal (two), poor sleep (one) and decreased appetite (one).

Conclusion

As a conclusion of this review on therapies in DS, it can be said that up to now no pharmacological treatment exists that is able to significantly improve mental function or cognitive abilities in children with DS. This statement is the result of many controlled studies that have been conducted for over 20 years, as well as the result of the failure of a number of treatments that have been proposed in the same period.

We are confident that in the near future, scientific studies, both genetic and clinical, will clarify the still poorly known biological aspects of the syndrome, leading to effective treatments and prevention of the disabilities affecting people with DS.

References

Amil Dias J, Walker-Smith J (1990) Down's syndrome and celiac disease. J Pediatr Gastroenterol Nutr 13: 121–4.
Annerèn G, Gustavson KH, Sara V (1993) Down's syndrome during growth hormone therapy. J Intell Disabil Res 37: 381–7.
Barlow PJ, Sylvester PF, Dickerson JWT (1981) Hair trace metal levels in Down's syndrome patients. J Ment Defic Res 25: 161–8.
Barreca A, Rasore-Quartino A, Acutis MS (1994) Assessment of growth hormone insulin like growth factor-I axis in Down's syndrome. J Endocrinol Invest 17: 431–6.
Bentley D (1975) A case of Down's syndrome complicated by retinoblastoma and celiac disease. Pediatrics 56: 131–3.
Bidder RT, Gray P, Newcombe RG, Evans BK, Hughes M (1989) The effects of multivitamins and minerals on children with Down syndrome. Dev Med Child Neurol 31: 532–7.
Bonamico M, Mariani P, Danesi HM, Crisogianni M, Failla P, Gemme G, Rasore-Quartino A, Giannotti A, Castro M, Balli F, Lecora M, Andria G, Guariso G, Gabrielli O, Catassi C, Lazzari R, Ansaldi Balocco N, DeVirgiliis S, Culasso F, Romano C, SIGEP and Medical Genetic Group (2001) Prevalence and clinical picture of celiac disease in Italian Down syndrome patients: a multicenter study. J Pediatr Gastrenterol Nutr 33: 139–43.

Bonamico M, Rasore-Quartino A, Mariani P, Scartezzini P, Cerruti P, Tozzi MC, Cingolani M, Gemme G (1996) Down's syndrome and celiac disease: usefulness of gliadin and antiendomysium antibodies. Acta Paediatr 85: 1503–5.

Bucci I, Napolitano G, Giuliani C, Lio S, Minnucci A, DiGiacomo F, Calabrese G, Sabatino G, Palka G, Monaco F (1999) Zinc sulfate supplementation improves thyroid function in hypozincemic Down children. Biol Trace Elem Research 67: 257–68.

Castells S, Torrano C, Bastian W (1992) Growth hormone deficiency in Down's syndrome children. J Intell Disabil Res 36: 29–43.

Cominetti M, Rasore-Quartino A, Acutis MS, Vignola G (1985) Neonato con sindrome di Down e leucemia mieloide acuta. Difficoltà diagnostiche tra forma maligna e sindrome mieloproliferativa. Pathologica 77: 625–30.

Creutzig U, Ritter J, Vormoor J (1996) Myelodysplasia and acute myelogenous leukemia in Down's syndrome. A report of 40 children of the AML-BFM Study Group. Leukemia 10: 1677–86.

Epstein CJ (1999) The future of biological research on Down syndrome. In J Rondal, J Perera, L Nadel (eds) Down Syndrome: A Review of Current Knowledge. London: Whurr Publishers, pp. 210–22.

Fort P, Lifschitz F, Bellisario R, Davis J, Pugliese M, Richman R, Post EM, David R (1984) Abnormalities of thyroid function in infants with Down syndrome. J Pediatr 104: 545–9.

Franceschi C, Chiricolo M, Licastro F, Zanotti MM, Fabris V (1988) Oral zinc supplemention in Down's syndrome. Restoration of thymic endocrine activity of some immune defects. J Ment Defic Res 32: 169–81.

Garré ML, Relling MV, Kalwinsky D (1987) Pharmacokinetics and toxicity of methotrexate in children with Down's syndrome and acute lymphocytic leukemia. J Pediatr 111: 606–12.

Giuffrè L (1983) Miti e realtà della terapia farmacologica nella sindrome di Down. In F Dagna Bricarelli, C Inglese, A Moretti, A Rasore-Quartino (eds) Aspetti Epidemiologici, Genetici, Clinici, Riabilitativi e Sociali della Sindrome di Down. Genova: CEPIM, p. 265.

Harrel RJ, Capp RH, Davis DR (1981) Can nutritional supplements help mentally retarded children? Proceedings of the Nat Acad of Sci USA 78: 574–8.

Hasle H, Clemmensen IH, Mikkelsen M (2000) Risks of leukemias and solid tumors in individuals with Down's syndrome. Lancet 355: 165–9.

Hoffenberg EJ, Haas J, Drescher A, Barnhurst R, Osberg I, Bao F, Eisenbarth G (2000) A trial of oats in children with newly diagnosed celiac disease. J Pediatr 137: 361–6.

Holmes LB (1999) Concern about Piracetam treatment for children with Down syndrome. Pediatrics 103: 1078–9.

Jackson CUE, Holland AJ, Williams CA, Dickerson YWT (1988) Vitamin E and Alzheimer's disease in subjects with Down's syndrome. J Ment Defic Res 32: 479–84.

Lobaugh NJ, Karaskov V, Rombough V, Rovet J, Bryson S, Greenbaum R, Haslam RH, Koren G (2001) Piracetam therapy does not enhance cognitive functioning in children with Down syndrome. Arch Pediatr Adol Med 153: 442–8.

Luke A, Sutton M, Scholler DA, Roizen NJ (1996) Nutrient intake and obesity in prepubescent children with Down syndrome. J Am Dietet Assoc 96: 1262–7.

Miller M, Cosgriff JM (1983) Hematologic abnormalities in newborns with Down's syndrome. J Med Genet 16: 173–8.

Pueschel SM, Pezzullo JC (1985) Thyroid dysfunction in Down's syndrome. Am J Dis Child 139: 636–9.

Pueschel SM, Pueschel JK (1992) Biochemical Concerns in Persons with Down's Syndrome. Baltimore: Paul H Brookes Publishing Co Inc.

Rasore-Quartino A, Cominetti M (1994) Clinical follow-up of adolescents and adults with Down syndrome. In L Nadel, D Rosenthal (eds) Down Syndrome: Living and Learning in the Community. New York: Wiley-Liss, pp. 238–45.

Rosner F, Lee SL (1972) Down's syndrome and acute leukaemia: myeloblastic or lymphoblastic. Report of forty-three cases and review of the literature. Am J Med 53; 203–14.

Salman M (2002) Systematic review of the effect of therapeutic dietary supplements and drugs on cognitive function in subjects with Down syndrome. Eur J Paediatr Neurol 6: 213–19.

Smith GF, Spiker D, Peterson CP, Cicchetti D, Justine P (1984) Use of megadoses of vitamins with minerals in Down syndrome. J Pediatr 228–34.

Storm W (1990) Hypercarotenemia in children with Down's syndrome. J Ment Defic Res 34: 283–6.

Turkel H (1975) Medical amelioration of Down's syndrome incorporating the orthomolecular approach. J Orthomol Psych 4: 102–15.

Weathers C (1983) Effects of nutritional supplementation on IQ and certain other variables associated with Down syndrome. Am J Ment Def 88: 214–17.

Weinstein HS (1978) Congenital leukaemia and the neonatal myeloproliferative disorders associated with Down's syndrome. Clin Haematol 7: 147–56.

Yang Q, Rasmussen SJ, Fridman JM (2002) Mortality associated with Down's syndrome in the USA from 1983 to 1997: a population-based study. Lancet 359: 1019–25.

SECTION III
COGNITION AND
LANGUAGE ASPECTS

Chapter 14
Episodic memory across the lifespan of adults with Down syndrome

D. Devenny, P. Kittler, M. Sliwinski,
S. Krinsky-McHale

Introduction

Episodic memory involves the storage and retrieval of events that occur in a particular time and place (Tulving, 1983). In general, it is memory for personally experienced past events that enables individuals mentally to travel back to the past and to re-experience these events while still being aware of the present. Episodic memory is late in developing, is probably unique to humans, and is vulnerable to changes associated with normal ageing and to neuronal dysfunction associated with dementia.

Adults with Down syndrome (DS) show changes in cognitive functioning beginning in their fifth decade of life that resemble the age-associated changes observed in older adults without intellectual disabilities (ID). Specifically, declines in memory and new learning have been documented in longitudinal studies (Devenny et al., 1996, 2000; Haxby and Shapiro, 1992; Oliver et al., 1998) and cross-sectional studies typically have found poorer performance by older participants with DS on a variety of measures of memory, learning, language and visuospatial organization (Thase et al., 1984; Haxby, 1989; Vicari et al., 1995).

In addition to cognitive changes, studies of older adults with DS have shown parallel age-associated changes in adaptive behaviour (Silverstein et al., 1988; Collacott, 1993; Rasmussen and Sobsey, 1994; Zigman et al., 1996) and increased frequency of biological markers of ageing such as cataracts (Prasher, 1994), hypothyroidism (Prasher, 1995) and hearing loss (Buchanan, 1990; Evenhuis et al., 1992). The overall consensus emerging from these and other studies appears to be that age-associated changes in adults with DS are detected earlier than is characteristic of the general population, but not usually before 50 years of age (Zigman et al., 1987; Das and Mishra, 1995; Devenny and Krinsky-McHale, 1998; Holland et al., 1998).

Because small changes in episodic memory are typical of normal ageing in the general population, performance on tasks that depend on this type of memory could be useful in identifying the onset and rate of age-associated decline among these individuals with DS.

Study design

We have been conducting a longitudinal study over the past 15 years of adults with DS and with unspecified intellectual disability (ID) in which we examine changes in memory and cognition associated with normal ageing and with dementia. All participants entered the study at a time when they were healthy and were not suspected of declines by their caregivers. Additional criteria for entering the study included IQ scores of at least 30, no serious uncorrected sensory impairments, no recent onset of seizures and participation in a workshop or day programme. Participants were tested every 18 months on a battery of tests that included measures of episodic, working, implicit and semantic memory, and measures of new learning, attention, visuospatial organization, motor ability and orientation to person, place and time.

Participants in the present report include 58 adults with DS and 44 with unspecified ID (Table 14.1) who are currently healthy and who are not showing signs of decline based on our test battery and reports from caregivers. We excluded 10 individuals who have shown significant memory declines in recent years (two with unspecified ID, eight with DS) because some of these individuals may be preclinical for Alzheimer's disease. We also excluded individuals who have a diagnosis of dementia (six adults with DS) or who have a history of medical conditions (e.g. multi-infarcts, depression) that could produce declines in functioning. We also excluded five participants in the unspecified ID group with IQ scores higher than 78 because we wanted the groups to be comparable in overall ability. While the two groups did not differ on IQ scores, there was a significant difference in age ($t = 5.05$, $df = 110$, $p < .001$). This age difference was appropriate because precocious ageing has been identified in older adults with DS (Haxby and Shapiro, 1992; Devenny et al., 1996;

Table 14.1 Participant characteristics. Means, with standard deviations in parentheses, of age at recent test time and IQ

Aetiology group	N	Age	IQ
Down syndrome	58	46.8 (7.6)	54.4 (11.4)
Unspecified ID	44	56.9 (11.6)	57.0 (10.4)

Silverman et al., 1998). The cross-sectional data come from the most recent cycle of testing. The longitudinal data span an average of 5.3 years, and include all administrations of our measure of episodic memory, the Cued Recall Test.

Episodic memory

We measured episodic memory with the Cued Recall Test, a list-learning task that was adapted from Buschke (1984). A list-learning task requires attention to items presented in the context of the immediate testing situation, including the recognition of meaning, categorization and the exclusion of unrelated items. The demands of the task present an immediate context in which the items on the list are retrieved. This test consisted of 12 items and each item was associated with a unique category. During the learning phase pictures of the items were presented four at a time and the category was named at the time of the initial presentation of each item (Figure 14.1). For example, the examiner would say: 'Show me something that flies'. The participant was required to point to the helicopter and to name it. If the participant said 'airplane' the examiner provided the correct label. Once all the pictures on a card were named, the card was removed and the participant was asked to name all four items. If any items were omitted the card was re-presented.

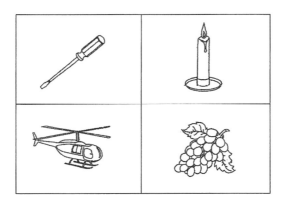

Figure 14.1 Card one of the Cued Recall Test.

The testing phase for recall of the items consisted of three trials. On each trial there was an opportunity for free recall. After free recall of the items, for each item not recalled, the unique cue was provided. (The test items were chosen to be relatively low frequency exemplars of the categories in order to minimize obtaining the correct response by guessing.) If the cue was not sufficient to aid retrieval, then the name of the item itself was given. (See Devenny et al., 2002 for additional details of testing procedures.)

Free recall

To examine episodic memory we analysed the total score of the three trials on the free recall portion of the test. Free recall is traditionally associated with the type of list-learning tasks that are representative of episodic memory, while the cued recall score is associated with recognition memory. We compared the performance on free recall between the aetiology groups with an analysis of covariance in which aetiology was a between-subjects variable and age and IQ were continuous variables. Using General Linear Modelling we also tested an aetiology by age interaction. The findings indicated a significant main effect of IQ in which higher IQ was associated with better performance $(F(1,97) = 5.39, p = .02)$ and a main effect of age in which older participants had poorer scores $(F(1,97) = 6.09, p = .02)$. There was also a significant main effect of aetiology in which individuals with unspecified ID had better overall performance than those with DS $(F(1,97) = 4.13, p = .05)$. Of most interest to us was the significant aetiology by age interaction $(F(1,97) = 7.41, p = .01)$ in which adults with DS showed significant age-associated differences in performance, while adults with unspecified ID did not (Figure 14.2).

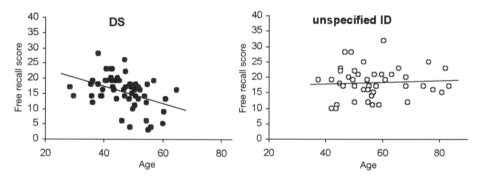

Figure 14.2 Free recall score as a function of age for participants with Down syndrome (DS) and with unspecified intellectual disability (ID).

In order to examine the performance on free recall across trials we constructed four age groups for each aetiology group. Because the participants with unspecified ID were older, we used different cut-off points to construct these age groups. In an analysis of covariance, with aetiology and age group as between-subjects variables and IQ as a continuous variable and trial as a repeated measure, we found the same significant main effects of aetiology, age group and IQ and a significant aetiology by age group interaction. There were also significant effects of trial, the interaction of trial by aetiology, and a three-way interaction of trial by age group by aetiology $(F(6,186) = 2.35, p = .03)$. Adults with unspecified ID in each age group showed improvement across trials, indicating that they were learning with repeated presentations of the test items. While adults with DS in the two younger age groups also showed an increase in scores across the trials, adults with DS over 50 years of age showed no evidence of learning across trials.

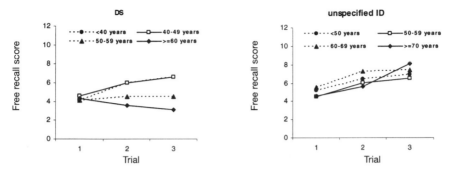

Figure 14.3 Free recall scores by trial for age groups for adults with DS and unspecified ID.

Cued recall

We repeated the above analyses using the total score as the dependent measure. Total score is the sum of the free recall score and the number of items retrieved after the category cue was provided. In the analysis of covariance with IQ and age as continuous variables and aetiology as a between-subjects variable, only IQ was significant ($F(1,97) = 11.75, p = .001$) such that higher IQ scores were associated with better performance. When we examined performance across trials with participants divided into age groups we again found a significant effect of IQ ($F(1,93) = 12.03, p = .001$) and a significant effect of trial ($F(2,93) = 10.69, p < .001$) in which participants improved across trials. There were no aetiology or age group differences on this measure.

Implicit memory

We wanted to determine if these findings related to age-associated differences were specific to episodic memory or whether they represented a global deterioration in memory. We chose implicit memory as a contrast because it is viewed as a distinct system from explicit memory (an example of which is episodic memory). Implicit memory refers to the influence or facilitation of a specific experience on memory without the support of deliberate or effortful retrieval processes (Graf and Schacter, 1985; Schacter, 1987).

We measured implicit memory within the framework of the same Cued Recall Test. After the three retrieval trials were completed, we presented the participant with a blank card divided into quadrants. We then gave the participant the four pictures that were on the first card of the learning trials and asked that they be replaced in their previous positions. This procedure was repeated for the two remaining cards. This is an implicit memory task of spatial location because during the learning phase the participant was not asked to remember the position of the test items.

Participants performed well on this task (DS: M = 8.3; unspecified ID: M = 8.2). An analysis of covariance with IQ and age as continuous variables and aetiology as a between-subjects factor showed no differences in performance related to aetiology, IQ or age.

Longitudinal findings of episodic memory

To understand individual change across time on the free recall score we applied general linear mixed models with correlated errors to longitudinal data that spanned an average of 5.3 years. The approach involved fitting random coefficients models (Laird and Ware, 1982) to each measure to estimate level of performance, the rate of age-based change (fixed effects), and individual differences in level and rate of change (random effects). The key predictions involved testing the fixed age effects (linear and quadratic) for the two aetiology groups for significant differences. The following model was evaluated for each of the relevant dependent measures after adjusting for IQ:

$$Y_{ij} = \beta_0 + \beta_1 Age_{ij} + \beta_2 Age^2_{ij} + \beta_3 Aetiology_i + \beta_4 Aetiology_i XAge_{ij} + \beta_5 Aetiology_i XAge^2_{ij}$$

where Y_{ij} is the score for the jth testing time on subject i on the relevant variable, Age_{ij} is the age for subject i at time j, $Aetiology_i$ is a dummy variable coded as ID = 0 and DS = 1, and the remaining terms carry the interaction between aetiology groups and the linear and quadratic age effects. This equation describes only the fixed effects, but random intercepts, random slopes and their covariance were included in the analysis. To facilitate interpretation of the intercepts and slopes, we centred age at 45 years, a value close to the average age at baseline ($X = 43.3$ yrs).

The results indicated that the group with DS exhibited strong evidence of accelerating decline ($\beta_4 = -0.02$, SE = 0.007). Figure 14.4 indicates that memory performance in the group with DS was relatively stable until early in the fifth decade, at which point an abrupt and rapid loss of memory occurred. In contrast, the results indicated that the group with unspecified ID declined at a rate of −0.26 items per year (SE = 0.09). There was no evidence for accelerating decline in this group, and in fact there was some evidence of deceleration in rate of loss ($\beta_2 = 0.008$, SE = 0.003), indicating learning and a practice effect.

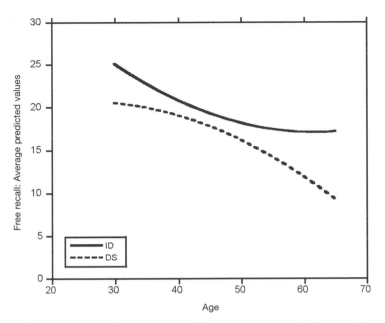

Figure 14.4 Average predicted values of change across time in free recall score based on longitudinal data for adults with DS and with unspecified ID.

Discussion

Our findings indicate that adults with DS have substantial age-associated declines in episodic memory that appear to accelerate during the fifth decade even though these individuals were selected to be a 'healthy' group. This decline was not associated with intellectual disability, *per se*, as their peers with unspecified ID showed only a small, linear decline over the same ages. This pattern of results appears to be specific to episodic memory, as measured by free recall, as there were no age or aetiology differences on a measure when the cued recall component was added to the score. For these healthy adults, although the category cues provided only partial information about the items, there was sufficient information associated with the cue to facilitate the retrieval of additional words. In addition, healthy older adults with DS were able to compensate for their age-associated declining free recall ability by utilizing the category cues to prompt retrieval. This finding suggests a possible strategy for supporting memory in older adults. By providing a context to aid retrieval, it may be possible to improve everyday memory functioning in older adults with DS.

Similarly, there were no group or age differences on a measure of implicit memory. This finding is consistent with previous studies (Carlesimo et al., 1997; Vicari, this volume) which have shown that individuals with DS have performance on implicit measures consistent with their overall level of mental ability. Studies of individuals from the general population have shown that implicit memory is less sensitive to age-associated decline than is episodic memory (Light and Singh, 1987; Graf, 1990; Mitchell, 1993). From our current study it appears as if this is also true for individuals with DS and their peers with unspecified ID.

In adults with DS, the effects of ageing on the memory system are imposed on an organization with a developmental history characterized by deficits in auditory short-term memory (Hulme and Roodenrys, 1995; Wang, 1996; Jarrold and Baddeley, 1997; Jarrold, this volume) that appear to be greater than the overall cognitive impairment. In addition, 'ageing' in these individuals has some unique features. Adults with DS develop the neuropathology of Alzheimer's disease beginning early in life. Located on chromosome 21 is a gene for the production of amyloid precursor protein, a transmembrane glycoprotein that gives rise to β-amyloid. Because individuals with DS have a third copy of chromosome 21 there is an over-expression of amyloid precursor protein that results in the accumulation of extracellular deposits of β-amyloid protein, called plaques, beginning in their third decade of life (Hof et al., 1995; Hyman et al., 1995). These plaques are deposited initially in the amygdala and hippocampus, followed by depositions in the association areas of frontal, temporal and parietal cortex (Mann et al., 1986; Mann, 1993). These deposits continue to accumulate throughout adult life and by the time individuals with DS enter their sixth decade they are presumed to have additional neuropathological features of Alzheimer's disease, including neurofibrillary tangles and neural cell loss (see Mann, 1993 for review). This accumulation of neurofibrillary tangles shows a slow accumulation over an estimated 19-year period with an accompanying loss of neurons (Wegiel et al., 1996). The limbic system, including the hippocampal gyrus, is a key component in the consolidation of memory and is critical to episodic memory. It is also an area of the brain that is vulnerable to early accumulation of neuropathology and to neuronal cell loss.

In spite of the presence of significant neuropathology associated with Alzheimer's disease, in our experience, very few adults with DS develop dementia before the end of their sixth decade. We believe this is not because we have missed detecting dementia. The adults with DS in our study who are healthy show good orientation to person, place and time and do not show declines on many of our cognitive or functional measures.

The findings in this report suggest that there is a long period of time in which subtle declines in episodic memory are occurring. One of the implications of these findings is that adults with DS, while appearing to live healthy, adaptive lives, may be having unusual difficulty integrating their experiences into their autobiographical memory. When treatment for memory enhancement becomes available, it will be important to consider adults with DS as a high-risk group that are candidates to receive intervention early in their adult life.

Acknowledgements

This research was supported by funds from the Office of Mental Retardation and Developmental Disabilities of the State of New York and by a grant from the National Institute on Aging of NIH AG 14771. We gratefully acknowledge the contributions of our project coordinator, Catherine Marino, BSN. We would also like to thank the participants, their families and the many agencies that cooperate with us for their support of our research.

References

Buchanan LH (1990) Early onset of presbycusis in Down syndrome. Scand Audiol 19: 103–10.

Buschke H (1984) Cued recall in amnesia. J Clin Neuropsych 6: 433–40.

Carlesimo GA, Marotta L, Vicari S (1997) Long-term memory in mental retardation: evidence for a specific impairment in subjects with Down's syndrome. Neuroychologia 35: 273–9.

Collacott RA (1993) Epilepsy, dementia and adaptive behavior in Down's syndrome. J Intell Disab Res 37: 153–60.

Das JP, Mishra RK (1995) Assessment of cognitive decline associated with aging: A comparison of individuals with Down syndrome and other etiologies. Res Devel Disab 16: 11–25.

Devenny DA, Hill AL, Paxtot O, Silverman WP, Wisniewski KW (1992) Ageing in higher functioning adults with Down syndrome: an interim report in a longitudinal study. J Intell Disab Res 40: 241–50.

Devenny DA, Krinsky-McHale S (1998) Age-associated differences in cognitive abilities in adults with Down syndrome. Topics in Geriatric Rehabilitation 13: 65–72.

Devenny DA, Krinsky-McHale SJ, Sersen G, Silverman WP (2000) Sequence of cognitive decline in dementia in adults with Down's syndrome. J Intell Disab Res 44: 654–65.

Devenny DA, Silverman WP, Hill AL, Jenkins E, Sersen EA, Wisniewski KE (1996) Normal ageing in adults with Down's syndrome: a longitudinal study. J Intell Disab Res 40: 208–21.

Devenny DA, Zimmerli EJ, Kittler P, Krinsky-McHale SJ (2002) Cued recall in early-stage dementia in adults with Down syndrome. J Intell Disab Res 46: 472–83.

Evenhuis HM, van Zanten GA, Brocaar MP, Roerdinkkholder WHM (1992) Hearing loss in middle-age persons with Down syndrome. Am J Ment Retard 97: 47–56.

Graf P (1990) Life-span changes in implicit and explicit memory. Bull Psychon Soc 28: 353–8.

Graf P, Schacter DL (1985) Implicit and explicit memory for new associations in normal and amnesic subjects. J Exp Psychol Learn Mem Cog 11: 501–18.

Haxby JV (1989) Neuropsychological evaluations of adults with Down's syndrome: patterns of selective impairment in non-demented old adults. J Ment Def Res 33: 193–210.

Haxby JV, Shapiro MB (1992) Longitudinal study of neuropsychological function in older adults with Down syndrome. In L Nadel, CJ Epstein (eds) Down Syndrome and Alzheimer Disease. New York: Wiley-Liss, pp. 35–50.

Hof PR, Bouras C, Perl DP, Sparks L, Mehta N, Morrison JH (1995) Age-related distribution of neuropathologic changes in the cerebral cortex of patients with Down's syndrome. Arch Neurol 52: 379–91.

Holland AJ, Hon J, Huppert FA, Stevens F, Watson P (1998) Population-based study of the prevalence and presenation of dementia in adults with Down's syndrome. B J Psychiatry 172: 493–8.

Hulme C, Roodenrys S (1995) Practitioner review; verbal working memory development and its disorders. J Child Psychol Psychiatry 36: 373–98.

Hyman BT, West HL, Rebeck W, Lai F, Mann MA (1995) Neuropathological changes in Down's syndrome hippocampal formation: effect of age and apolipoprotein E genotype. Arch Neurol 52: 373–8.

Jarrold C, Baddeley AD (1997) Short-term memory for verbal and visuospatial information in Down's syndrome. Cognit Neuropsychiatry 2: 101–22.

Laird NM, Ware JH (1982) Random-effects models for longitudinal data. Biometrics 38: 963–74.

Light LL, Singh A (1987) Implicit and explicit memory in young and older adults. J Exp Psychol Learn Mem Cog 13: 531–41.

Mann DMA (1993) Association between Alzheimer disease and Down syndrome: neuropathological observations. In JM Berg, K Karlinsky, AJ Holland (eds) Alzheimer Disease, Down Syndrome, and their Relationship. Oxford: Oxford University Press, pp. 711–92.

Mann DMA, Yates PO, Marcyniuk B, Ravindra CR (1986) The topography of plaques and tangles in Down's syndrome patients of different ages. Neuropath Appl Neurobiol: 12; 447–57.

Mitchell DB (1993) Implicit and explicit memory for picture: multiple views across the lifespan. In P Graf, MEJ Masson (eds) Implicit Memory: New Directions in Cognition, Development, and Neuropsychology. Hillsdale, NJ: Erlbaum, pp. 171–90.

Oliver C, Crayton L, Holland A, Hall S, Bradbury J (1998) A four year prospective study of age-related cognitive change in adults with Down syndrome. Psychol Med 28: 1365–77.

Prasher VP (1994) Screening of medical problems in adults with Down syndrome. Down's Syndr Res Pract 2: 59–66.

Prasher VP (1995) Age-specific prevalence, thyroid dysfunction and depressive symptomatology in adults with Down syndrome and dementia. Int J Geriatr Psychiatry 10: 25–31.

Rasmussen DE, Sobsey D (1994) Age, adaptive behavior, and Alzheimer's disease in Down syndrome cross-sectional and longitudinal analyses. Am J Ment Retard 99: 151–65.

Schacter DL (1987) Implicit memory: history and current status. J Exp Psychol Learn Mem Cog 13: 501–18.

Silverman W, Zigman WB, Kim H, Krinsky-McHale S, Wisniewski HM (1998) Aging and dementia among adults with mental retardation and Down syndrome. Topics in Geriatric Medicine 13: 49–64.

Silverstein AB, Herbs D, Miller TJ, Nasusta R, Williams DL (1988) Effects of age on the adaptive behavior of institutionalized and noninstitutionalized individuals with Down syndrome. Am J Ment Retard 92: 455–60.

Thase ME, Tigner R, Smeltzer DJ, Liss L (1984) Age related neuropsychological deficits in Down's syndrome. Biol Psychiatry 19: 571–85.

Tulving E (1983) Elements of Episodic Memory. Oxford: Clarendon Press.

Vicari S, Nocentini U, Caltagirone C (1995) Neuropsychological diagnosis of aging in adults with Down syndrome. Developmental Brain Dysfunction 7: 340–8.

Wang PP (1996) A neuropsychological profile of Down syndrome: cognitive skills and brain morphology. Ment Retard Dev Disab Res Rev 2: 102–8.

Wegiel J, Wisniewski HM, Dziewiatkowski J, Popovitch ER, Tarnawski M (1996) Differential susceptibility to neurofibrillary pathology among patients with Down syndrome. Dementia 7: 135–41.

Zigman WB, Schupf N, Lubin RA, Silverman WP (1987) Premature regression of adults with Down syndrome. Am J Ment Def 92: 161–8.

Zigman WB, Schupf N, Sersen E, Silverman W (1996) Prevalence of dementia in adults with and without Down syndrome. Am J Ment Retard 100: 403–12.

Chapter 15
Short-term memory and long-term learning in Down syndrome

C. JARROLD

The term 'verbal short-term memory' refers to the ability to actively hold verbal information in mind. Traditionally, one would test the capacity of an individual's verbal short-term memory using a span task, in which increasing amounts of verbal information are presented for subsequent recall, with an individual's span corresponding to the maximum number of verbal items that they can correctly remember. For example, in a digit or word span task an individual is presented with a series of digits or words that they hear, and then have to repeat in correct serial order. Adults' spans using such procedures are typically around seven items (Miller, 1956). The processes underpinning successful performance on such tasks have received considerable attention from psychologists (Baddeley, 1986), partly because digit and word span tasks are, on the face of it, fairly simple assessments. In addition, neuropsychological patients have been identified who appear to suffer from a specific impairment in verbal short-term memory functioning (Vallar and Papagno, 1995). Studies with such patients have suggested that verbal short-term memory may play an important role in aspects of language acquisition and comprehension.

For example, Baddeley et al. (1988) assessed an adult neuropsychological patient, PV, who had suffered a left hemisphere lesion that resulted in impaired verbal short-term memory performance (Basso et al., 1982). Baddeley et al. found that PV was also impaired in a vocabulary learning task. In this task, PV was presented with a series of known words in her native language (Italian), as well as being told their equivalent translation in an unfamiliar language (Russian). When re-presented with the known words, PV was singularly and consistently unable to provide their translations, in contrast to controls who, over a series of trials, successfully learnt these associations. This kind of finding, as well as evidence on the relationship between children's verbal short-term memory and vocabulary acquisition, suggests that an individual's verbal short-term memory plays an important role in learning novel phonological forms during the process of vocabulary acquisition (Baddeley et al., 1998).

A second area where verbal short-term memory may be important is in the 'on-line' comprehension of spoken utterances. Intuitively, one might expect that a record of a spoken utterance is held in verbal short-term memory by a listener, in case they need to refer back to the start of the utterance in order to disambiguate or confirm its meaning. In fact, experimental evidence shows that verbal short-term memory does play a role in making sense of spoken sentences, albeit a limited one. Vallar and Baddeley (1984) assessed the effect of PV's verbal short-term memory deficit on her ability to comprehend speech. They found that PV was able to judge that sentences in which terms were semantically mismatched (e.g. 'Lettuce is the kind of person that one rarely meets in the schoolroom') did not make sense. However, she struggled to judge the sense of sentences in which semantically related terms were switched (e.g. 'One could reasonably claim that sailors are often lived on by ships of various kinds'). This suggests that listeners use semantic information to determine the gist of a sentence, a process that need not necessarily involve verbal short-term memory. However, verbal short-term memory is presumably required when a verbatim record of an utterance needs to be held in mind, as would be the case when the relative ordering of semantically related words is crucial to the sense of a sentence.

Verbal short-term memory in Down syndrome

The fact that verbal short-term memory may be involved in language development and language comprehension is relevant to the study of Down syndrome (DS), because individuals with DS tend to show relatively poor verbal short-term memory performance (Jarrold et al., 1999). For example, Kay-Raining Bird and Chapman (1994) assessed the digit spans of 47 children and young adults with DS, and compared them to those of a similar number of typically developing children of an equivalent level of general intelligence. They found that while this comparison group had spans of between 3 and 6 digits, individuals with DS tended to have spans of 3 or 4 digits, and on average performed less well on this task. Although there are examples of individuals with DS who show good verbal short-term memory performance (Vallar and Papagno, 1993), subsequent studies have confirmed that, on average, DS is associated with impaired verbal short-term memory performance.

In our own, recent, work (Jarrold et al., 2002) we have explored the causes of this poor performance, to determine whether this truly reflects impaired verbal short-term memory, or rather is caused by difficulties in other areas. First, we have investigated whether short-term memory problems in DS are specific to the verbal domain, by comparing digit spans with a measure of short-term memory for spatial locations. Second, we have examined whether hearing difficulties cause problems in typical digit span tasks, which involve auditory presentation of the to-be-remembered items, by assessing whether individuals are helped by also seeing a visual representation of the digits that they hear. Third, we have looked at whether speech difficulties associated with DS cause problems for individuals when they are required to respond to a traditional digit span task by providing all the items in the presented list. To do this we have compared this standard serial recall method with a test in which the items are re-presented either in the same or a different order, and the participants' task is to judge whether the second list was the same or different to the first (see Gathercole et al., 2001).

In this study we compared the performance on these various short-term memory tasks of 19 individuals with DS, aged between 10 and 17, with that seen for two sets of controls. These were individuals with moderate learning difficulties and typically developing children, both matched to the individuals with DS for level of receptive vocabulary. The results indicated that individuals with DS tended to be impaired when asked to remember verbal, but not spatial information. This impairment was not dramatically reduced by providing visual support when digits were presented, nor was it removed by asking individuals to recognize a switch in the order of a list. This suggests that DS is associated with a specific deficit in verbal short-term memory, and one that is not purely a reflection of problems of hearing and speech that are known to be associated with the condition.

Implications for vocabulary and language comprehension in Down syndrome

If this is the case, then given the evidence of the role of verbal short-term memory in aspects of language development and comprehension outlined above, one would expect individuals with DS to have consequent difficulties in vocabulary development and spoken language comprehension. Indeed, there is evidence for relative problems in these areas in DS (Chapman, 1995), but are these the direct result of a verbal short-term memory deficit?

We have explored the role of verbal short-term memory in vocabulary development in DS using a variant of the task employed with PV by Baddeley et al. (1988) (see above). Twenty-one individuals with DS were compared to 22 individuals with moderate learning disability of a similar level of non-verbal ability on a task in which individuals had to provide a verbal label associated with novel pictures of unknown objects. In one condition, these objects were paired with known verbal labels (they were described as mechanical parts of a *bus*, a *car*, a *train* etc.), while in another they were linked to non-word labels (parts of a *bip*, a *cus*, a *tran* etc.). Individuals were presented with two items whose labels they had to learn in the initial stages of each condition, and progressed to a maximum of six items depending on the success on the initial items presented. The results of this study showed that both groups found it easier to learn associations with known verbal labels. Individuals with DS performed as well as the controls on this task, and, in particular, were equally affected by having to learn novel, non-word labels.

This finding runs counter to what one would predict if verbal short-term memory problems were adversely affecting vocabulary learning in DS; individuals should be particularly impaired in their ability to learn the form of novel phonological items. However, this result is consistent with other evidence suggesting that vocabulary skills in DS are somewhat stronger than this 'verbal short-term memory account' would predict. Rondal (1995) has reported the case of Françoise, an individual with DS with relatively poor verbal short-term memory performance, yet relatively strong language skills including vocabulary. This kind of evidence has led Laws (1998) to suggest that 'the link between vocabulary and phonological memory in Down syndrome is not as well established as it is in normal development'.

Turning to the other possible implication of a verbal short-term memory deficit, one might expect individuals with DS to have difficulties in comprehending spoken utterances that place demands on this system, namely relatively long sentences where word order is crucial to meaning. One study that provides some tentative evidence for this suggestion was performed by Hartley (1982). In fact the expressed aim of this work was to assess grammatical comprehension in DS, and to that end Hartley employed the Token Test, a task in which the participant has to touch a series of differently shaped and coloured 'tokens' in response to a verbal prompt (e.g. 'Touch the red circle'). While the early trials of this task arguably place limited demands on verbal short-term memory, later trials consist of longer utterances in which multiple and potentially interchangeable tokens need to be touched in the correct order (e.g. 'Touch the small red circle and the big blue square'). Here, verbal short-term memory is more likely to be required in order to maintain a correct, verbatim record of this kind of utterance.

This test was given to 17 children with DS, whose performance was compared to that shown by controls with moderate learning difficulties and typically developing children of a comparable level of receptive vocabulary. Despite this matching, individuals with DS tended to perform less well, particularly on longer and more complex items. While this might reflect a particular problem in grammatical understanding of DS, it is equally possible that this results from the increased load on verbal short-term memory associated with these items. Clearly, further work is needed to test this suggestion directly.

Conclusions

There is considerable evidence that DS is associated with a deficit in verbal short-term memory. Consequently, there is reason to suspect that this may have an adverse impact on both language development and language comprehension in the condition. As yet there is relatively little experimental work testing these two hypotheses. What evidence there is suggests that vocabulary in DS is actually stronger than one would expect given individuals' poor verbal short-term memory performance. This may be because individuals are able to find ways of compensating for problems in representing the phonological forms of new words. Vocabulary learning does involve more than simply learning the sound that is associated with an item – one must learn the meaning or semantics of that label as well – and it is possible that individuals with DS place a relatively greater emphasis on this more semantic aspect of vocabulary learning.

As noted above, much more work is needed to determine whether individuals with DS suffer from problems in the comprehension of spoken utterances as a result of problems in verbal short-term memory. This is certainly possible, although these problems may well be limited to cases where individuals have to make sense of relatively long sentences that contain multiple semantically related terms. Nevertheless, there are likely to be educational implications of a problem of this form, as sentences of this kind are often used to convey instructions or directions (e.g. 'Please put your book on the shelf and your pencil on the desk'). If individuals with DS do have difficulty in maintaining a verbatim record of spoken utterances in verbal short-term memory, then they are likely to benefit from having such information broken up into a series of shorter sentences, each containing fewer discrete pieces of information.

References

Baddeley AD (1986) Working Memory. Oxford: Oxford University Press.

Baddeley A, Gathercole S, Papagno C (1998) The phonological loop as a language learning device. Psychol Rev 105: 158–73.

Baddeley A, Papagno C, Vallar G (1988) When long-term learning depends on short-term storage. J Memory Lang 27: 586–96.

Basso A, Spinnler H, Vallar G, Zanobio ME (1982) Left hemisphere damage and selective impairment of auditory-verbal short-term memory. Neuropsychologia 20: 263–74.

Chapman RS (1995) Language development in children and adolescents with Down syndrome. In P Fletcher, B MacWhinney (eds) Handbook of Child Language. Oxford: Blackwell, pp. 641–63.

Gathercole SE, Pickering SJ, Hall M, Peaker SM (2001) Dissociable lexical and phonological influences on serial recognition and serial recall. Q J Exp Psychol 54A: 1–30.

Hartley XY (1982) Receptive language processing of Down's syndrome children. J Ment Def Res 26: 263–9.

Jarrold C, Baddeley AD, Phillips C (1999) Down syndrome and the phonological loop: The evidence for, and importance of, a specific verbal short-term memory deficit. Down's Syndr Res Pract 6: 61–75.

Jarrold C, Baddeley A, Phillips CE (2002) Verbal short-term memory in Down syndrome: A problem of memory, audition, or speech? J Speech Lang Hear Res 45: 531–44.

Kay-Raining Bird E, Chapman RS (1994) Sequential recall in individuals with Down syndrome. J Speech Hear Res 37: 1369–80.

Laws G (1998) The use of nonword repetition as a test of phonological memory in children with Down syndrome. J Child Psychol Psychiatry 39: 1119–30.

Miller GA (1956) The magical number seven, plus or minus two: some limits on our capacity for processing information. Psychol Rev 63: 81–97.

Rondal JA (1995) Exceptional Language Development in Down Syndrome. Cambridge: Cambridge University Press.

Vallar G, Baddeley AD (1984) Phonological short-term store, phonological processing and sentence comprehension: a neuropsychological case study. Cognit Neuropsychol 1: 121–41.

Vallar G, Papagno C (1993) Preserved vocabulary acquisition in Down's syndrome: the role of phonological short-term memory. Cortex 29: 467–83.

Vallar G, Papagno C (1995) Neuropsychological impairments of short-term memory. In AD Baddeley, BA Wilson, F Watts (eds) Handbook of Memory Disorders. Chichester: John Wiley & Sons, pp. 135–65.

Chapter 16
Implicit long-term memory in individuals with intellectual disabilities

S. VICARI

Neuropsychological research has permitted the definition of different cognitive profiles among subjects with intellectual disabilities (ID) of differing aetiologies. For example, numerous authors have stressed that the typical language profile for persons with Down syndrome (DS) consists of poor production with greater compromise of morphosyntax than of lexical abilities, but relatively preserved comprehension (Vicari et al., 2000b). Williams syndrome (WS) is another genetic condition; it is less common but equally characterized by ID and typified by a number of severe medical anomalies, such as facial dysmorphology and abnormalities of the cardiovascular system (Frangiskakis et al., 1996). Children with WS often show marked impairment in certain visual-spatial abilities (especially praxic-constructive) and relative preservation of both productive and receptive language, at least concerning the phonological elements (Pezzini et al., 1999). Also different cognitive profiles were described in subjects with comparable intellectual deficits or even with the same aetiopathological picture (Pezzini et al., 1999).

All these observations seem to support a theoretical approach that considers ID not as a mere slowing of normal cognitive development, but as distinct, individual profiles, which can be qualitatively specified. In line with this theoretical point of view (which also suggests the need for strongly individualized rehabilitation treatment protocols), many recent studies emphasize the need for better definition of not only the impaired cognitive abilities in each subject but, just as importantly, the respective strengths, or relatively preserved abilities in children with ID. The importance of this approach was shown in several recent studies of memory, especially implicit memory in subjects with ID.

The neuropsychological studies reported in the literature suggest insufficient development of the mnesic function in ID at different levels of articulation. Although there are some exceptions, for example, children

142

with WS (Vicari et al., 1996), multiple deficits have been identified in short-term memory function. The peripheral systems of articulatory reiteration and the central systems that direct information processing seem to be deficient in these subjects.

Long-term memory (LTM) has also been extensively investigated in persons with ID both in the explicit and in the implicit component. Explicit memory concerns intentional recall or recognition of experiences or information. Implicit memory is manifested as an improvement in performance in perceptual, cognitive and motor tasks, without any conscious reference to previous experiences. Explicit memory deficits in persons with ID have been extensively documented. According to recent studies, people with ID should show a relative preservation of implicit memory due to the diffuse impairment of mnesic abilities.

In a recent study (Carlesimo et al., 1997), we described LTM abilities in persons with DS and in others with ID of unknown aetiology, comparing them with normal subjects of similar mental age. The performance of the normal subjects in explicit memory tests was significantly better than the children with ID of unknown aetiology, and the latter were better than those with DS. On the other hand, the performances of the three groups did not differ in an implicit memory test (repetition priming); both ID groups performed as well as mental age matched controls. These results seem to confirm a dissociation between explicit and implicit memory in subjects with ID. However, there are many limits in the studies reported thus far on this issue: results are often contradictory and methodological limits include the use of populations with ID of often undefined aetiology. Furthermore, the selection criteria used for the control group (chronological age, mental age), and the limited number of tests used for evaluating especially implicit memory (almost always visual priming tests) are other significant methodological limits. This last point is particularly interesting and has important implications for both theoretical and applied issues. Specifically, if the presumed facility demonstrated by persons with ID in repetition priming tests were confirmed, for example, in procedural learning tests, this would suggest substantial preservation of implicit memory functions, and thus would support the theoretical distinction between implicit and explicit memory. From a more applied perspective, these findings would suggest the possibility of using techniques based on automatic learning in the rehabilitation of these subjects.

Studies of explicit and implicit memory

Two recent studies have been carried out which concern the different aspects of implicit and explicit memory in two groups of persons with ID (DS and WS) compared to normal subjects matched for mental age (i.e. with a comparable global cognitive level of functioning).

Our aims were, first, to verify the hypothesis that persons with ID would have impaired explicit memory abilities compared to controls, but that the groups do not differ significantly in implicit memory abilities; second, to determine whether this profile is characteristic of all ID people or, alternatively, distinct profiles may be described in different aetiological groups of ID.

Participants

Performances of three groups of people were examined. The first consisted of 14 individuals with free trisomy 21 DS (Chronological age: M=21 years; SD=2.42. Mental age: M=6.5 years; SD=0.76). The second consisted of 12 persons with WS (Chronological age: M=14.7 years; SD=2.8. Mental age: M=6.5 years; SD=0.8). The deletion on chromosome 7 was confirmed in all the subjects by FISH (fluorescent *in situ* hybridization). Thirty-two children with normal cognitive abilities, of comparable mental age, evaluated with the L-M form of the Stanford-Binet Intelligence Scale formed the control group. The DS and WS groups did not differ in mental age but were significantly different in their chronological age. For this reason, a direct comparison between these two special populations was not allowed and distinct control groups were identified for each experimental group (DS and WS).

Neuropsychological tests

Consistent with our hypothesis, the neuropsychological battery included tests for evaluating implicit memory (Tower of London, Fragmented Pictures Test, Serial Reaction Time Test, Word Stem Completion), episodic explicit memory tests for verbal material (free recall of a list of unrelated words) and episodic explicit memory tests for visual-perceptual material (explicit recognition of material studied in the Fragmented Pictures Test). All the tests used in the present study have been described in previous papers (Vicari et al., 2000b, 2001; Vicari and Carlesimo, 2002).

The subjects were tested individually; administration of the entire protocol required two sessions of approximately 1 hour each, on 2 successive days.

Results

Results obtained by DS subjects and their controls in the implicit memory tasks are reported in Table 16.1. In all the tasks considered, DS and normal controls do not differ. In particular, a similar pattern within the two groups is observed both in the Serial Reaction Time (SRT) and Tower of London (TOL) test.

Concerning the WS group, results were quite different. Indeed, although WS individuals were similar to normal controls in the priming

Table 16.1 Results of implicit memory tests for Down syndrome subjects and controls

Implicit memory task	DS	MA	*p*
Serial Reaction Time (V-IV trials)	+102.7	+162.5	n.s.
Tower of London (II-I testing session score)	M = 2.8 (4.5)	M = 3.2 (1.9)	n.s.
Fragmented Picture Test	M = 3.64 (5.1)	M = 6.3 (3.7)	n.s.
Word Stem Completion	M = 4.9 (2.9)	M = 5.65 (2.4)	n.s.

n.s. = not significant

repetition tasks (for verbal as well as for visual material) they failed to show the similar pattern of normal controls both in the SRT and TOL (Table 16.2).

Table 16.2 Results of implicit memory tests for Williams syndrome subjects and controls

Implicit memory tasks	WS	MA	*p*
Serial Reaction Time (V-IV trials)	+62	+219	.01
Tower of London (II-I testing session score)	M = 1.2 (2.6)	M = 3.2 (1.5)	.05
Fragmented Pictures Test	M = 3.9 (2.9)	M = 4.8 (3.2)	n.s.
Word Stem Completion	M = 5.3 (3.7)	M = 5.9 (2.5)	n.s.

n.s. = not significant

The results for the explicit memory tasks show that DS individuals are always poorer than the normal controls (Table 16.3).

Table 16.3 Results of explicit memory tests for Down syndrome subjects and controls

Explicit memory task	DS	MA	*p*
Free recall	M = 35 (8.2)	M = 45.3 (6.4)	.001
Words recognition	M = 25.6 (5.2)	M = 29 (1.1)	.05
Pictures recognition	M = 24.8 (5.4)	M = 28 (0)	.01

The performances of WS individuals, however, do not differ from those of normal controls (Table 16.4).

Table 16.4 Results of explicit memory tests for Williams syndrome subjects and controls

Explicit memory task	WS	MA	*p*
Free recall	M = 42.9 (6.8)	M = 47.1 (6.6)	n.s.
Words recognition	M = 28.7 (1.05)	M = 29.2 (1.03)	n.s.
Pictures recognition	M = 27.3 (1.02)	M = 28 (0)	n.s.

n.s. = not significant

The principal result of our study was the distinct memory patterns in persons with DS and with WS. With regard to explicit memory abilities, subjects with DS obtained lower performance scores than the individuals with WS and normal MA matches. In contrast, WS subjects showed a similar performance profile to the normal controls. In the implicit memory domain the pattern of the results was the reverse. Although we observed comparable results between the two experimental groups in repetition priming tasks, only participants with DS were comparable to the MA control group in the ability to learn new procedures. On the contrary, WS subjects were severely impaired in these tasks.

Conclusions

The discrepant performance profiles shown by children with DS and WS suggest that the procedural learning deficit exhibited by WS individuals (as well as the deficit in explicit memory of DS subjects) is not the expression of the global cognitive impairment affecting ID people but, rather, that it is a peculiarity of the WS group. It presumably results from some specific characteristics of their anomalous brain development. Concerning our study, any attempt to identify which neuroanatomical structure is specifically involved in the implicit memory impairment displayed by WS subjects must necessarily be based on qualitative analogies of their deficit with that displayed by adult neurological patients: Huntington's disease with a degenerative loss of neurons at the level of basal ganglia, and cerebellar patients (Molinari et al., 1997).

WS children's brain development is characterized by both a remarkable atrophy of the basal ganglia (Jernigan and Bellugi, 1990) and a neurochemical alteration (reduction of the neurotransmitter N-acetylaspartate) in the cerebellum (Rae et al., 1998), thus suggesting a neurobiological substrate for the impaired maturation of procedural learning.

In our opinion, there are two reasons for attributing a dominant role to the volumetric reduction of basal ganglia. First, the performance profile exhibited by WS children resembles Huntington's disease patients more than cerebellum-damaged patients. Second, DS subjects, despite severe atrophy of cerebellum, show normal procedural learning of both visuo-motor and cognitive tasks, thus undermining the role of cerebellar circuit maturation in the development of skill learning. Further studies, directly evaluating the possible correlation between morphovolumetric and spectroscopic indices of brain function and the ability of WS subjects to learn visuo-motor and cognitive procedures, are needed to understand better the relative contribution of basal ganglia and abnormal cerebellar development in the impaired maturation of procedural memory in these subjects.

References

Carlesimo GA, Marotta L, Vicari S (1997) Long-term memory in mental retardation: evidence for a specific impairment in subjects with Down's syndrome. Neuropsychologia 35: 71–9.

Frangiskakis JM, Ewart AK, Morris CA (1996) LIM-Kinase-1 hemizygosity implicated in impaired visuospatial constructive cognition. Cell 86: 59–69.

Jernigan TJ, Bellugi U (1990) Anomalous brain morphology on magnetic resonance images in Williams syndrome. Arch Neurol 47: 529–33.

Molinari M, Leggio MG, Solida A (1997) Cerebellum and procedural learning: evidence from focal cerebellar lesions. Brain 120: 1753–62.

Pezzini G, Vicari S, Volterra V, Milani L, Ossella MT (1999) Children with Williams syndrome: is there a single neuropsychological profile? Dev Neuropsychol 15(1): 141–55.

Rae C, Karmiloff-Smith A, Lee MA (1998) Brain biochemistry in Williams syndrome. Evidence for a role of the cerebellum in cognition. Neurology 51: 33–40.

Vicari S, Bellucci S, Carlesimo GA (2000a) Implicit and explicit memory: a functional dissociation in persons with Down syndrome. Neuropsychologia 38: 240–51.

Vicari S, Bellucci S, Carlesimo GA (2001) Procedural learning deficit in children with Williams syndrome. Neuropsychologia 39: 665–77.

Vicari S, Carlesimo GA (2002) Children with intellectual disabilities. In A Baddeley, B Wilson, M Kopelman (eds) Handbook of Memory Disorders. Chichester: John Wiley & Sons, pp. 501–18.

Vicari S, Carlesimo GA, Brizzolara D, Pezzini G (1996) Short-term memory in children with Williams syndrome: a reduced contribution of lexical-semantic knowledge to word span. Neuropsychologia 34(9): 919–25.

Vicari S, Caselli MC, Tonucci F (2000b) Early language development in Italian children with Down syndrome: asynchrony of lexical and morphosyntactic abilities. Neuropsychologia 38: 634–44.

Chapter 17
Language in adults with Down syndrome

J.A. RONDAL

Introduction

People with Down syndrome (DS) live markedly longer these days than was the case early in the 20th century and before. According to Baird and Sadovnick (1995; see also Dupont et al., 1986; Jancar and Jancar, 1996), estimates give a life expectancy beyond 68 years for over 15% and 55 years for over 50% of DS persons. Strauss and Eyman (1996) estimate the life expectancy in people with DS to be around 55 years on average. Further progress can probably still be expected.

These gains in longevity have brought about an increased interest in the adult and ageing years of DS people. About three decades ago, however, the possibility of a marked susceptibility of DS individuals to a degenerative condition known as Alzheimer disease (AD) was signalled, as well as a tendency towards earlier anatomophysiological and neuropsychological ageing in comparison with non-handicapped (NH) and mentally handicapped (MH) people of other aetiologies. Recent estimates suggest an onset of AD or AD-like disease in 25–45% of DS persons beyond 55 years (Zigman et al., 1997) and 20% before 50 years (van Buggenhout et al., 2001). Age is probably not the sole and may not even be the primary cause of senile dementia, however (Brion and Plas, 1987; Oliver et al., 2000). Aged persons with severe intellectual disabilities (ID) may suffer from (treatable) pseudodementia sometimes misdiagnosed as a depressive state (Campbell-Taylor, 1993; Florez, 2000).

Additionally, the question remains of an earlier onset of neuropsychological decline in DS adults unrelated to AD (Brown, 1985), but more marked than in other ID individuals of other aetiologies (Thompson, 1999). Van Buggenhout et al. (2001) report a significant increase in the proportion of DS persons presenting additional health problems when over 50 years of age (e.g. hearing and sight losses, epilepsy, hypothyroidism). Although there are few data available on this topic, it would appear that ageing DS adults are well aware of their increased functional limitations (e.g. lowering of cognitive and physical performance, loss of sensorial acuity, skin problems, additional dental and health problems) with men seeming to resent these signs more than women (Hannecart and Haelewyck, in press).

Predisposition towards earlier ageing in DS may be associated with overexpression of genes located on chromosome 21, distinct from the gene coding for amyloid preprotein (which resides in the proximal part of the long arm of chromosome 21 and supplies one key factor to AD neuropathology). Similarly, the clinical phenotype of DS can be modulated by genes on chromosomes other than chromosome 21 (Royston et al., 1994), but these genes remain to be identified (Wisniewski and Silverman, 1996). Research is needed to assess the abilities of DS people in their forties, fifties and beyond, and to measure as precisely as possible declines in neuropsychological functioning.

Studies of language evolution in adults with Down syndrome

Few specific data have been published regarding the language evolution of adult and ageing DS people. My co-workers and I have collected series of data relevant to this subject (Comblain, 1996; Rondal and Comblain, 1996, 2002; George et al., 2002). The same instrument for analysing morphosyntactic aspects of language (BEMS; Batterie pour l'Evaluation de la Morpho-Syntaxe; Comblain, 1995) was used with cohorts of DS subjects of different chronological ages (CA) allowing cross-sectional comparisons. Each group included seven subjects (females and males). They were compared on the receptive subtests of the BEMS, assessing nominal coreference in the case of personal pronouns, definite and indefinite articles, temporal morphological inflections, negative sentences, reversible and non-reversible passive sentences, sentences with coordinate clauses, sentences with temporal, causal, conditional or consequential subordinate clauses, and sentences with relative subordinates in *qui* (grammatical subject) or *que* (direct grammatical object).

Table 17.1 lists the definitional characteristics of the three CA samples of DS subjects (Comparison I). Table 17.2 displays the group means and standard deviations for the eight subtests of the BEMS.

A one-way MANOVA for non-repeated measures carried out simultaneously on the eight dependent variables for the three CA groups revealed no significant statistical difference (at the conventional $p < .05$ level) in the receptive morphosyntactic functioning of DS individuals from adolescence to mature adulthood, i.e. over a time interval of 32 years. Regarding language production, no direct comparison of the younger and the older

Table 17.1 Definitional characteristics of the samples of DS subjects (comparison I)

	Adolescents (n=7)	Younger adults (n=7)	Older adults (n=7)
CA			
Mean	16;7 years	26;9 years	44 years
SD	22 months	32 months	38 months
VI	14;5–19;6 years	23;4–30;1 years	40;5–46;7 years
MA			
Mean	4;4 years	4;7 years	4;4 years
SD	8 months	9 months	6 months
VI	3;8–5;6 years	3;6–5;3 years	3;9–5;4 years

CA: chronological age; SD: standard deviation on the mean; VI: variation interval around the mean; MA: mental age. The differences between mean MAs across CA groups were not statistically significant (one-way ANOVA for unrelated samples).

Table 17.2 Group means and standard deviations from the BEMS subtests in three samples of DS subjects (comparison I)

BEMS subtests	Adolescents	DS SUBJECTS Younger adults	Older adults
1. Nominal coreference	43 (8)	48 (35)	51 (15)
2. Articles	30 (6)	34 (8)	36 (17)
3. Temporal inflections	40 (4)	43 (6)	40 (15)
4. Negatives	57 (24)	38 (37)	36 (35)
5. Passives	57 (17)	48 (42)	52 (29)
6. Coordinates	64 (13)	70 (7)	64 (27)
7. Subordinates	43 (21)	31 (25)	51 (20)
8. Relatives	77 (20)	71 (25)	73 (18)

Data are expressed in percentage of correct responses. Standard deviations are given in parentheses.

adults was possible because, this time, the same set of language productive measures was not used for comparing the adolescent and the younger adult groups (in what were actually two studies) (see Comparison II below for the productive measures used). The paper by Rondal and Comblain (1996) contains the productive data resulting from the comparison of the same DS adolescents and younger adults as in the present report. Accordingly, no significant change was observed as to mean length of utterance (MLU) – a valid if global index of expressive morphosyntax – and expressive referential lexicon (TVAP: Test de Vocabulaire Actif et Passif; TVP: Test de Vocabulaire Productif). Although we do not have specific data at hand to support our conclusion, it is unlikely that marked changes in productive language take place in the interval of time between 30 and 40 years in DS people. No significant change has been documented in the receptive abilities of the same DS people and no significant productive or receptive change has been revealed either by our analyses of the language of DS persons between 40 and 50 years (see below).

As indicated in reviews of specialized literature (Rondal and Comblain, 1996; Rondal and Edwards, 1997), marked language progress does not seem to take place, at least in the phonological and the grammatical aspects, beyond mid-adolescence. Significant progress may still be observed beyond that age in the conceptual and the pragmatic aspects of language (e.g. vocabulary, conversational and more generally commu-nicative abilities, and discourse organization) (Chapman, 1999; Berry et al., 1984). Henceforth, it is obviously necessary to distinguish between language components and avoid global maturational hypotheses of the type proposed by Lenneberg (1967) and Fowler (1990), according to which no marked language improvement (at all) is possible beyond early adolescence. Lenneberg and Fowler's characterizations may indeed not be appropriate. I have suggested and justified that it makes more theo-retical and empirical sense to restrict the maturational susceptibility to the formal components of language, i.e. phonology and grammar.

We have also conducted a 4-year longitudinal study with 12 DS subjects aged between 37 and 49 years (six women and six men). The language functions (receptive as well as productive) were assessed for every subject at 1 year intervals during the first 2 years. Four subjects did not maintain their participation beyond the second year. For the others, the study was continued for another 2 years using the same evaluation procedure. For eight subjects (four women and four men) a measure of cerebral metab-olism rate (CMR) for fluorodeoxyglucose (18FDG) was made every year using the PET (positron emission tomography) scan technique and yield-ing 31 reconstructed plans from the emission scans (see George et al., 2002). For seven of these eight subjects (one died in the meantime), the cerebral imagery investigation was continued for 2 more years with one examination taking place every year.

Table 17.3 displays the group means and standard deviations resulting from the analyses of the language of these seven DS adults. The BEMS was used to assess receptive morphosyntax. A receptive lexical task (picture designation) adapted and modified after the test of Bishop and Byng (1984) was given too. Productively, a task of verbal (semantic) fluency was applied. Subjects were requested to supply orally the largest possible number of animal names in one minute. A home-made test of lexical labelling (picture denomination) was administered. It counted 127 items divided into five semantic categories (fruits, clothes, vegetables, kitchen tools and objects, and animals). The phonetic length (one, two or three syllables) of the items was controlled as well as the frequency of appear-ance of these items in the language (frequency tables for the French language). The subjects were allowed 20 seconds to answer. After this time, a phonemic cue was provided (the first phoneme of the target word was supplied by the examiner). In the case of further error or absence of response, syllabic help was given (the first syllable of the target word was

Table 17.3 Group means and standard deviations from the receptive and the productive tasks in older DS adults at 1 year intervals during 4 years (comparison II)[1]

		DS SUBJECTS/TIME		
RECEPTIVE TASKS	1	2	3	4
BEMS				
1. Nominal coreference	51 (15)	29 (9)	39 (17)	40 (15)
2. Articles	36 (17)	23 (7)	27 (11)	28 (16)
3. Temporal inflections	40 (15)	35 (8)	32 (10)	34 (7)
4. Negatives	36 (35)	45 (35)	34 (29)	30 (20)
5. Passives	52 (29)	48 (18)	43 (10)	36 (21)
6. Coordinates	64 (27)	48 (26)	50 (13)	57 (10)
7. Subordinates	51 (20)	47 (14)	39 (13)	37 (15)
8. Relatives	73 (18)	68 (10)	55 (12)	46 (14)
Lexical designation[2]	19 (5)	18 (5)	19 (5)	20 (5)
PRODUCTIVE TASKS				
Verbal fluency	10 (5)	9 (4)	8 (3)	8 (3)
Lexical labelling				
TOTAL[3]	144 (17)	137 (33)	135 (28)	137 (33)
Fruits	25 (6)	24 (4)	23 (5)	25 (9)
Clothes	28 (5)	26 (5)	28 (4)	27 (6)
Vegetables	25 (11)	24 (8)	21 (8)	21 (6)
Kitchen tools & objects	33 (4)	31 (8)	30 (8)	32 (6)
Animals	33 (9)	31 (12)	33 (10)	1 (11)
Narrative text about pictures (verbal recall)				
Ideas[4]	3 (1)	3 (1)	2 (2)	3 (2)
Words[5]	10 (4)	10 (6)	7 (5)	8 (6)
Report (morphosyntactic & semantic aspects)[6]	25 (13)	28 (15)	28 (20)	23 (13)

[1]BEMS data are expressed as percentage of correct responses. Other data are raw scores of correct responses. Standard deviations are given in parentheses; [2]Maximum correct score is 40; [3]Maximum correct scores is 254; maximum correct scores for the semantic categories: fruits 56, clothes 48, vegetables 46, kitchen tools & objects 52, and animals 52; [4]Each global idea from the original story correctly recalled was worth 0.5 point; [5]Number of words per utterances in the story recall; [6]Global index integrating separate scores for the use of causal relations, anaphoric pronouns replacing thematic nouns functioning as sentence subjects, the correct working of chronology in the story, the production of complex sentences, and the number of tenses used in the story recall (maximum no. 100).

provided by the examiner). The aim was to separate a possible difficulty with word retrieving from a genuine ignorance of the target name. Lastly, the test 'Récit sur images' (narrative text about pictures; verbal recall; adapted from Chevrie-Müller, 1981) was administered. This test takes into account the number of global ideas, words and several formal and semantic characteristics of the narratives as they are freely recalled by the subjects.

None of the one-way (four age levels) multiple analyses of variance (MANOVA) on the eight dependent variables from the BEMS, analyses of variance (ANOVA) on the lexical designation scores, ANOVA on the verbal fluency data, MANOVA on the five dependent variables of the task of lexical labelling, and ANOVA on the total denomination scores, yielded a significant result, failing therefore to corroborate the hypothesis of a language change in the DS subjects across the 4-year study.

The CMR data were analysed as follows. The left and right frontal, parietal and temporal cortices of each subject were examined and the visual metabolic images from the associative cortical regions were evaluated in a semi-quantitative way on a scale from zero (normal metabolism) to two (severe metabolic reduction) (Hoffman et al., 1996; Pickut et al., 1997). As expected, no CMR image proved normal in any DS subject and there was significant inter-individual variability. Globally, metabolic reduction was more marked at the level of the left hemisphere. Along the time dimension, there was a gradual decrease in global CMR for each two cerebral hemispheres and for each of the seven DS persons (average global CMR for the right hemisphere at times 1 and 3, respectively 1.57 and 3.58; average global CMR for the left hemisphere at times 1 and 3, respectively 2.50 and 5.50). The average decreases, however, were due to large decreases in three of the DS subjects. Analysing the performance of these three subjects in the language tasks over the same interval of time, no indication of deterioration emerged that could be meaningfully related to the lowering in CMR. It is possible that global brain metabolism (particularly within the left cerebral hemisphere) is diminished substantially in some DS subjects without, at least temporarily, any clear negative consequence on language functioning.

As our series of data suggest, no major change seems to take place in the language of DS individuals between late adolescence and 50 years of age. This is worth noting as functional modifications of language and memory have been indicated as the first signs of earlier ageing and degenerative diseases. Jodar (1992), for example, suggested that in normal ageing, lexical and verbal comprehension in general are preserved, whereas verbal fluency, lexical labelling, and more generally the capacity for verbal production tend to decline.

What may happen beyond 50 years or so in DS people is unknown at present because of the lack of systematic data. Hints may be derived from the limited literature in existence pending verification through more extensive studies. A study by Das et al. (1995) suggests that there is little to no change in non-verbal reasoning, memory, language (receptive and expressive vocabulary), planning and attention, perceptual-motor and adaptive skills, until close to 60 years. However, the same authors indicate that the older DS subjects in their cohorts (i.e. those slightly beyond 60 years) were actually performing more poorly than those in younger groups particularly in tasks requiring planning and attention. This can probably be put in relation with Ribes and Sanuy's (2000) observation of a slight decline in expressive language (particularly vocabulary) in some of their DS subjects beyond 38 years; Prasher (1996) also suggested the existence of an age-associated functional decline in short-term memory, speech, practical skills, activity and general interests in approximately 20% of the

DS persons aged 50–71 years; Moss et al. (2000) suggested a significant inverse relation between age and several aspects of auditory linguistic comprehension in a sample of DS adults of between 32 and 65 years of age.

Cross-sectional studies, of course, are limited in their ability (validity) to demonstrate time changes as they compare different subjects at different ages, mixing together inter-individual and age-related variances. Regarding DS individuals, the problem is complicated by a cohort difference: i.e. younger DS subjects have generally been the targets of early cognitive intervention (at least in the developed countries) whereas older DS individuals generally have not been. It could be hypothesized that early intervention has the potential effect of upgrading development in many DS subjects therefore rendering the comparisons with older cohorts difficult or even invalid. A few longitudinal studies have been conducted. Devenny et al. (1992) and Burt et al. (1995) did not observe significant changes in the cognitive functioning of DS individuals aged between 27 and 55 years and 22 and 56 years in the two studies, respectively, over time intervals of 3 to 5 years. Devenny et al. (1996) report only four cases of cognitive involution in 91 DS subjects followed for several years beyond the age of 50.

The above observations do not suggest rapid and marked age-related decline in the cognitive and language functioning of DS subjects beyond 50 years, apart from the episodic occurrence of progressive deterioration.

Unfortunately, such marked progressive deteriorations do take place in the language and cognitive functioning of some DS persons (even before 50 years). As commonly thought, they may signal incipient AD or an AD-like pathology. One particular follow-up study throws some beginning light on the course of such outcomes, mainly from a language perspective. About 10 years ago, I found myself in a position to analyse the language and cognitive levels of a DS woman, named Françoise, presenting exceptional language abilities for a DS person (Rondal, 1995). Two years ago, the day centre where Françoise spends several days a week requested a neuropsychological examination motivated by her depressed behaviour, lack of initiative and possible memory losses. Dr Michel Ylieff, a neuropsychologist from the University of Liège, a specialist in the clinical aspects of ageing, agreed to carry out a re-examination of some of Françoise's cognitive functions. Comparing his data with those of Rondal (1995), Ylieff (2000a) signalled a marked lowering of Françoise's episodic memory and ability to deal with visuospatial and graphic material. Pending further neurological and neuroradiological examinations, he suggested a localized pathology of the right cerebral hemisphere possibly linked with incipient brain degeneration. If this were the case, the first clinical expression of the neuropathology would affect the less well developed cognitive domains, i.e. spatial functions in the case of Françoise. Regarding oral language, one labelling test yielded a global score closely corresponding to the estimated NH population mean. No morphosyntactic evaluation was attempted. However, based on three personal encounters with Françoise needed to complete the testing and including informal conversations, Ylieff's impression (Ylieff, 2000b) was that Françoise's overall language was intact, which was also the opinion of the staff of the day centre. At age 46 (at the time), therefore, no major lowering in Françoise's functional language seemed attested, even if she was experiencing additional difficulties in weaker mental functions as a consequence of a possible accelerated ageing or degenerative process.

In collaboration with Mouna Elbouz and Michel Ylieff, I have retaken the analysis of Françoise's (now 47 years old) cognitive and overall language abilities. It appears that cognitive and behavioural deterioration has deepened quite substantially over the relatively short time interval between Ylieff's assessment and the more recent one, in all psychological aspects investigated.

Considering language, the overall deterioration this time is manifest in all the structural aspects evaluated in comparison with Rondal's systematic assessment of 8–10 years ago (serving now as a baseline). Table 17.4 summarizes a limited number of the comparative measures used in this latest study (a full report on the evolution of Françoise's linguistic and cognitive abilities over time is in preparation).

As may be seen in Table 17.4, receptive lexicon, although it has deteriorated, is still relatively preserved (at least by comparative standards with typical adults with DS). However, Françoise has noteworthy difficulties in finding her words as can be seen in the numerous dysfluencies which characterize her present-day conversation. She is keenly aware of this limitation and at times expresses her regrets at not being able to find her words anymore.

The only productive aspect of her language that seems to have held up so far is grammatical morphology. In the three samples of spontaneous, conversational speech that we have recorded recently, no error was documented in that respect. Françoise's reading ability once assessed at primary school grade three or close to it (Rondal, 1995), has now degraded to the point of being nil except for a limited number of current words and two- or three-word expressions with functional signification (e.g. *toilette* (toilet), *entrée* (entrance), *sortie* (exit), *arrêt de bus* (bus stop) etc.). Likewise her writing ability has deteriorated significantly. She is no longer able to write her first name, family name or date of birth. Instead she tries to comply with the instruction to do so by covering parts of the sheet with unconventional letter-like signs arranged diagonally across the page.

Finally, Françoise's auditory-vocal short-term memory span is now limited to two items (compared to four 10 years ago).

The immediate conclusion of this most unfortunate evolution over a time period of roughly 10 years, is that no matter what level of language functioning a person with DS may have reached during his or her development, profound deterioration may take place and substantially reduce the functional benefits accumulated. It is not obvious that, as tentatively suggested in a previous publication (Rondal and Comblain, 2002), more

Table 17.4 Comparative evaluation of Françoise's oral language abilities over time

LANGUAGE ABILITY	TIME / FRANÇOISE'S AGE	
	1989–1991 32–36 years	2002 47 years
1. Articulation 1.1 Segmental	Fully correct	Between 40 and 70% of correct repetitions of non-words (logatomes) containing up to four syllables; 0% correct repetition beyond that level; 60% correct repetition of balanced monosyllables; error types: omission, addition, substitution of consonantic sounds, various perseveration
1.2 Suprasegmental	Fully correct	Incorrect prosody in longer utterances (see dysfluencies)
2. Dysfluencies	Virtually absent	Numerous speech dysfluencies (word and phrase repetitions, false starts, hesitations, undue pauses, broken utterances)
3. Approximate speech rate (in number of words per second)	3.3 words (12 to 15 phonemes)	1 word (4 to 5 phonemes) and less
4. Receptive lexicon 4.1. TVAP 5–8[1]	28 correct designations out of 30 16 correct designations out of 30	24 correct designations out of 50
4.2. TRT[2]	48 correct designations out of 50	
5. Productive morphosyntax Mean length of utterance[3]	12.34	6.91
6. Receptive syntax 6.1. Relative clauses introduced by *qui* (who)	Correct interpretation 31/32	Correct interpretation 1/16
6.2. Causative subordinate clauses	32/32	5/32
6.3. Temporal subordinate clauses	46/48	0/16
6.4. Passive sentences		
6.4.1. Non-reversible	31/32	5/32
6.4.2. Reversible	32/32	7/32

[1]TVAP : Test de Vocabulaire Actif et Passif; [2]Test des Relations Topologiques ; [3]Computed in number of words plus grammatical morphemes (see Rondal, 1995).

highly developed cognitive functions would resist the degenerative process better and for longer possibly because of their better established representation in the circuitry of the brain devoted to them. Françoise's contemporary very low receptive ability with advanced syntactic structures (e.g. passives, relatives, temporal and causal subordinate clauses, as shown in Table 17.4) by comparison with the situation 10 years ago, seems to militate against such a hypothesis. On the other hand, and regarding the productive side of language functioning this time, it seems clear that so far she has retained her grammatical morphological ability virtually intact (no error in this domain was observed in her spontaneous conversational speech). Pending a dissociation between syntax and grammatical morphology, there have been several observations in the literature on normal adults with AD that the grammatical aspects of language tend to be spared in the early stages of the condition (Appel et al., 1982; Kempler et al., 1987; Murillo Ruiz, 1999), including the syntactic processing capacity once it is evaluated separately from processing load (e.g. longer sentences and sentences with more propositions which are problematic in these subjects) (Waters et al., 1995).

References

Appel J, Kertesz A, Fishman M (1982) A study of language functioning in Alzheimer's patients. Brain Lang 17: 73–91.

Baird P, Sadovnick A (1995) Life expectancy in Down syndrome. Lancet 2: 1354–6.

Berry P, Groenweg G, Gibson D, Brown R (1984) Mental development of adults with Down's syndrome. Am J Ment Defic 89: 252–6.

Bishop D, Byng S (1984) Accessing semantic comprehension: methodological considerations and a new clinical test. Cognit Neuropsychol 1: 223–43.

Brion S, Plas J (1987) Etat actuel de l'approche histopathologique des démences. Psychologie Médicale 19: 1235–42.

Brown W (1985) Genetics of aging. In M Janicki, H Wisniewski (eds) Aging and Developmental Disabilities: Issues and Approaches. Baltimore, MD: Brookes, pp. 185–94.

Burt D, Loveland K, Chen Y-W, Chuang A, Lewis K, Cherry L (1995) Aging in adults with Down syndrome: report from a longitudinal study. Am J Ment Retard 100: 262–70.

Campbell-Taylor I (1993) Communication impairments in Alzheimer disease and Down syndrome. In J Berg, H Karlinsky, A Holland (eds) Alzheimer Disease, Down Syndrome and their Relationship. New York: Oxford University Press, pp. 175–93.

Chapman R (1999) Language development in children and adolescents with Down syndrome. In J Miller, M Leddy, L Leavitt (eds) Improving the Communication of People with Down Syndrome. Baltimore, MD: Brookes, pp. 41–60.

Chevrie-Müller C (1981) Epreuves pour l'examen du langage: Batterie composite. Paris: Editions du Centre de Psychologie Appliquée.

Comblain A (1995) Batterie pour l'évaluation de la morpho-syntaxe. Liège: Laboratoire de Psycholinguistique de l'Université de Liège (unpublished).

Comblain A (1996) Mémoire de travail et langage dans le syndrome de Down. Doctoral thesis in Psychology (Logopedics), Université de Liège, Belgium (unpublished).

Das J-P, Divis B, Alexander J, Parrila R, Naglieri J (1995) Cognitive decline due to aging among persons with Down syndrome. Res Dev Disabil 16: 461–78.

Devenny D, Hill A, Patxot O, Silverman W, Wisniewski H (1992) Ageing in higher functioning adults with Down's syndrome: an interim report in a longitudinal study. J Intell Disab Res 36: 241–50.

Devenny D, Silverman W, Hill A, Jenkins E, Sersen E, Wisniewski H (1996) Normal ageing in adults with Down's syndrome: a longitudinal study. J Intell Disab Res 40: 208–21.

Dupont A, Vaeth M, Videbech P (1986) Mortality and life expectancy of Down's syndrome in Denmark. J Ment Defic Res 30: 111–20.

Florez J (2000) El envejecimiento de las personas con sindrome de Down. Revista Sindrome de Down 17: 16–24.

Fowler A (1990) Language abilities in children with Down's syndrome: evidence for a specific syntactic delay. In D Cicchetti, M Beeghly (eds) Children with Down Syndrome: A Developmental Perspective. New York: Cambridge University Press, pp. 302–28.

George M, Thewis B, van der Linden M, Salmon E, Rondal JA (2002) Elaboration d'une batterie d'évaluation des fonctions cognitives de sujets âgés porteurs d'un syndrome de Down. Revue de Neuropsychologie, in press.

Hannecart M, Haelewyck MC (in press) Le vieillissement commence par la vie: approche exploratoire de la perception du vieillissement et de la qualité de vie chez les personnes présentant un handicap mental. Journal de la Trisomie 21.

Hart A (1988) Language and dementia: a review. Psychol Med 18: 99–112.

Hoffman J, Hamson M, Welsh K, Earl N, Raine S, Delong D, Coleman R (1996) Interpretation variability of 18FDG-positron emission tomography studies in dementia. Investigation in Radiology 31: 316–22.

Jancar J, Jancar P (1996) Longevity in Down syndrome: a twelve year survey (1984–1995). Italian Journal of Intellectual Impairment 9: 27–30.

Jodar M (1992) Envejecimiento normal versus demencia de Alzheimer. Valor del lenguaje en el diagnostico differencial. Revista de Logopedia, Foniatria y Audiologia 12: 171–9.

Kempler D, Curtiss S, Jackson C (1987) Syntactic preservation in Alzheimer's disease. J Speech Hear Res 30: 343–50.

Lenneberg E (1967) Biological Foundations of Language. New York: Wiley.

Moss S, Tomoeda C, Bayles K (2000) Comparison of the cognitive-linguistic profiles of Down syndrome adults with and without dementia to individuals with Alzheimer's disease. J Med Speech-Lang Pathol 8: 69–81.

Murillo Ruiz B (1999) Estudio de la evolucion del lenguaje en la demencia Alzeimer. Barcelona: ISEP Editorial.

Oliver C, Crayton L, Holland A, Hall S (2000) Cognitive deterioration in adults with Down syndrome: effects on the individual of caregivers and service use. Am J Ment Retard 105: 455–65.

Pickut B, Saerens J, Marien P, Borggreve F, Goeman J, Vandevivere J, Vervaet A, Diercks R, de Keyn P (1997) Discrimination use of SPECT in frontal lobe-type dementia versus (senile) dementia of the Alzheimer's type. J Nucl Med 38: 929–34.

Prasher V (1996) Age-associated functional decline in adults with Down's syndrome. Eur J Psychiatry 10: 129–35.

Ribes R, Sanuy J (2000) Declive cognitivo en memoria y lenguaje: indicadores del proceso de envejecimiento psicologico en la persona con sindrome de Down. Revista Sindrome de Down 17: 54–9.

Rondal JA (1995) Exceptional language development in Down syndrome. Implications for the cognition language relationship. New York: Cambridge University Press.

Rondal JA, Comblain A (1996) Language in adults with Down syndrome. Down Syndrome 4(1): 3–14.

Rondal JA, Comblain A (2002) Language in ageing persons with Down syndrome. Down Syndrome 8(1): 1–19.

Rondal JA, Edwards S (1997) Language in Mental Retardation. London: Whurr.

Royston M, Mann D, Pickering-Brown S, Owen F (1994) Apolipoprotein E., e2 allele promotes longevity and protects patients with Down's syndrome from dementia. Neuro Report 5: 2583–5.

Strauss D, Eyman R (1996) Mortality of people with mental retardation in California with and without Down syndrome, 1986–1991. Am J Ment Retard 100: 643–51.

Thompson S (1999) Examining dementia in Down's syndrome. Decline in social abilities in DS compared with other learning disabilities. Clin Gerontol 20: 23–44.

van Buggenhout G, Lukusa S, Trommelen J, de Bal C, Hamel B, Fryns J-P (2001) Etude pluridisciplinaire du syndrome de Down dans une population résidentielle d'arriérés mentaux d'âge avancé: implications pour le suivi médical. Journal de la Trisomie 2: 7–13.

Waters G, Caplan O, Rochon E (1995) Processing capacity and sentence comprehension in patients with Alzheimer's disease. Cognit Neuropsychol 12: 1–30.

Wisniewski H, Silverman W (1996) Alzheimer disease, neuropathology and dementia in Down syndrome. In JA Rondal, J Perera, L Nadel, A Comblain (eds) Down Syndrome: Psychological, Psychobiological and Socio-educational Perspectives. London: Whurr, pp. 43–52.

Wisniewski H, Silverman W (1999) Down syndrome and Alzheimer disease: variability in individual vulnerability. In JA Rondal, J Perera, L Nadel (eds) Down Syndrome. A Review of Current Knowledge. London: Whurr, pp. 178–94.

Ylieff M (2000a) Evaluation neuropsychologique de Françoise (document confidentiel). Liège, Université de Liège, Service de Psychologie de la Santé, Unité de Psychologie Clinique du Vieillissement.

Ylieff M (2000b) Personal communication with JA Rondal.

Zigman W, Schup N, Haveman M, Silverman W (1997) The epidemiology of Alzheimer disease in intellectual disability: results and recommendations from an international conference. J Intell Disabil Res 41: 76–80.

Chapter 18
Developing the language skills of adults with Down syndrome

C. Jenkins, J. MacDonald

Introduction

This chapter begins by briefly discussing the existing research relating to the language of adults with Down syndrome, including the studies of language intervention with this group of people. The next part will describe a research study carried out over 2 years with a group of adults with Down syndrome. Finally, it attempts to draw together the existing research with the findings of the study to make suggestions about how we might promote continuing language development into adulthood.

Research and theories

Once one begins to look for studies involving adults with Down syndrome it becomes clear that there is very little research in this area. There are some notable exceptions, such as the work of Rondal and colleagues (e.g. Rondal and Comblain, 1996) and Chapman's research with older adolescents and young adults (Chapman et al., 1992; Chapman, 1999). One obvious reason for the shortage of research is that until recent times most people with Down syndrome have not been expected to live beyond late adolescence or at best early adulthood. Thankfully, medical and social advances over the last few decades have not only greatly increased life expectancy but also the health of people with Down syndrome, enabling them to participate more actively in many areas of life.

If there is little research into the nature of the language problems experienced by this group of people, there is even less into the effectiveness of interventions. As Buckley (1995) pointed out: 'There is an urgent need for speech and language intervention for people with Down's syndrome to be evaluated.' It is possible that little structured intervention is happening because of preconceptions that it will not be effective. This then becomes a self-fulfilling prophecy – people's language skills do not progress and it is therefore inferred that intervention with adults is not a good use of resources. Buckley (1995) adds: 'Too much of the literature seems to suggest that the usual difficulties are an inevitable consequence of the syndrome, particularly the poor grammar, yet there is no justification for this view until intensive interventions have been thoroughly investigated and evaluated.'

Two theories in particular have suggested that there are predetermined limits to progress. The hypothesis that there is a critical period for language development (Lenneberg, 1967) implies a time limit on development, while Fowler's (1990) proposal of a 'syntactic ceiling effect' suggests a limit to the complexity of language achievable. However, a considerable amount of research in this area by Chapman and colleagues (Chapman et al., 1992; Chapman, 1999) provided evidence that syntactic development does continue beyond early adolescence in people with Down syndrome. Chapman stressed the importance of collecting both narrative and conversational samples and found that not only did length of sentences increase with age but the longer sentences were likely to be more complex.

Small-scale studies of structured language and speech intervention have been carried out by Leddy and Gill (1999) with adults with Down syndrome, with encouraging results. They conclude, 'Although some individuals plateau in adolescence, others continue to learn well into adulthood.' For practitioners working with adults with Down syndrome it has been necessary to look at the small number of interventions with teenagers (e.g. Buckley, 1993, 1995) and try to relate them to adults.

An intervention to develop the language skills of adults with Down syndrome

Rationale

The study described here originated from the idea that it might be possible to link two of the findings from previous research studies and apply them in a way which could provide evidence for an effective intervention strategy to develop the speech and language skills of people with Down syndrome in adulthood. The first of these findings came from the research over a number of years by Buckley and colleagues at the University of Portsmouth (Buckley, 1993, 1995; Byrne et al., 1995; Buckley et al., 1996) on the use of reading as a strategy for developing speech and language skills, initially of young children with Down syndrome, and the subsequent application of this approach to adolescents.

The second premise on which this study is based, that it is possible for people with Down syndrome to acquire reading skills beyond adolescence, was proposed by Fowler et al. (1994) and Farrell (1996).

The rationale for the study also drew on research findings which indicated that there are differences in the processing of language by people with Down syndrome (Chua et al., 1996). This is linked to difficulties with auditory processing and memory, over and above those associated with a generalized cognitive delay resulting from a learning disability (MacKenzie and Hulme, 1987; Marcell and Weeks, 1988). Other studies have capitalized on the relative strengths of visual memory and processing, using visual media to support and facilitate learning (Powell and Clibbens, 1994).

Participants, materials and procedure

This study took place in two stages over 2 years. Twenty-eight people with Down syndrome were recruited to take part in the study. The participants' ages ranged from 19 to 49 years with a mean age of 37 years. All participants attended one of two Social Services Day Centres for people with learning disabilities (Table 18.1).

Table 18.1 Participant details

| | Age (years) N-28 | | Gender N-28 | | Residence N-28 | |
	Mean	Range	Male	Female	Family	Group home
All participants	37	19–49	16	12	20	8
Centre 1	36	19–49	8	10	15	3
Centre 2	40	28–49	8	2	5	5

Criteria for participation in the study were a minimum verbal comprehension level of at least three 'information-carrying words' on the Derbyshire Language Scheme (Masidlover and Knowles, 1982) and a maximum reading age of less than 8 years.

Following baseline assessments of language comprehension and expression, auditory and visual memory, non-verbal reasoning, phonological awareness and reading, participants were randomly assigned to one of two matched groups, the Reading Group or the Language Group. For the first year (Stage 1) both groups took part in teaching sessions involving a structured language programme based on Language through Reading (Hutt, 1986), together with some components of the Derbyshire Language Scheme. Picture materials were used with both groups, but in addition, these were supported by written materials for the Reading Group only. The baseline assessments were repeated at the end of the first year with the 25 people who had completed Stage 1.

For the second year of the study (Stage 2) the Language Group continued with the language programme, but with additional reading materials. The original intention was that the Reading Group would not continue to participate actively in the programme for Stage 2, but the maintenance of skills acquired would be monitored. This plan was changed at the end of

Stage 1 and Reading Group participants were able to choose whether or not to continue. Twenty-one people remained in the study at the end of Stage 2 and the baseline and Stage 1 assessments were repeated.

Teaching took place in small groups of two to four participants and each person attended two sessions each week. One session was with the researcher and the other with a volunteer tutor from the Day Centre staff. Tutors received initial training and regular monitoring during the study.

Results

Language

There were no significant differences between the groups at any stage of the study or for the Language Group in the two different conditions (language only and reading), suggesting that reading did not have an effect in this situation. However, there were significant gains for both groups in language comprehension and expression. These gains in expressive language included elements of morphosyntax, such as plurals, past tense endings and possessive/s/. There were also significant increases in the range of linguistic structures and the use of auxiliary verbs, pronouns and prepositions, as shown in Table 18.2.

Table 18.2 Language scores, means and (sds) for all participants (N=21), Baseline to Stage 2

	Baseline	Stage 2	Significance p
Language comprehension (TROG)	3.90** (2.05)	5.19** (1.99)	.000
Language expression (STASS total)	44.39* (15.78)	47.42* (17.91)	.041
Auxiliary verbs	25.86* (23.30)	38.77* (29.66)	.002
Prepositions	45.46** (22.85)	76.79** (23.64)	.000
Pronouns	35.54* (21.40)	42.49* (21.14)	.006

TROG – Test for the Reception of Grammar; STASS – South Tyneside Assessment of Syntactic Structure;
*significant – $p < .05$;
**highly significant – $p < .001$

Both groups also made significant gains in non-verbal reasoning and phonological awareness over the 2-year intervention.

Reading

Five of the participants who completed the study were able to score on a standardized reading test in the baseline assessments. Although the aim of the study was to use the written word as a medium to teach language, rather than to teach reading, three participants developed sufficient reading ability during the intervention to score on a standardized test. Seven other participants were able to recognize words used in the teaching programme outside that context (see Table 18.3).

Table 18.3 Reading scores

	Existing readers (n-5)		New readers (n-3)		Scheme readers (n-7)
	Test words (mean)	Scheme words (mean)	Test words (mean)	Scheme words (mean)	Scheme words (mean)
Baseline	14.8 (range 9–23)		0		
Stage 2	18.8 (range 10–26)	58.2 (range 37–73)	3 (range 2–5)	14.7 (range 8–21)	2.2 (range 1–5)

Test words – words recognized from standardized test;
Scheme words – words recognized from those used in teaching programme

Age and progress

There was no relationship between age and progress in any of the measures used in this study. The older participants were also able to develop new language skills.

Implications for language intervention with adults with Down syndrome

The results of this study suggest that it is possible for adults with Down syndrome to enhance their language skills, both in comprehension and expression. However, these gains followed a structured language teaching programme. This of course has resource implications for those providing education and therapy services. It has previously been possible to argue that there is no evidence that intervention is effective, but while there is little or no intervention, there will be no evidence. It may, however, be feasible to look at different ways of providing intervention. The language programme developed for this study was used by tutors from the resource centres attended by the participants. They had a range of training and experience. It should therefore be possible to support a variety of workers, other than speech and language therapists, to carry out this type of intervention.

Although the use of reading did not influence language skills in this study, there were other benefits from using the reading materials. Some people with Down syndrome did show the potential to develop new reading skills. As Fowler et al. (1994) point out, 'Even a limited amount of reading skill served to enhance both self-esteem and employability of persons with Down syndrome. It would be a pity not to provide them with the opportunity.'

Leddy and Gill (1999) noted that the older adults who participated in their programme appeared to be 'passive communicators who did not know how to play the communication game'. However, the adults in this study were as eager to communicate and to learn as their younger colleagues. Moreover, as there was no link between age and progress in the findings, there would appear to be no reason to exclude people from interventions on the grounds of age alone.

It is important to use teaching strategies that enable people to succeed, such as errorless learning techniques (Wishart, 1993) and the use of prompts which can be faded as people become more confident and competent. People with Down syndrome who have reached adulthood are likely to have experienced a considerable amount of failure in their lives, much of it associated with difficulties in communication. They need to feel that they can achieve success in communication and moreover that communication is an enjoyable and satisfying experience.

According to Leddy and Gill (1999), 'The future is promising for adults with Down syndrome.' The responsibility lies with us as researchers, service providers and individual professionals to ensure that the promise becomes a reality.

Acknowledgements

Thanks are due to the people with Down syndrome who gave up their time to participate in the study and the Resource Centre staff who acted as tutors. Professor John MacDonald and Professor Sue Buckley provided me with very valuable advice and support for which I am extremely grateful. I should also like to express my appreciation to the Research Committee of the NHS Executive, South and West for funding this research.

References

Buckley S (1993) Developing the speech and language skills of teenagers with Down's syndrome. Down's Syndr Res Pract 1(2): 63–71.

Buckley S (1995) Improving the expressive language skills of teenagers with Down's syndrome. Down's Syndr Res Pract 3(3): 110–15.

Buckley S, Bird G, Byrne A (1996) Reading acquisition by young children with Down's syndrome. In B Stratford, P Gunn (eds) New Approaches to Down Syndrome. London: Cassell, pp. 268–79.

Byrne A, Buckley S, MacDonald J, Bird G (1995) Investigating the literacy, language and memory skills of children with Down's syndrome. Down's Syndr Res Pract 3(2): 53–9.

Chapman R (1999) Language development in children and adolescents with Down syndrome. In JF Miller, M Leddy, LA Leavitt (eds) Improving the Communication of People with Down Syndrome. Baltimore: Paul H Brookes, pp. 41–60.

Chapman R, Schwartz SE, Kay-Raining Bird E (1992) Language production of older children with Down syndrome. 9th World Congress of the International Association for the Scientific Study of Mental Deficiency.

Chua R, Weeks D, Elliott D (1996) A functional systems approach to understanding verbal-motor integration in individuals with Down's syndrome. Down's Syndr Res Pract 4(1): 25–36.

Farrell M (1996) Continuing literacy development. In B Stratford, P Gunn (eds) New Approaches to Down Syndrome. London: Cassell, pp. 280–99.

Fowler A (1990) Language abilities in children with Down syndrome: evidence for specific syntactic delay. In D Cicchetti, M Beeghly (eds) Children with Down Syndrome. A Developmental Perspective. New York: Cambridge University Press, pp. 302–28.

Fowler AE, Doherty B, Boynton LS (1994) The basis of reading skills in young adults with Down syndrome. In D Rosenthal, L Nadel (eds) Down Syndrome: Living and Learning in the Community. New York: Wiley-Liss, pp. 182–96.

Hutt E (1986) Teaching Language-disordered Children: A Structured Curriculum. London: Edward Arnold.

Leddy M, Gill G (1999) Enhancing the speech and language skills of adults with Down syndrome. In JF Miller, M Leddy, LA Leavitt (eds) Improving the Communication of People with Down Syndrome. Baltimore: Paul H Brookes, pp. 205–13.

Lenneberg EH (1967) Biological Foundations of Language. New York: Wiley.

MacKenzie S, Hulme C (1987) Memory span development in Down's syndrome, severely subnormal and normal subjects. Cognit Neuropsychol 4: 303–19.

Marcell MM, Weeks SL (1988) Short-term memory difficulties and Down's syndrome. J Ment Def Res 32: 153–62.

Masidlover M, Knowles W (1982) The Derbyshire Language Scheme. Alfreton: Derbyshire County Council.

Powell G, Clibbens J (1994) Actions speak louder than words: signing and speech intelligibility in adults with Down's syndrome. Down's Syndr Res Pract 2(3): 127–9.

Rondal J, Comblain A (1996) Language in adults with Down's syndrome. Down's Syndr Res Pract 4(1): 3–14.

Wishart J (1993) Learning the hard way: avoidance strategies in young children with Down's syndrome. Down's Syndr Res Pract 1(2): 47–55.

SECTION IV
PSYCHOSOCIAL, EDUCATIONAL AND PROFESSIONAL ASPECTS

Chapter 19
Sex and contraception in Down syndrome

H. GOLDSTEIN

Introduction and background

The topic of sexual relations has been increasingly discussed regarding adolescents and adults with Down syndrome (DS), probably due to the more open-minded attitudes in Europe during the past decades regarding sex and sexual relations. European culture has changed since World War 2, and together with increasing welfare in the health and social sector, the well-being of our patients and citizens has a high priority. This focus on quality of life for various patients with handicaps includes the right to sex. In particular, the way of life has changed for mentally handicapped citizens.

In Denmark, and probably most of Europe, many individuals with DS get better medical and social care, and, if possible, they are not institutionalized. They often live with their parents, siblings or other caregivers or in smaller community settings, where their privacy has improved. This means there is a possiblity to meet a boyfriend or girlfriend, and obviously the possiblity of, and wish to have, sexual relations.

As a result of these rather new circumstances, at least seen through the glasses of medical history, we have to be open-minded regarding the possibility of offspring, the need for contraception and the danger of sexual exploitation. There is a need for improved sex education for DS individuals as well as their caregivers, but this is not covered in this chapter. Such education is always based on national culture, building upon secular and religious attitudes.

It is unknown whether these new social conditions have, in fact, created more frequent sexual intercourse with DS individuals. Epidemiological surveys dealing with these questions still have to be conducted in a scientific, systematic way.

An important, and maybe the first, question to be asked is: Are individuals with Down syndrome fertile or not?

Fertility

Males with Down syndrome

Are DS males fertile? A review of the scientific literature forces us to accept that our knowledge is rather limited. More than 40 years ago, it was found by Stearns et al. (1960) that males with DS had poor quality sperm, if any production at all. Later Campbell et al. (1982) found that, in general, males with DS had smaller testes than controls, and they were softer when examined. Campbell et al. also stated that the FSH and LH values of these patients were elevated significantly, which means that their possibility of producing high quality sperm was reduced.

Very few cases of males with DS being a father have been reported. The first case was published in Journal of Medical Genetics in 1989 by Sheridan et al., and in spite of this case report, our knowledge of DS male fertility remains insufficient.

Females with Down syndrome

Medical knowledge of the fertility of DS females is more adequate. This may, however, be due to the fact that the medical speciality of gynaecology is so well developed, and no real medical speciality on male genitals exists.

Is the DS female fertile, and if so, at the same level as the non-DS female? There are several ways of investigating if ovulation occurs or not. Table 19.1 shows at least five aspects which need to be discussed in order to give a valid answer.

Table 19.1 Characteristics of fertility for females with Down syndrome

Menarche and menstrual cycles
Body temperature curves
Physical findings: external and internal genitalia
Serum hormone levels
Reported pregnancies

Menarche, menstrual cycles and body temperature curves

At least six scientific papers deal with the onset of menstruation, i.e. menarche. The results of these papers are summarized in Table 19.2.

Table 19.1 Age of menarche for females with Down syndrome: results of various studies

Study	Age of menarche (years)
Øster (1953)	13.9
Salerno et al. (1975)	18.3
Bellone et al. (1980)	13.1
Goldstein (1988)	13.6
Scola and Pueschel (1992)	12.5
Angelopoulou et al. (1999)	12.2

Three of the papers, Goldstein (1988), Scola and Pueschel (1992) and Angelopoulou et al. (1999), state that there is no significant difference between the onset of menstruation for DS women and non-DS women. The paper by Bellone et al. (1980) states a significantly later menarche in DS women than controls. Some papers find that the menstrual cycle of DS women is shorter than controls and some find that the menstrual cycle is normal.

We cannot conclude very much on ovulation when only considering the menstrual cycle and length. Therefore, some authors (Scola and Pueschel, 1992; Cento et al., 1996) used the method of finding a possible biphasic body temperature curve showing an elevated body temperature when ovulation occurs. They examined, however, only DS women with regular menstruation, and both papers used a very small number of women. There seems to be a real difference between the results.

At least three papers (Goldstein, 1988; Scola and Pueschel, 1992; Cento et al., 1996) find that the length of the menstrual cycle is similar among women with and without DS, although a few papers state that more cycles are without ovulation among DS women than among controls.

Hormone levels in serum

Probably the best method for finding out about ovulation is testing hormone levels, in particular progesterone in the luteal phase. A significant elevation of progesterone in the serum in this period is a strong indicator that ovulation has occurred.

Other hormones play a role in the evaluation, such as oestrogen, which participates in building the endometrium, and LH and FSH which participate in the mechanism of ovulation and ripening of the follicles in the ovary. However, elevated progesterone in the luteal phase of regularly menstruating women is probably the best sign of ovulation. From the literature (Cento et al., 1996; Angelopoulou et al., 1999), there seems to be evidence that ovulation occurs in many menstrual cycles among DS women, although not at the level of normal controls.

Internal and external genitalia

Although one may find that there are hormone levels compatible with ovulation, this is not the same as genitals compatible with normal sexual relations, pregnancy and delivery.

Some decades ago, several reports found that women with DS had smaller genitals than controls. One study by Højager et al. (1978) used pathological examinations to state that ovaries in DS women are smaller and abnormal compared to controls of the same age. However, a recent Greek study (Angelopoulou et al., 1999) found no difference between genitals among DS women and controls. The use of ultrasonography is extremely important and has been used in a recent Danish study by Ejskjær et al. (personal communication). The study finds most genitals normal by abdominal ultrasonography.

Pregnancy

It is possible for DS women to become pregnant, although the endocrinological findings may tell us that the likelihood of pregnancy is reduced. How much it is reduced is unknown; it is also linked to the frequency of sexual intercourse.

It is nearly 100 years since the first case report on pregnancy in a DS woman was published (Pogue, 1917). Until 1990, 31 pregnancies were reported in the literature, and such reports are not of any interest any longer. The risk/chance of pregnancy is present, and any physician dealing with DS patients should be aware of this fact.

Conclusion

It can be concluded that males with DS are rarely fertile, while women with DS seem to be more fertile.

Offspring

The above conclusion raises the delicate question of offspring for DS individuals, in particular women. It is not a new question, and the final answer probably does not exist. But the question can be analysed from at least four angles:

- The woman with DS
- The parents/caregiver of the DS woman
- The current interest of society
- The possible unborn child

Of course, there are several other ways of looking at this question, both from a social and from an ethical point of view.

The woman with Down syndrome

The central person is, however, the woman with DS, and whenever this problem is discussed, the question of the rights of the woman is raised. In Western culture most persons will emphasize that the DS woman has the same right as anybody else to reproduce. She also, however, has the same right to use contraception and choose not to reproduce. From a more philosophical point of view it can be stated that although the woman has the right to reproduce like anybody else, it does not mean that it is appropriate or wise to use this right.

Caregivers

The problem of possible offspring is probably different if parents and caregivers are asked. They may have difficulties in accepting, for example, that the unborn child may be raised in an inappropriate way and will suffer for the rest of its life. The point of view of parents or, for example, siblings of a DS individual may be based on rational thinking rather than legal or ethical rights. One may note that the discussion in which parents are very active is regarding the possible sterilization of their children; where non-parental caregivers are often strongly outspoken against sterilization, parents or siblings can often vary in their views.

This problem has been discussed for at least 50 years and probably more; the question was raised in a German medical journal from 1974 (Lenz) on the fertility of a 12-year-old DS girl. The mother had requested that her daugther be sterilized. The German gynaecologist at the time answered that, due to the reduced possibility of pregnancy, a sterilization could not be justified.

The interest of society

Another view is of the current interest of society. At the beginning of the 20th century, there was the attitude that Western societies should not include DS and other mentally handicapped citizens, if possible. Coercion was used in order to protect society by sterilizing mentally handicapped individuals.

It is a fact that coercion in medicine has been used many times. During the last two decades coercion has been used in some countries with regard to the HIV virus. Also in most countries we find coercion to some extent when we deal with serious psychiatric diseases. As a principle, coercion should not be used regarding sterilization of DS individuals, neither to protect society, the individual or anybody else.

The unborn child

We cannot deal with possible offspring of DS women without asking if the unborn child has any rights. The answer is no. Like any other person in this world, the unborn child of a DS individual does not choose its parents. One may ask if an individual can bring its parents to court, accusing them of being responsible for its birth. The legal, ethical and other aspects of such a question are not covered by this chapter.

Contraception

As long as it seems possible that at least the DS woman is fertile, contraception is a need, regardless of rights of reproduction. What are the demands for a contraceptive device for a DS woman? Are demands for contraceptive devices for DS women different to those of non-DS women? At least three qualities of a contraceptive device must be considered:

- The device should be as safe as possible
- The device must have minimal side effects
- The device should create no problems of compliance

There is no reason why safety and possible side effects should be different for DS females than for controls, but easy compliance is extremely important when dealing with females with DS. The contraceptives market is large, and, when dealing with mentally handicapped patients, the physician should focus on contraception which needs no daily action from the female herself. This means that any form of birth-control pill or the diaphragm should be excluded. The physician is, therefore, left with three serious possibilities, the intrauterine device (IUD), the progesterone rod and the progesterone injection.

If the female is menstruating regularly, the IUD with cupper is probably the most useful, since it does not disturb the regular cycles, although bleeding may be somewhat stronger. The rod and the injection often create irregular bleeding or no bleeding at all. These disturbances from regularity may create problems of understanding for the DS female. She has learnt that bleeding comes every month, and will need more biological education if using these methods.

It can be concluded that a regular IUD is preferred; if this is not possible, the progesterone rod should be tried. The progesterone injection can be given, but it cannot be removed, and possible side effects will last at least a few months.

References

Angelopoulou N, Souftas V, Sakadamis, A, Matziari C, Papameletiou V, Mandroukas K (1999) Gonadal function in young women with Down syndrome. Int J Gynecol Obstet 67: 15–21.

Bellone E, Tanganelli E, LaPlaca A, Danen C (1980) Menarca e fisiopatologia menstruale nella sindrome di Down. Minerva Gincol 32: 579–88.

Campbell WA, Lowther J, McKenzie I, Price WH (1982) Serum gonadotrophins in Down's syndrome. J Med Genet 19: 88–99.

Cento RM, Ragusa L, Proto C, Alberti A, Romano C, Boemi G et al. (1996) Basal body temperature curves and endocrine pattern of menstrual cycles in Down syndrome. Gynecol Endocrinol 10: 133–7.

Goldstein H (1988) Menarche, menstruation, sexual relations and contraception of adolescent females with Down syndrome. Eur J Obstet Gynecol Reprod Biol 27: 343–9.

Højager B, Peters H, Byskov AG, Faber M (1978) Follicular development in ovaries of children with Down's syndrome. Acta Paediatr Scand 67(5): 637–43.

Lenz W (1974) Fertilität mongoloider Frauen. Deutsche Medizinische Wochenschrift 99: 2193.

Øster J (1953) Mongolism. Copenhagen: Danish Science Press Ltd.

Pogue ME (1917) Brief report of 29 cases of mongolian idiocy, with special reference to etiology from standpoint of clinical history, with presentation of three cases. Illinois Med J 32: 296–8.

Salerno LJ, Park JK, Giannini MJ (1975) Reproductive capacity of the mentally retarded. J Reprod Med 14: 123–9.

Scola PS and Pueschel SM (1992) Menstrual cycles and basal body temperature curves in women with Down syndrome. Obstet Gynecol 79: 91–4.

Sheridan R, LLerna J, Matkins S, Debenham P, Cawood A, Bobrow M (1989) Fertility in a male with trisomy 21. J Med Genet 26: 294–8.

Stearns PE, Droulard KE, Sahhar FH (1960) Studies bearing on fertility on male and female mongoloids. Am J Ment Defic 65: 37–41.

Chapter 20
Mental disability and sexuality

F. VEGLIA

Introduction: models and discrepancies

There are not any special 'techniques' or specific answers to the many questions that a disabled person puts to the sexologist. We have to be satisfied with reasonable opinions, based on the experience of a few experts in this field, that are still temporary and incomplete.

In this chapter, I will briefly explain a theoretical model and a method of intervention which enable the application of sexology to handicap psychology and education.

Any sexual and affective behaviour can be subject to the interference of disabilities thus making it, at least partially, non-adaptive. The main deficits affect cognitive, meta-cognitive, affective, interpersonal and, occasionally, motor skills.

The following are the problems which appear most frequently in the sexual life of people suffering from mental insufficiency or psychiatric disorders:

- Deficit in the regulation of physical approach and contact. Contact with someone else's body is not appropriate to the situation, takes place unpredictably, and appears intrusive, vicious, coercive or is inappropriate to patterns and choice of the parts of the body to touch; or the contact was not negotiated
- Deficit in the regulation of social behaviour and intimacy: public stripping and exhibitionism. Quite often the act of stripping does not express sexual content, but is rather used to draw attention, to spite someone, or it might just be used to feel more comfortable or for self-gratification; in this case we should differentiate it from exhibitionism, a form of paraphilia consisting of being able to reach sexual arousal

only when showing genitals to people who certainly will not wish to engage in a relationship

- Deficit in the regulation of social behaviour and intimacy: public masturbation. Public masturbation can result, for people with more severe disabilities, from their inability to recognize the appropriate time and place, while people with milder disabilities can send messages to the people around them conveying sexual, aggressive or challenging content; it can instead be an indication of severe mental autarchy
- Deficit of the necessary skills for masturbation. We might observe either a meta-cognitive deficit of goal setting, emotion sequencing and control, or a deficit of the finer motility (let us consider, for instance, the difficulties connected with the stimulation of the clitoris) or the interference of any learning disorder or of the side effects of many psychiatric medications on the orgasm mechanism
- Compulsive masturbation. This is not usually a sign of sexual dysfunction but it is a symptom of either emotional distress (anxiety, depression, boredom are the most frequent inner states) or difficulties connected with the internal control mechanism
- Deficit of the necessary skills for an appropriate use of the genital apparatus. The lack of both explanatory and procedural knowledge and the difficulty in sequence building or appropriate goal representation can cause important dysfunctions connected with personal hygiene, autonomous management of menstruation or attempts at sexual gratification that might be wrong or indeed cause harm such as, for example, masturbating with objects that could easily cause bodily harm or excessive and self-injurious stimulation of the genital organs
- Deficit of the necessary skills for courting and difficulty in finding and choosing a partner
- Deficit in the regulation of seductive behaviour with exposure to the risk of sexual abuse. Patients suffering from psychosis or mental retardation usually show inability to make hypotheses and previsions on the inner state and intentions of other people, often associated with the lack of filters or inhibitions; all these aspects make them particularly sexually vulnerable
- Deficit of anger management causing the risk of violent sexual acting-out which can be both self-harmful and assaultive
- Issues related to performed hetero- or homosexual behaviours due to impaired cognitive, meta-cognitive, motor skills, poor impulse control and lack of interpersonal skills
- Issues related to sexual dysfunction and coital difficulties
- Issues related to unacknowledgement of the right to expression of sexuality, to marriage, parenthood or contraception for disabled persons
- Issues related to establishing love relationships and pair life projects
- Homosexuality induced by the compulsory and prolonged cohabitation with people of the same sex or denying of any heterosexual behaviour

The sexuality of disabled persons raises difficult issues and causes the emergence of some dramatic discrepancies in our educational approach. Currently, educational projects are guided by the fundamental principle of giving disabled persons the greatest autonomy possible, given their disabilities. However, the application of this principle to the sexual life of disabled persons is constantly disregarded: educational interventions rarely aim at facilitating autonomous expression of their sexuality.

When we deal with sexual issues, there are, apparently, no convincing arguments for not giving back all the possible freedom to disabled persons: the most probable reasons for the reversal of this trend are to be found in our fears.

As a matter of fact, the model that refers to the greatest autonomy possible provides that its procedures for application are organized according to a precise hierarchy. When we have to deal with problematic sexual behaviours, we normally try first of all to provide training on the missing skills and knowledge; only when this attempt seems to be insufficient or when one of our agency users is exposed to the risk of causing harm to him or herself or to other people, do we decide to suppress, restrict or contain his or her behaviour.

Since almost every problem related to the sexual life of individuals with disabilities is due to some kind of deficit, a good rehabilitation plan should first of all provide for the training of new skills and, secondly, if necessary, for the suppression of inappropriate behaviours. In the field of sexuality, however, the logical sequence is once more reversed and instead of proposing educational interventions we often design restrictive interventions. It is clear that this second problem is a consequence of the first: since we do not feel up to dealing with the sexuality of disabled individuals we necessarily have to intervene to suppress it.

Another discrepancy is related to the choice of the ground on which we want to work. Commonsense tells us that it is better to cultivate the rich ground first and later, if we have time, the less fertile fields. The sexuality of mentally disabled persons is, in most cases, spontaneously active and definitely a healthy aspect of their life, since it is controlled by parts of the brain which are normally not affected by damage: therefore there are plenty of good reasons for using it. Nonetheless it is almost always deliberately neglected. Although sexuality is a biologically healthy aspect, impaired cognitive, affective, relational and behavioural skills can interfere with it and, consequently, it might result in inappropriate behaviours or show many difficulties. This is, however, the actual reason why we take care of disabled individuals.

Yet, the idea of allowing, teaching and facilitating the use of an appropriate sexuality might seem so dangerous, involved or even unrestrainable that, most of the time, we fail to cultivate this fertile ground. If we had to make a decision for ourselves, we would hardly prefer to learn, with a great effort, the use of cutlery, shoe laces or methods to bind books rather than the appropriate use of our body to express desire, love, arousal or to share sexual pleasure. When we make decisions for other people, however, we find it is more reassuring taking care of thousands of other issues rather than arousing or managing the dangerous world of their sexuality.

The main issue seems to be our own sexual life. Any educational intervention challenges us as human beings and requires that we are willing to share meanings and emotions, that we are aware of our cognitive and affective mechanisms, that we take on the responsibility of making decisions for other people. It is actually much more difficult to share the daily sufferings of disabled persons than the joy and surprise produced by a caress; it is much more dangerous to allow two patients to cross the street than to sleep in the same bed. Nonetheless, sex keeps on frightening us.

Between sexual education and suppression

Some people are compelled to deal with their life within the limits imposed by some physical or mental disability. This apparently obvious concept has become, with difficulty, part of the scientific culture. Some 'experts' still assert that 'disabled people are human beings'. This is of course much better than still having doubts about it but is nonetheless an unfortunate statement, since it assumes that the category 'disabled' connotes those people as being thought of as other than 'human beings'.

Obviously, what disabled people have in common with everyone else is that part of the ontological dimension that many believers call soul, which if it exists, cannot be investigated by the biological sciences. Furthermore, what they also have in common with so-called 'normal people' (those showing less visible and impairing disabilities) is a brain that tries, as much as possible, to survive, to maintain a reasonable control over the body and the external environment, to engage in positive relationships with other human beings, to make reliable hypotheses, to give events a meaning, to have an impact on events with some degree of freedom, to develop some knowledge and awareness, to share this experience with someone else and telling a story, placing all this in the flow of time.

The sexuality of persons with disabilities is a normal disabled sexuality. Obviously, disabilities, especially mental ones, do not enable people to live a normal life, at least considering it from a statistical point of view. A considerable percentage of normally intelligent people can learn many things which are, on the contrary, precluded to a small minority of persons with disabilities. However, this does not mean that the brain of a disabled person has modified its general logic, its motivational system, its biological, evolutionary and personal goals. If we consider its functional limits, disabilities and lack of skills, it is clear that disabled persons will use extraordinary strategies to solve personal and interpersonal problems. According to the seriousness of their disabilities, they might become so extreme and bizarre that other people cannot understand them. Again, this does not mean that the brain has lost the typical functioning of the human being.

Unfortunately descriptive diagnostics, being easier and more cursory than the explanatory one, easily leads people into error and to confuse the form with the content of the disorder. It is, in fact, unreasonable to replace attempts at functional understanding of mental disorder with the statistical definition of categories of disabled individuals, recurrent symptoms and useful techniques to make their life as similar as possible to a presumed normal existence.

Rather than normalizing disabled persons, we would be better off bringing our attitude towards them and their sexuality back to normal.

For all the reasons mentioned above, we strongly oppose any sexology designed especially for disabled persons. We have a more beneficial normal (and clinical) sexology, thought of and designed for human beings in general.

Those who work with disabled individuals need to know the fundamentals of psychological, educational and rehabilitative interventions and to master a reasonable theory on sexuality. Many particular applications will derive from this.

In many cases it is necessary to provide something more than just one-to-one supervision to the disabled person. The sexual supervisor also needs to know how to interact with relatives and caregivers, who usually have direct knowledge and the needed relational skills to address the problem and support it in practice.

Furthermore, caregivers quite often look directly for sexual supervision. They are in fact often involved in complicated relationships with their patients, in which sexuality becomes a source of distress, ambiguity and conflict. Many individuals with disabilities fall in love or sexually desire their caregivers. They often are the same age, might be attractive and be compelled, on professional grounds, to touch them daily in any part of their bodies.

It also happens that a caregiver or a nurse might be sensitive, for instance, to the seductiveness of a beautiful psychotic patient who, free from filters normally used in social relations, is able to send direct, intense and perfectly aimed sexual signs.

The sexual supervisor should be able to address similar issues without any dramatization and, instead, give them a precise ethical, clinical and educational definition. Although love between two people has always been to some extent mysterious and therefore unquestionable, a sexual relationship between a clear-headed and aware person and someone confused by affection disorders or meta-cognitive deficits gives way to the strong suspicion of abuse. In a similar way an eventual love relationship would always be unbalanced and it would be necessary to look into the motivations that push a normally intelligent person to engage in such an atypical relationship: is it due to perversion, a need to dominate other people, hyperactivity in looking after people or is it just inscrutable love?

The sexual supervisor should be able to lead the caregiver to become self-aware and aware of his or her own sexuality. The supervisor should help the caregiver to read critically all the signs, which are unexpectedly sent every day by those people he or she takes care of.

Issues related to disturbed sexuality in the family are even more complicated and, in some cases, tragic. Unsatisfied sexual desires might provoke very deep anxiety states in people who do not have any skill to delay, give a meaning to or 'sublimate' the most urgent drives. This acute suffering, that might become manifest in aggressive, hypomaniac, depressive, dissociative aspects, pushes some parents, especially mothers of psychotic or severely disturbed patients, to have sexual relationships with them. We are not talking of incest, but rather of a form of compassion that must not and cannot be judged; it only requires help. It is an excessive burden for the psychological balance of a mother and we are not certain that sleeping with her could be really profitable for her son, even though he is impaired with respect to any other form of sexual life.

An equally piercing helplessness is felt, even if for different reasons, by those parents who see their son or daughter in love with a normal person, knowing that his/her dream will never come true. This attempt to prevent future despair and disappointment is one of the main reasons why parents try to deny sexuality to their children.

It is clear that none of these problems can be addressed with predefined technical solutions: half secret 'use' of prostitutes, planned sexological nursing, summer camps for people with disabilities, chemical castration, suppression, sexual surrogates are some of the intervention attempts already employed in different countries without producing any convincing and definitive model.

The sexual expert should know how to listen, understand and arrange the issue in the context of a reasonable scientific hypothesis, personalize, historicize and then finally explore the possible ways of coping with the issue. It is normal that we are not able to solve all the problems which are taken on for supervision. Unfortunately this becomes the rule with persons with disabilities: understanding their distress, giving suffering a meaning and sharing problems is something important that we can offer to those who suffer.

Suppression of inappropriate sexual behaviour

Interventions designed to increase knowledge are strictly connected with repressive ones: we need at least to understand on what grounds a behaviour is problematic, for whom it is problematic, what is the cause or what is the expressed meaning, which strategies we master to modify it, and which of them produce the best outcomes with the least distress possible for people who undergo them.

We must above all consider that we might teach the individuals an alternative sexual behaviour. Treatment of non-adaptive sexual behaviours is actually more complicated during assessment and design than at the concrete stage.

Masturbation performed compulsively, for instance, or at inappropriate times, places and ways, exhibitionism, intrusiveness and abuse are all sexual behaviours which are generally considered quite disturbing.

However, we must remember that suffering and the feeling of constraint due to a lack of autonomy make the quest for pleasure and personal satisfaction, typical of any human being, even more pressing. Sexual gratification is a powerful organizer of self-knowledge and self-image. Those behaviours, that we promptly judge as non-adaptive are quite often the best answer possible to the distress felt by people with disabilities. Caregivers may feel extremely distressed when they decide that the brief, ill-assorted gratification derived from inappropriate or disturbing behaviours must be eradicated. It is often something difficult to elaborate for them. Therefore, before any intervention, we should remember that:

• We should try to understand the logic behind any behaviour. It sometimes follows the rule of 'everything immediately' or 'less bad'. This logic might be negative if used to accomplish complicated projects while it is often useful to survive and to satisfy the most urgent needs
• Considering that any behaviour is meaningful, it is not possible to extinguish any behaviour without replacing it with a more appropriate one that satisfies the same needs
• Preventing anyone from using a certain behaviour without proposing any other alternative is, in any case, a cruelty which may create rage and deep anxiety in those who experience it
• If we want to set up alternatives, we necessarily have to convey new skills
• Any intervention restricting individual initiative or repressing inappropriate behaviours is meaningful only in the context of an educational project aimed at developing the person's self-determination and the greatest autonomy possible allowed by his or her disability
• Decisions about the problematic nature of inappropriate behaviours should precede any treatment and be grounded on rigorous criteria, shared by the whole working group

Should anyone decide to intervene to reduce the intensity or frequency of either an offensive sexual behaviour or harmful self-stimulation, it would be profitable to apply the Least-restrictive Treatment Model, designed by Foxx (1986) and adapted by Veglia (1991), for managing non-adaptive sexual behaviours.

The correct application of this model requires the rigorous knowledge and use of the following rules:

• Assess the baseline of inappropriate behaviour performed by the person
• Review available literature on the treatment, with the goal of determining the most effective treatment procedures to reduce or eliminate the inappropriate behaviour

- Within the most effective treatment procedures, choose the least restrictive one
- Continue ongoing collection of objective and reliable data to determine the actual effectiveness of the applied treatment
- Exposure of an individual to a more restrictive treatment is acceptable only if ongoing data show ineffectiveness of a previous procedure
- Should it be necessary to use extremely restrictive programmes, all concerned parties should share the decision-making process

Procedures used to manage sexual issues of individuals with disabilities can normally be used with any other person or to solve any other sex-related problem. However, it is necessary to choose them with competence since not every known technique is appropriate for the treatment of the different non-adaptive behaviours.

Differential reinforcement of alternative behaviours, differential reinforcement of appropriate behaviours (not very restrictive), differential reinforcement of incompatible behaviours, satiation, negative practice, termination, physical restraint, timeout and hypercorrection are some of the primary procedures.

Application of reinforcement of appropriate behaviours is particularly important, since it maintains the intrinsic connection between suppression of behaviours and development of new skills. When applied to sexuality, this normally effective, synthetic and elegant intervention conceals great difficulty for the caregiver. In fact, since there are no specific needs to be satisfied, the most effective reinforcement is sharing events and emotional states with other people, especially those important for our life. Reinforcing a more appropriate sexual behaviour (though not yet perfectly 'normal') means publicly showing joy, satisfaction and gratification for expressions of sexuality which people normally do not completely accept and understand themselves. On the other hand, more restrictive procedures can be delivered within the context of emotional detachment and keeping safe distances.

An in-depth knowledge of educative methods and, obviously, competence in the field of sexology are therefore necessary to give professional advice on reducing inappropriate sexual behaviours.

Methodology of sexual skills teaching: the example of masturbation

Masturbation is one of the most frequent meeting points between the educative approach based on teaching new skills and the approach based on the modification or suppression of inappropriate behaviours. Being able to masturbate appropriately in an adequate place and time, is normally an excellent alternative to many other behaviours which are usually experienced as extremely problematic.

I am going to discuss this applicative issue as an emblematic example of the knowledge and operations necessary to articulate an educational and rehabilitative intervention into the sexual behaviour of a person with disabilities.

Exploring one's own body, experiencing the related gratification, finding out the most sensitive parts, feeling the drive to stimulate them, learning gradually more and more sophisticated ways to increase arousal, usually taking peers as models, are all behaviours that make up the path that leads to learning how to masturbate.

Although this behaviour might seem egoistic, it constitutes a useful premise to learn how to make love. We might say it allows one to become familiar with an important aspect of body language; and, above all, to teach someone who desires us, how to approach our body. If it were unknown to us, it could be much more difficult to get on well with someone else, especially if we had some disabilities.

Since masturbation is an intentional behaviour, except for compulsive events and the strong biological drive that controls it in determined periods of our life, it must also be assessed from the perspective of ethics. Before designing any intervention, an educative environment, given the set of principles it refers to, should deal with and define this aspect of the issue.

A group of caregivers might have decided, after a frank reflection, that masturbation could be, for some of their service's users, an appropriate behaviour to reply to sexual desire. It might be a definitive solution for some of them; some others might use it temporarily while awaiting access to sexual relationships; masturbation should obviously take place in the appropriate way, time and place. If, for instance, the above mentioned group of caregivers had made this decision, they might have to deal with a consequent quite complicated problem.

Many people with disabilities try insistently to masturbate without, however, succeeding in experiencing any gratification or attaining orgasm. If they are particularly inexperienced, they might sometimes even self-injure or insert items, built for other purposes, in their vagina. Desire to experience sexual gratification is expressed normally, but cognitive and motor deficits related to their disability might cause constant failures which have a negative impact on their mood. If any time we make love, some events that we cannot understand prevent us from performing and finishing the experience of gratification, we would certainly become quite nervous, depressed or even aggressive. Therefore it should not astonish us if the continuous failure to experience gratification makes our patients restless. It is not masturbation that upsets them, as someone said, ideologically simplifying the issue, but rather being unable to masturbate appropriately.

Following the thread of the argument, in similar cases it would be necessary to:

- Perform a task analysis aimed at precise definition of prerequisites, skills and behaviour sequence necessary to masturbate successfully

- Verify which of the above are already present and which must be taught
- Define strategies to facilitate learning of any lacking skill
- Set goals carefully since certain medication or CNS lesions might prevent individuals with disabilities from attaining orgasm
- Set up a step-by-step learning process, based on task, chained responses, help, correct use of gratification and eventually use of one's own behaviour as a model
- Identify places and times in everyday life where the learning process can be physiologically inserted
- Relate masturbation to the normal stage of desire and arousal to avoid separating it from the normal physiology and psychology of pleasure
- Choose only one caregiver who will provide the training on masturbation
- Verify that the caregiver has the appropriate features and skills to work on this topic and that he or she is supported by the working group
- Teach the appropriate masturbation behaviour, tailoring the intervention to the ongoing outcomes
- Teach the appropriate time, place and opportunities in which masturbation can be used
- Work towards autonomy and self-determination, giving privacy, which has been necessarily violated to provide education, back to the disabled person

Performing the task analysis and thus reflecting on masturbation, we will soon realize that it is not as simple as we would believe.

Masturbation requires being able to collect sensory and proprioceptive signals coming from genital organs, giving them attention, having a discrete fine motor ability, being able to connect events through cause–effect relationships, using intentional behaviours that partially self-reinforce and in turn require the skill of designing beyond short-term actions. In other words, it requires one to know one's own body, to know how it reacts when stimulated, to learn how to touch it with delicate and fine movements (especially in the case of vulva and clitoris stimulation), to keep on performing the action waiting for the orgasm-related sensations which are still remote, being aware that those sensations will be the outcome of carrying on the action and of the attention on changes in the level of pleasure. These are by no means simple cognitive and behavioural operations and many people with disabilities are unable to activate them. Many normally intelligent people quite often show the same disabilities.

At a more complicated level of cognitive organization we may observe other hindrances to masturbation such as, for instance, difficulty in abandoning oneself to pleasure-related sensations fearing to lose control, interference of performance anxiety, fear of harming oneself, feelings of guilt, fear of being caught or of negative social opinion.

A decision to teach masturbation should be supported by a careful assessment of the present situation. Necessary data to design the intervention might be obtained through an interview if the patient has a mild disability or through direct observation in more serious instances.

As in any other intervention on sexuality we need to know exactly what happens at each stage of the behaviour that we want to modify or teach, otherwise we might seriously embarrass the patient or, what is more, the caregiver who performs the observation. Therefore we should wonder what is most serious, the momentary embarrassment or the impossibility to intervene? I believe that using a little bit of experience, good taste, and sense of situations we are able to know whatever we need without causing any particular problem. It is, however, necessary not to fear sex.

The caregiver that intervenes to teach a disabled person how to masturbate should have the following features:

- Good skills in sexology
- Expertise in using teaching techniques
- Clarity about the nature and ethical implications of the behaviour he or she is going to teach
- A defined motivation for intervention totally consistent with his or her own set of values and beliefs and at least compatible with those used by the working group
- An in-depth knowledge of his or her own sexual experiences
- Ability to manage emotions in a sophisticated way, especially those emotions related to sexuality
- A positive relationship with his or her own body and a secure approach to that of others
- Ability to exclude any morbid interest towards the patient or the learning situation
- Knowing it is not the case that the patient has any sexual interest or has fallen in love with him or her
- Ability to play a well accepted educative role causing sympathy and peacefulness without possibly being the primary caregiver or substituting for parents
- Can use problem-solving to correct possible mistakes but is not afraid to make mistakes
- Can lead by the patient's feedback, tailor the intervention to the person rather than the 'case', and thus avoid technicalities and anonymity

Intervention can be applied only when all the above described conditions are fulfilled; this is in a very limited number of instances.

The ethical aspect of the issue is however difficult to solve, especially if referring to Catholic morality. It is an almost unexplored area where the only certainty is that we cannot go on acting as if the profound suffering of an unexpressed and disabled sexuality does not exist (Veglia 1991).

Sexual education for persons with disabilities

Sexual education for individuals with disabilities cannot therefore be considered as optional; on the contrary it is an integral part of any intervention aimed at modifying their behaviour. It would be even better if it could become a proposal, a project developing sexuality for the users of our services even when they do not express any problems. It is a fundamental aspect of human life and, unless we have specific reasons, we should not disregard it when we think about the future of someone we have at heart or we take care of.

To cope with some of the specific issues of sexual education for people with disabilities we need to define the meaning of some educative principles and so-called normal sexuality.

In reality, sex defies any definition. Any attempt at classification seems immediately reductive. On the one hand this allows us to feel free in giving our sexual life a very personal meaning, while on the other, if we want to address the issue, we necessarily have to agree on a shared view.

The most common perspective is that of biology. Sexuality is an excellent trick of nature to push us towards reproduction, recombining our genetic endowment. It is a quite expensive project (let us think of how many resources we use to court someone) that focuses on differences to gain a better adaptation to the environment.

In reality, experiences related to the act of coupling are much more complicated than a simple reproductive event and depend, for instance, on our opinions about life, who creates it, what responsibilities we have towards our children or how we can look for a glimmer of immortality through their existence. Making love for some people makes a difference: for those who believe in God, procreation requires divine intervention, while a male and a female are enough for a positivist.

Already at the beginning of the 1960s, the United Nations acknowledged in principle the right to sexuality, even to procreation, for all human beings independently from the typology or seriousness of their disability. More recently, the *Standard Rules on the Equalization of Opportunities for Persons with Disabilities*, elaborated in 1993 by the UN, acknowledge the right to sexual life, procreation, parenthood and to have the same access as others to available services for the education of their children. Some individuals with disabilities do not even consider it an issue; while, on the other hand, it might be necessary to make every possible effort to dissuade other people with disabilities from exercising it, although in full respect of their basic right. Finally, for those affected by milder mental disabilities we are often on the threshold of an ineffable mystery.

Also within the perspective of biology, sex might be considered as a special way of being together designed by Nature or God to give a further good reason to build a stable and lasting relationship necessary to offer a mother and a father to a defenceless and slow-growing progeny. A belief shared today both by science and the Catholic religion is that sex is also a way to exchange reciprocal pleasure and love and this idea also offers wide opportunities for individuals with disabilities.

Self-eroticism itself, considered from a developmental point of view, might be a transitory way (although it might be definitive in some instances) to learn sexuality and gradually approach a shared experience. However, if we forget the reproductive goal, there are a variety of ways to exchange love and pleasure that are appropriate to anyone, including individuals with disabilities who can at least partially interact with other people or with themselves.

A second perspective considers sex as a form of knowledge. It is not a new idea, it has rather been rediscovered: 'to know one another' in the Old Testament meant to make love. Through sexuality we can know ourselves and other people in a way that is as valuable and deep as it is tacit, immediate and difficult to express in words. And exactly for this reason it is more comprehensible for those with deficits which impair their language and reasoning. It might be easier to talk about it using the metaphor of caressing, which refers to all the possible caresses that a man and a woman (or two people of the same sex) can exchange using hands, mouth, vagina, penis and any other part of the body.

A caress is given with the body and, in its simplest form, consists in touching another body to experience pleasure. Putting one's hand between someone else's legs gives quite exciting sensations. We can feel pleasure if someone touches us in this way but we will soon feel as if we were just an object and we will even think that some people establish a price to let other people touch them. We probably expect something more. In fact, the body we touch with a caress is a special place where we can meet other people: in this way we would touch someone with our hand. Fingers, among the rest, speak a universal language and enable us to communicate messages through the old language of signs, telling what we are not able to say with words. Through caresses, we can communicate emotions, affections and feelings with an unbelievable precision; we can even express what we are thinking in our imagination. Saying with words to a woman, 'I want to touch you and make you mine because you are the one that I love and I am happy, and I will always desire you as much as I did while I was waiting for you' is quite difficult and somewhat awkward while we can communicate it perfectly with our hands.

The caresses that individuals with disabilities can give are moving, silent, full of shared meanings and pleasure. Although mental deficits quite often make their reasoning difficult, can anyone say that they are completely lacking in thought and knowledge? Should anyone have met and embraced a person suffering from serious mental handicap, they would have grasped in that hug intentions, emotions, meanings and sharing, therefore, knowledge incarnate.

How can we deliberately deny sexual caresses to people with disabilities? They may make mistakes and seem to forget that caresses are nicer if they express the whole person in one unique gesture. They sometimes are rude, arrogant, reductive, awkward or seem to touch objects more than persons and might even insult each other. What about us? Are our caresses always the integrated expression of our whole being? Have we ever touched someone else without love, have we ever experienced pleasure while keeping distance from the partner, or taken some satisfaction without saying anything? If persons with disabilities have more difficulty in setting up good caresses, then it is our duty at least to try to teach them.

The overall strategy that we will use to give experiences of sexual caresses back to persons with disabilities will consist of patient work of reconstructing meta-cognitive, emotional and interpersonal skills, within the limits of their disabilities.

And finally, sex might be considered as a story. When telling people about our love experiences, we often say 'I had a story with Marco' which is quite different from saying 'I had sex with Marco', a typical expression to describe occasional sexual intercourse. Giving a time perspective to caresses enables us to set up a project and to experience sexuality as a story made up of images, gestures, characters. Making love then becomes a way to recognize each other and to choose each other again, to talk about the reciprocal love and share its meaning. The desire of seeking the other person through his or her body will then still be active when we get old and the pleasure for young flesh becomes genuine passion for the older. Over time, in the course of the story, the body will be transfigured and become beautiful, even the apparently awful body of many persons with disabilities. With the simplicity of their stories, many disabled persons have overcome their caregivers' relationships in terms of faithfulness, duration and sometimes even richness of meaning.

Shared experiences, reciprocal knowledge and story give sex a meaning. Caregivers intervening to teach, correct and rehabilitate must know the caresses they want to take care of and are compelled to partial violation of their patients' privacy to protect them from abuse. It is necessary to accompany sexual desire with awareness, intentionality (a positive way of being in the relationship), the ability to modulate emotions and a trace of meaning. If these features are totally lacking, caresses might become quite questionable. On the contrary, should there be little traces, they would show that we are on the right track.

For the sexual education of persons with disabilities we would be better to refer to a model for 'normal' people, tailoring it, with partial changes, to the peculiar situation of each patient.

The cognitive, meta-cognitive and interpersonal deficits of disabled persons quite evidently require an emotion-provoking relationship between trainer and trainee. While a normally intelligent person is able to correct inevitable mistakes and lack of teaching cognitively and almost in real time, the person with disabilities should be able to make good use of the emotional and affective knowledge channel, which is usually readily available and functions better. Emotions, in fact, motivate learning, enabling the individual to receive constant feedback from what happens inside themselves and in other people and take part meaningfully in the process of knowing the world. The problem is that when teaching sexual education we come in touch with sexual emotions and we are not used to sharing them in the educative context. If we say in words that what we are talking about is really beautiful, our state of mind should be on the same wave-length of sexual pleasure. The best way we can experience it is by talking about a beautiful movie, which is running before our eyes, where we could be the protagonist or the satisfied audience. If we could hire 'actors' with disabilities in our minds, and test the consistency and quality of our emotions, we would then be reliable. The screenplays of such 'movies' require a good knowledge of oneself and one's own sexuality.

The contents we want to transmit through this emotion-provoking relationship should be determined by an arbitrary decision within a variety of possible issues about human sexuality. Since there is no objective and neutral method for providing sexual education for individuals with disabilities, I usually prefer to talk to them only about the ideas on sexuality that will take bodily form in the caresses their hands will give. There is a question that, in my opinion, should help us constantly in choosing the information we want to transmit to them: 'Is what I want to teach them useful, will it help them to know each other, to court, choose, caress and better enjoy the love of each other?'

The words we use to explain male and female bodies, their functioning in the experience of pleasure, how we can make use of them by ourselves or with someone else, then issues about sexual health, love and relationships should be simple, domestic and familiar, and everyone should understand them, even if they have not had a chance to study. A cold, distant, difficult scientific language is useful only if we do not want to provoke any emotions while pretending to talk about the pleasure of love. The use of a familiar lexicon requires precision, fantasy and a little bit of happiness; the effect will certainly be positive and above all, it will enable everyone to talk sincerely, at least when they need to.

When we deal with individuals with mental disabilities, words are not the right instrument for approaching reality and knowing the world. The only genuine alternative is the direct experience on one's own body or on a model's: exactly what we do with any other kind of learning. For some reasons related to respecting other people's privacy it is not easy to use our own or someone else's body as a teaching instrument; however if we respect some fundamental deontological and methodological rules, it turns out to be the only sensible way to make knowledge possible, overcoming, at least partially, the limits imposed by the disability.

Any information we succeeded in transmitting would be totally useless unless the person who received it could give it a meaning. In reality, for any new knowledge there are always four different meanings. The first is a logical meaning: what I learned should constitute a logical and goal-orientated sequence of thoughts and behaviours. The second is ethical because I should use it to do good things, and aesthetic because I should be able to do beautiful things. Above all, it has a personal meaning because my caress should be recognized as unique and unrepeatable: it probably is not the expert gesture of a masseur but it is a touch incarnated by me and my personal history. The essence of caresses is, in reality, to go to bed with the genuine history of a special person. Although logic might be lacking, ethics, aesthetics and personal meanings can always be found wherever intention and awareness, even if with no words at all (and it might be even better), are preserved. Experience of the field and many theoretical principles allow us to believe that the core of these meanings might be proposed to many persons with disabilities even if with some obvious difficulties.

Let us try to imagine that we want to talk to a disabled girl about her vulva and vagina and help her know them. Although maintaining a scientific rigour, we should avoid using medical language and choose only those contents that will be fundamental for her caresses and experiences; we should find a way to let her learn by experience and then allow her to give, for instance, her labia a functional, ethical, aesthetical and personal meaning. A special way to experience herself as beautiful, good and able to carry those sweet, warm, tender folds of skin in her body and maybe, one day, to offer them and meet someone else.

Many people seem to believe that making love means having coitus with another person, preferably of a different sex, and thus attaining orgasm. A similar behaviour is probably too complicated for some persons with disabilities and it could turn out to be disappointing and reductive.

Our distorted and stereotyped perspective on sexual relationships often induces us to consider them as not really appropriate for disabled persons. We had better give any gesture back its original value, setting aside the meaning it must assume in the chain of compulsory and necessary behaviours. Making love means trying to share some pleasure with someone else.

Pleasure is not only a physical sensation. It is an experience that comprises all the meanings, emotions and sensations that we experience, sometimes in an unexpressed way, feeling complicity and abandoning ourselves in the arms of another person. It is communication, spectacle and creativity. Schemes make it fade, playing regenerates it, it expands beyond the body and passes its limits and boundaries.

Knowing the rules of the game and having developed the necessary skills, making love might be a limited experience for people with disabilities, although not as reductive as it often is for normally intelligent persons.

Although gestures and thoughts of mentally handicapped persons might have limits, it does not mean that their experience of love will have limits as well (Veglia, 1991).

The word incarnate

Human sexual behaviour is largely learned.

Meanings that we can give to love gestures and the opportunity to transform them into a language are beyond the reproductive goal of the sexual experience.

This is the argument that has led us so far; it has formed the basis of our theoretical and methodological model for many years and it has been widely confirmed by research and everyday practice.

The body is a finer instrument than the word because it can communicate countless nuances, it allows establishment of immediacy and reciprocity with someone else and it has the inimitable property of incarnating and manifesting emotions.

The emotional, dialogical and unitive use of the body is allowed by biological programmes that organize and guide behaviour; however, in the course of life it intertwines with the development of individual awareness. Experience, learning, events and the countless meanings given to reality make up the structure of the dialogue between bodies.

Even very complicated contents can be transmitted through these elementary, analogical and extremely versatile codes. The simplicity of its syntax, the innate basis of forming sentences, the possibility of avoiding problems related to choosing words, make body language extremely appropriate for persons with mental disabilities.

Since sexual life is mainly based on non-verbal language, it could even be a privileged field of experience for people with disabilities if compared to other forms of communication that make them face their deficits much more dramatically.

People with severe disabilities will not transmit any concept through their bodies, but rather pure emotions. Although many people could complain about it or think it is reductive and use it as an excuse to deny sexuality to persons with disabilities, we, and other people too, prefer not to express definitive judgements on the ineffable mystery of human mind and being. We wish to think that the experiences of pleasure and love are not necessarily the outcome of knowledge based on word and concept elaboration. And we would like to enable disabled persons to experience sexuality in an atmosphere of love, in any silent, emotional or inscrutable way they can. Anyone who has tried to communicate with persons with disabilities knows, even though it might be difficult to find the words to talk about it, that their caresses and hugs are full of deep emotions and reciprocal understanding (Veglia, 1991).

However, as with any other language, body language should be learned, to develop and become real speech even if in its more elementary forms. Quite often disabilities make learning difficult and caregivers who agree on the importance of sexual life for persons with disabilities, should facilitate it using all their human and professional skills.

Bibliography

Baldaro Verde J (1987) La sessualità dell'handicappato. Roma; Il Pensiero scientifico.

Bara BG (1990) Scienza cognitiva. Torino: Bollati Boringhieri.

Bruner J (1990) The Culture of Education. Cambridge: Harvard University Press (tr. It. La cultura dell'educazione. Milano: Feltrinelli, 1997).

Damasio AR (1995) L'errore di Cartesio. Emozione, ragione e cervello umano. Milano: Adelphi.

Dixon H (1990) Anch'io ... L'educazione alla sessualità nell'handicappato. Trento: Erickson.

Foxx RM (1986) Increasing Behaviors of Severely Retarded and Autistic Persons, Decreasing Behaviors of Severely Retarded and Autistic Persons. USA: Research Press (tr. It. Tecniche base del metodo comportamentale, Trento: Erickson).

Veglia F (1991) Una carne sola: insegnare la sessualità agli handicappati. Milano: Angeli.

Veglia F (1992) Il discorso sul metodo. In AA. VV. Disabilità e apprendimento. Torino: Omega.

Veglia F (1996) I disturbi sessuali. In BG Bara (ed.) Manuale di psicoterapia cognitiva. Torino: Bollati Boringhieri.

Veglia F (1999) Storie di vita. Narrazione e cura in psicoterapia cognitiva. Torino: Bollati Boringhieri.

Chapter 21
Siblings in the family of a person with Down syndrome

J. PERERA

We all know from experience that in the development and maturation of a person, the family has a decisive influence and that within the family, siblings play an important role. Since Lobato (1954) published his work on 'Brothers, sisters and special needs', many articles have been published concerning the role of siblings in the family with a person with disability, and Down syndrome (DS) in particular.

In my opinion, the role of siblings has changed radically in the last 10 years due to two fundamental factors:

1. The greater life expectancy of persons with DS
2. The change of the family 'model' in our developed society

The impact of the birth of a child with Down syndrome on the family

Since the 1960s, studies have been undertaken on the impact that the birth of a child with DS has on the family group. These studies started by investigating the reactions of the mother to the birth of a child with DS, emphasizing the frequent attitude of overprotection, once the initial shock had been overcome. Later studies started to consider the father as an independent element (Kazan and Marvin, 1984) with reactions of depression and low self-esteem, while also studying the marital reaction and its response. Both parents generally pass from shock to acceptance, following a sequence of determined behaviours that we can generally classify in three phases (Garrard and Richmond, 1963):

* Emotional disorganization
* Period of reintegration (mobilization of defences)

• Phase of mature adaptation

Over the last 10 years, it has been considered necessary to analyse family relationships from the perspective of a new family model. More dynamic and realistic, the model is based on four sub-systems in continuous interaction: marital, parental, sibling and extra-family. This interaction between the four sub-systems is the key element in evaluating whether the family nucleus is sufficiently stimulating and appropriate to force the global development of the child with DS.

In general, we can say that no evidence exists to support the notion that having a baby with DS automatically produces negative effects in the family system and sub-systems (marital, parental, sibling and extra-family), or in any particular one. Occasionally, it can even be positive, and the relationships established can be enriching, for both siblings and parents. Evidence does not exist that suggests that couples with children with DS have a greater tendency to separate. Indeed, many are strengthened by the experience of having a child with this condition (Kazan and Marvin, 1984).

It is logical that conflicts will occur in the family, many of which can be eliminated if they are identified and discussed with greater sincerity.

The parents of a baby with DS are not conscious that their social life has become restricted, that things get harder as the child grows up and that they depend on his or her level of independence and of the family possibilities. Consequently, we must consider that the marital response is never going to be uniform, but will depend on a series of factors such as:

• The severity of the mental handicap
• The age and gender of the baby. The birth of a boy with DS appears to produce a greater negative effect (Farber, 1971)
• The quality of the marital relationship prior to the birth
• The relationship with the community, support systems and other ecological variables (Crnic et al., 1983)

How does the birth of a child with Down syndrome affect siblings?

It is evident that the new family situation that is produced by the birth of a child with DS fully affects siblings. Generally, it is the siblings, even though they may have been born later and are younger, who adopt the senior role. Women also exercise the role of substitute mothers, with the negative consequences this can have on their normal personal and social development; sometimes they will adopt positions of dedication and sacrifice in life, and ultimately comprise a high risk group for behavioural problems (Crnic et al., 1983).

The negative behaviour that can appear in siblings of subjects with DS can include:

• Attention-seeking behaviour
• Fear of becoming disabled

- Feelings of blame, pity and negligence
- Excessive worry about the future (McCullough, 1981)

However, the majority of studies on siblings agree in indicating that the interaction between siblings is similar in families with no handicapped children and families with handicapped children (Corter et al., 1992). The sibling without disability always assumes the role of big sister or brother, and the sibling with DS, the role of little brother or sister. The interaction between siblings will also depend on the behavioural characteristics of the mother (Stocker et al., 1989).

In general, we can deduce that children with DS present a better and greater level of function in their development when the interactive style of the family unit fulfils certain prerequisites (Mahoney et al., 1992):

- Accepts and values the actions that the child is capable of carrying out
- Provides the child with the possibility of controlling the activities in which he or she is involved

In 1999, van Riper presented the results of a study carried out in Ohio, on how children respond to the experience of living in a family that has a child with DS. The results demonstrated that, for many siblings, the experience of living in a family that has a child with DS can be a positive and enriching one. As a group, the siblings in this study had a higher than average self-image. In addition, the mothers' reports typically indicated that these siblings were socially competent, with fewer incidences of behavioural problems.

Four family-based variables (vulnerability of the family, perception of the family, the family's resources and communication in the family to solve problems) were significantly associated with the well-being of the siblings.

The majority of siblings indicated that their life had changed or was somewhat different as a consequence of having a brother or sister with DS. However, they indicated that this had helped them and had taught them many important things.

Programmes of investigation concerning families of children with Down syndrome

Two extensive programmes of investigation concerning families of children with DS, have been carried out by Gath and Cunningham. Both were started at the beginning of the 1970s in England, and both investigators have continued to update their results over the years.

The results from Gath's first works concerning siblings (Gath, 1973, 1974) indicated that siblings of children with DS, especially older sisters, may have a greater risk of developing behavioural problems. In her later work (Gath, 1985), she suggested that the improvement in the provision of services may have diminished the 'weight of attention' that previously went to the siblings. She also indicated that her results did not support earlier predictions made by researchers and healthcare professionals, that siblings of children with DS would suffer from the lack of parental care and attention.

Gath (1985) observed that when things are going badly in a family, the very existence of a child with DS brings the vulnerable areas that exist in the family to the fore. These include personality disorders, immaturity and precarious relationships. She went further in claiming that it is unfair to the child with DS to consider that these problems are inevitable consequences of the increase in tension originating in the raising of a child with DS. She ended by claiming that many families of children with DS are capable of functioning in a healthy fashion and that a significant number of families have progressed in life precisely because of that which had initially seemed like an intolerable weight.

In 1996, Cunningham published a revision of his five studies. According to him, the predominant impression of the families and of their child with DS is one of normality. The majority of families did not present pathology as a consequence of having a child with DS. In fact, the data indicated the positive effects for many families with a member with DS. Their levels of psychological and physiological alteration were lower than those described by families with children with other disabilities (Sloper and Turner, 1993). The divorce rate among the Manchester group was below the national average and only 14% of parents indicated that having a child with DS had had a prejudicial effect on their marriage. The majority of parents indicated that their lives had changed for the better after the birth of their child with DS.

Once the child reached adolescence, the mothers in the Manchester study had a reduction in the perception of satisfaction with life (Cunningham, 1998). This reduction was associated with a reduction in the real and perceived satisfaction with social support. There was also a tendency for more mothers to perceive the adolescent with DS as having a negative impact on the family. According to Cunningham, this can be due to the fact adolescents with DS can impose greater restrictions on family life than adolescents with no disability.

The main result from the data concerning siblings collected by Cunningham, was that of positive adaptation (Cunningham, 1998). Approximately 80% of siblings indicated that they had maintained a positive relationship with their parents and with their brother or sister with DS. They also showed positive or neutral feelings concerning the effect of having a sister or brother with DS. In addition, siblings had positive perceptions regarding their own worth. A very high proportion (95%) of siblings were actively involved in assisting the child with DS, and this seemed to have a positive impact on the relationship between the siblings. More than half (60%) of siblings indicated that they had no more domestic responsibilities than their friends. The majority of mothers in the Manchester group thought that the experience of having a brother or sister with DS had had a positive effect on the other children in the family.

Cunningham (1998) emphasized that while the majority of the families in the Manchester study were functioning well, some were vulnerable and at risk. The factors that seemed to have the greatest impact on the well-being of these families, were the characteristics of the child with DS (e.g. mental capacity, behavioural problems) and the families' resources, especially those of a utilitarian nature (e.g. salary, house and employment).

Principal problems of the siblings of a person with a disability

This section will centre on the siblings, drawing from my own experience and after Meyer (1985).

It is a common experience that many siblings consider the fact of having a brother or sister with a disability to have been a beneficial factor: it has made them more understanding of the needs of people, more tolerant, more sensitive to the feelings of others, to value their own health, personal intelligence and their capacity for work and so on. We should not, however, forget the problems that others confront and it is to these that we must attend. Above all, we must accept that they can have problems, without parents or educators realizing. We need to identify these problems and see the way in which to attend to them and solve them (Florez, 1990).

Excess of identification

Some siblings wonder whether they have a degree of mental handicap, or whether they will present some type of pathology in the future. This can occur more when children are small, or when the sibling has a deficiency with few external signs.

A 'complex'

Some siblings have a fear that friends will identify them with their brother or sister with a disability. For this reason, siblings may show a certain resistance to inviting their friends home, although this could also be due to other reasons. There are ages at which this feeling can be more intense, and it is at its maximum when they feel the strong need to integrate themselves into a group: they adopt the forms and tendencies of those who comprise the group, with the fear of appearing different. They may fear being seen with their parents or being seen with their brother or sister with DS. Feelings of guilt can develop from the conflict between a certain feeling of shame and the indubitable love that they feel for their brother or sister.

Feelings of guilt

Feelings of guilt can be due to several reasons:

- Feeling superior to a sibling with DS
- Mocking a sibling with DS on occasion, despite this being usual behaviour between siblings
- Having been angered or even infuriated by some annoying behaviour of their sibling
- Thinking that they are abandoning their sibling and their parents when they leave home to study or for other reasons

Isolation

Isolation is more frequent and significant the smaller the families are. Here, the sibling of a person with a disability can feel isolated, incapable or fearful of sharing their problems with parents, friends, teachers or even other siblings with a disability.

The need for opportune and accurate information

Lack of information adds to isolation. This lack may concern the nature of DS and its consequences or the parents' plans for the future. Very frequently, these subjects are not discussed easily and sincerely in the family. The information needs to be adapted to the increasing ages and responsibilities of the children.

Worries about the future

Worries about the future include both the worry of the sibling for the health of his or her future children (will they also have Down syndrome?), and for their future life and that of their sibling. Will they have sufficient economic resources? When the parents die, who will assume responsibility for the care of the sibling? In what conditions? Again, the lack of communication between the sibling and his or her parents can cause enormous disquiet, anxiety and fears for the future. It is not good if the parents keep quiet and assume that the brothers or sisters, or one sibling in particular, will look after the other sibling with DS.

Resentment

Resentment can occur when too many and too serious responsibilities are put on the sibling for his or her age, or when they are punished or strongly reprimanded for making an error in the care of their sibling. On other occasions, the difference is too marked in the behaviour of parents, whose life ends up revolving almost exclusively around the child with DS. Attention, praise and conversations about the child with DS can convert him or her into the little idol of the home, resulting in little attention being given to the other children. Resentment can also occur, especially with older sisters of DS children, when siblings have had to assume great responsibility at the cost of truncating their own future.

Provision of care

On occasion, parents rely, almost always out of overriding necessity, on the siblings to care for the child with DS. This is logical and forms part of the education regarding solidarity. It can, however, become an abuse and an intolerable weight if the sibling is always relied upon, or when there are more siblings and the same one is always relied upon, or parents ask more of a child than he or she can give in terms of their age, abilities and so on.

Feeling of 'pressure'

Sometimes siblings feel pressure from their parents who force their non-deficient children to achieve educational success, as if it were they who have to compensate for the 'failure' that the deficient child represents.

Summary

Not all these feelings will be present in siblings, and they will be evident at different levels in different individuals. I know many brothers and sisters who, as I affirmed above, have matured extraordinarily and have benefited from the fact of having been raised next to a sibling with DS. However, I believe that we must be sensitive to those who do not find help for their very real problems.

Questions and answers regarding siblings

The life expectancy of people with DS has increased considerably in the last few years and today stands at an average of 55 years of age.

Do these new worries and responsibilities affect siblings?

How does one prepare siblings for when the person with DS outlives their parents?

Do parents have the right to demand that their children without disability take on responsibility for their sibling with DS (Perera, 2000)?

These questions are not easy to answer but they do suggest certain reflections and answers:

1. It is, in my opinion, the responsibility of the parents to procure and demand an education for their child with DS that will prepare them to be as autonomous and independent as possible, so that in the future, the child will not be a burden on his or her siblings. A fundamental

objective is to prepare them for a job and help them obtain one (Perera, 1996)

2. It is better to limit the siblings' responsibilities regarding care from childhood (Powell and Ogle, 1985). It is easy to rely on siblings to cooperate in direct care activities. It is normal in any family for the older siblings to help in some way to raise the younger ones, but these activities can multiply when there is a sibling who needs extraordinary care. It is important to achieve a balance based on sharing the different responsibilities and to also rely on people who are not members of the family. Remember that brothers and sisters always like to be thanked or recognized for their complementary participation in the care given to their sibling

3. It is advisable for parents to listen to siblings. Children know their disabled sibling in a different way to their parents. Theirs is a unique relationship. As they mature, siblings make their own observations, comments and suggestions concerning their brother or sister. Their opinions and interests must be closely listened to; and this careful listening also means that parents must attend to unspoken messages or behaviours. Asking the sibling to talk, or facilitating communication between parents and children in some other way, will let the sibling know that his or her ideas and suggestions are valued

4. Involving siblings from an early age in the decisions regarding their brother or sister with DS helps a lot. As they mature, siblings will want to involve themselves in an active way in decisions regarding their brother or sister. It is good that parents make them responsible in any of these ways:

   i. Inviting them to attend meetings at the school of their brother or sister
   ii. Commenting on future plans for them
   iii. Asking their ideas about treatment and service needs
   iv. Attending work sessions that professionals have with the disabled sibling
   v. Helping them to develop their own capacity to teach their sibling new abilities
   vi. Providing them with opportunities in terms of tutelage

5. It is appropriate to point out the special times of stress and to try to reduce the negative effects. Just like parents, siblings experience greater levels of stress at different times. From what we know, these moments can be when:

   i. Another child is born
   ii. The child with disability starts school
   iii. The sibling starts to have relationships
   iv. Friends reject the disabled sibling
   v. Friends ask questions about the sibling

vi.   The child with DS becomes seriously ill

vii. Problems relating to the deficient child are kept secret

viii. The parents die or separate

ix.   The siblings leave home or marry

These are usually the moments of greatest tension, often because of a lack of information, or communication or both, between the parents and the siblings of the disabled child. Stress can be minimized if possible problems are identified, discussed in a frank and open way and viable solutions are sought (Florez, 1991)

6. Be prepared for the future. It is important for parents to make a will, to be advised about the convenience of legally disqualifying their children, and to be informed about the resources their community offers DS people when their parents die: tutelary foundations, tutelary accommodation, and so on. It is advisable for parents to obtain, if possible, a controlled emancipation of their children with DS. This is the best way of preparing them for the future (Perera, 1995)

No parent has the right to ask their children without disability to assume responsibility for their sibling with DS for life. Many want to do so voluntarily. But let us not forget that every person, by the mere fact of being adult, has the right to their own life, to create their own family into which, obviously, completely outside elements will be incorporated that have no affective connection to the sibling with DS. I refer to the husbands or wives of brothers and sisters of the person with DS. Parents have the obligation to respect the siblings' freedom of decision with respect to their brother or sister with DS.

Consequently, the role of siblings is becoming increasingly important, necessary and decisive. But it is the parents who must talk to the siblings in order to prepare for the future of their child with DS, valuing the responsibility and involvement that the siblings can and want to assume in their care and attention.

References

Corter C, Pepler D, Stanhope L, Abramovitch R (1992) Home observation of mothers and siblings dyads compromised of Down's syndrome and nonhandicapped children. Canadian Journal of Behavioral Science 24: 1–13.

Crnic K, Friedrich W, Greenberg M (1983) Adaptation of families with mentally retarded children: a model of stress, coping and family ecology. Am J Ment Def 88: 125–38.

Cunninghan C (1996) Understanding Down Syndrome: An Introduction for Parents. Cambridge, MA: Brookline Books.

Cunninghan C (1998) Families of children with Down syndrome. Down Syndrome: Res Prac 4: 87–95.

Cunninghan C, Aumonier M, Sloper P (1982) Health visitor services for families with Down's syndrome infant-child care. Health Develop 8: 311–26.

Farber B (1971) Effects of a severely retarded child on the family. In E Trapp, P Himelstein (eds) Reading on the Exceptional Child. New York: Appleton-Century-Crofts.

Flórez J (1990) Los hermanos: motivo de atención. Síndrome de Down 7(4): 37–9.

Flórez J (1991) Los hermanos: motivo de atención II. Síndrome de Down 8(1): 3–5.

Garrad S, Richmond J (1963) Psychological aspects of the management of chronic diseases and handicapping conditions in childhood. In H Lief et al. (eds) The Psychological Basis of Medical Practice. New York: Harper & Row, pp. 370–473.

Gath A (1973) The school-age siblings of Mongol children. Brit J Psychiat 123: 161–7.

Gath A (1974) Sibling reactions to mental handicap: a comparison of brothers and sisters of Mongol children. J Child Psychol Psychiat 15: 187–9.

Gath A (1985) Parental reactions to loss and disappointment: the diagnosis of Down's syndrome. Develop Med Child Neurol 27: 392–400.

Gath A (1990) Down syndrome children and their families. Ann J Med Genet (Suppl 7) 314–16.

Gath A (1993) Changes that occur in families as children with intellectual disability grow up. Int J Disab Develop Educ 40: 167–74.

Kazan A, Marvin R (1984) Differences, difficulties and adaptation: stress and social networks in families with handicapped child. Family Relations 33: 67–77.

Lobato DJ (1954) Brothers, Sisters and Special Needs. Baltimore: P. Brooks Publishing.

Mahoney G, Robinson C, Powell A (1992) Focusing on parent–child interaction – the bridge to develop mentally appropriate practices. Topics in Early Childhood Special Education 12: 105–120.

McCullough M (1981) Parent and sibling definition of situation regarding trans-generational shift in care of handicapped children. Dissertation Abstract International 42: 16–18.

Meyer, M (1985) Sibhops. Washington: University of Washington Press.

Perera J (ed) (1995) Síndrome de Down. Aspectos específicos. Barcelona: Masson.

Perera J (1996) Social and labour integration of people with Down syndrome. In JA Rondal, J Perera, L Nadel, A Comblain (eds) Down Syndrome Psychological and Socio-educational Perspectives. London: Whurr Publishers, pp. 219–33.

Perera J (2000) People with Down syndrome: quality of life and future. In JA Rondal, J Perera, L Nadel (eds) Down Syndrome: A Review of Current Knowledge. London: Whurr Publishers, pp. 9–26.

Powell TH, Ogle PA (1985) Brothers and Sisters. A Special Part of Exceptional Families. Baltimore: Paul H. Brookes Publishing.

Sloper P, Turner S (1993) Risk and resilience factors in the adaptation of parents of children with severe physical disability. J Child Psychol Psychiat 34: 158–67.

Stocker C, Dunn J, Plomin R (1989) Sibling relationships: links with temperament maternal behavior and family structure. Child Development 60: 715–27.

van Riper M (1995) Links between family-provider relationships and well-being in families with children who have Down syndrome. Working models of family provider relationships. Unpublished dissertation. Univ. of Wisconsin-Madison.
van Riper M (1999) Living with Down syndrome: the family experience. Down Syndrome Quarterly 4(1): 1–11.

Chapter 22
Family involvement in the treatment of individuals with intellectual disability

L. NOTA

The importance of parents in facilitating children's cognitive and social development is unquestionable, although only over the last few decades have parents been recognized as having a considerable role in the prevention of their children's personal and social adjustment problems. This is far more significant if the parents have children with a disability, and must be taken into account by disability professionals and services in carrying out treatments (Glidewell, 1971; Patterson, 1986; Shriver et al., 1993; Cusinato and Framba, 1988; Cusinato, 1988; Cusinato and Tessarolo, 1993; Nota and Soresi, 1997; Soresi, 1998). In connection with this, a number of parent education and parent training 'projects' were set up at the end of the 1960s with the explicit aims of:

1. Increasing parental abilities in dealing with the daily problems of bringing up children with disabilities
2. Diminishing the probability of making educational 'errors' such as, for instance, strengthening problem behaviours and ignoring adequate ones, resorting excessively to punishments, following educational inconsistency, and so on
3. Increasing parents' abilities to collaborate with habilitation and rehabilitation operators

The need to look systematically after the family members of individuals with disabilities is described in the literature. There are clear and irrefutable 'objective' and 'subjective' indicators of the difficulties they are likely to encounter. Among the objective indicators is the significant reduction in the extra-family activities they actually carry out, the time devoted to their job and to leisure activities, and the decrease in social relationships (Farber, 1960; Helm and Kozloff, 1986). Among the subjective indicators there is an increased stress level, and decreased conjugal satisfaction and psychological well-being (Gallagher et al., 1983; Friedrich and Friedrich, 1981). Having a child with a disability actually involves giving care and attention as well as meeting 'unusual and additional' needs (Beckman and Pokorni, 1988).

The definition of disability itself, difficulty in performing daily activities, requires a number of observational operations that have to be carried out in the context of everyday life. Assessment of a disability requires the active involvement of the interpersonal context in which the disability is manifest (Soresi, 1995). Further, the choice of 'normalization' and inclusion models suggests that rehabilitation programmes cannot be activated through a 'separation' of the individual from his or her context. Although it can sometimes represent some sort of relief to the family, 'parentectomy' cannot be a solution to family problems and neither is it useful in diminishing the child's problems. On the contrary, it often results in the progressive estrangement of families from rehabilitation institutions and social agencies.

However, it must not be forgotten that requests for deinstitutionalization, 'normalization' and inclusion of individuals with disabilities cannot be efficaciously satisfied if these families are not given the support and social help needed to rationalize those problems that, because of their intensity, duration and frequency, the families cannot cope with alone.

Thus, in recent years there has been a significant evolution of the role allotted to the family in disability treatment and inclusion. Until a few years ago, parents and family members of individuals with disability were generally excluded from rehabilitation programmes and interventions, and were relegated to the role of mere spectators of what others (the experts) were doing; nowadays their involvement is gaining more and more importance, including the analysis of treatment efficacy. In particular, the 'prejudice', which caused family members to be excluded from the planning of treatments because of their lack of 'specific' knowledge and competence, has now been reassessed. However, if this awareness can be considered as acquired, the problem arises of the type of support one must guarantee the family and, further, the type of help parents must be given with the management of everyday practical problems. The presence of a child with a disability implies a series of financial, social and emotional problems. The achievement of successful intervention requires adherence to firm educational principles and 'competences' which can rarely be found in parents who are not adequately supported and 'trained' (Soresi and Meazzini, 1990; Soresi, 1993).

The requests that these parents make to disability professionals and services are about the ways to deal and cope with their children's inadequate behaviours and how to diminish their frequency, intensity and duration, and how to increase their children's abilities in different areas of development and learning. Moreover, they want to know what they can do to collaborate adequately with the experts in order to maximize the likelihood of success of the treatments the latter have planned. Although sometimes not adequately and clearly formulated, these are requests for participation and training; and this is what a great number of involvement programmes aim at favouring, as described in the literature. As an example, Figure 22.1 shows the structure of the Parent Training Programme that we usually propose. As can be seen from the contents of the didactic units, the programme aims to favour increasing observational abilities as well as the abilities necessary to manage difficult situations without delay and to activate efficacious cooperative relationships.

Figure 22.1 Schedule of a Parent Training Programme (from Soresi and Nota, 2003)

First Didactic Unit: All individuals are different
Second Didactic Unit: What are disabilities?
Third Didactic Unit: How to observe children's behaviours
Fourth Didactic Unit: How to increase abilities
Fifth Didactic Unit: Analysis of problem behaviours
Sixth Didactic Unit: How to cope with difficult situations
Seventh Didactic Unit: The competent and efficacious parent
Eighth Didactic Unit: The parent as a problem solver
Ninth Didactic Unit: Parents' and children's well-being
Tenth Didactic Unit: Educational bargaining
Eleventh Didactic Unit: Couple conflicts and educational inconsistency
Twelfth Didactic Unit: Communication styles in the family
Thirteenth Didactic Unit: How to communicate wishes and have one's rights respected
Fourteenth Didactic Unit: How to communicate criticism and obtain cooperation

Family and services for individuals with disability: a possible and necessary collaboration

Working with individuals with disabilities requires, on the one hand, rigorous and intersubjectively verifiable planning of habilitation and rehabilitation interventions, and, on the other, the search for and achievement of huge parental involvement. This may well result in conflicts and difficulties which must be dealt with; otherwise, it will be quite unlikely that efficacious habilitation, rehabilitation and inclusion programmes will be fulfilled.

Programming essentially means setting the goals to be achieved and choosing the conditions, instruments and strategies that have the highest likelihood of guaranteeing their achievement. A series of advantages for the individual benefiting from the intervention, that is to say the improvement of his or her health and well-being and quality of life, can be obtained thanks to the conscious and intentional choice of the interventions to be achieved. This can be guaranteed only by cutting out improvisation and chance and through meticulous planning.

When the focus is on the cooperation either between disability operators and parents or between different operators, it may be appropriate to analyse the methods used to activate the various operational decisions.

Greater awareness of this can lead to modification of interactions and a decrease in conflicts.

When considering the interaction that can exist between goal setting and intervention methods, we might find at least four different situations:

1. Disagreement between the individuals interested in programme realization as regards goals to be achieved and achievement modalities
2. Disagreement between the individuals interested in programme realization as regards goals to be achieved and agreement as regards possible achievement modalities
3. Agreement as regards goals to be achieved, but disagreement on achievement modalities
4. Agreement both as regards goals to be achieved and instruments and strategies to achieve them

These different situations are related to different decisional and relational processes and result in different consequences for the collaboration. Let us study each of these situations in more depth.

Disagreement as regards goals to be achieved and achievement modalities

This is the situation of most conflict: there is no agreement between service operators and parents, or between different operators, or between members of the same team or of the same family (mother and father, for instance) on the educational habilitation and rehabilitation goals, which are considered as the most urgent or appropriate to carry out. The parents, for example, may be more interested in increasing their child's ability to control his or her own aggressive reactions, whereas operators may think it more important to develop abilities considered necessary for work inclusion, or vice versa. Similarly, within the same team one operator may think it more urgent to increase some cognitive abilities (for example in relation to discriminant tasks) and another to increase non-cognitive abilities, related, for instance, to social and relational activities. In these situations the non-agreement is often not even spoken about, but its existence is proved by the very few contacts ever established between the different parties, the poor opinion they have of one another, the palpable tension between them when they are forced to meet and interact for bureaucratic or administrative reasons. Vis-à-vis such disagreement, it is apparent that cooperative relationships between family and service or between the various operators are very unlikely, as whatever one tries to do will be considered unimportant by the other and vice versa.

Significantly opposing positions can also arise as regards the methods used. For instance, in the case of reading, an operator may favour a syllabic approach and another a global one; in the case of social education some may emphasize the utmost expression of emotions and feelings and others may propose the use of specific communication techniques. These situations are likely to produce very poor relationships; more often than not reciprocal accusations are the norm, and there are attempts to devalue others' efforts as well as sabotaging what they are trying to achieve.

Disagreement as regards goals to be achieved and agreement as regards possible achievement modalities

In these cases agreement is generally recorded on the techniques to be used and there is appreciation of the professionals involved in the rehabilitation and habilitation programming. However, incomprehension and conflicts can be caused by the different level of priority attributed to the goals to be achieved. Conflicts can arise between families and services, but also between operators who may have different opinions. Such discrepancies and the ensuing conflicts can certainly reduce the actual possibility of cooperation and the commitment devoted to fulfilment of the aims of the programme.

Agreement as regards goals to be achieved and disagreement as regards achievement modalities

This situation is generally found when the type of habilitation or rehabilitation intervention to be carried out requires specific competencies which are not possessed by all those who are interested in decreasing the subject's disabilities. An instance is the case where the habilitation or rehabilitation intervention can be carried out with equipment available only in certain contexts (hospitals, for example) or requires professional abilities held only by specifically trained operators (physiotherapists and speech therapists, for example). When this happens, family members and operators, albeit sharing the goals, will necessarily carry out different interventions, not analogous to or overlapping those of the others.

Agreement both as regards goals to be achieved and achievement modalities

This is the best possible situation which results in particularly productive cooperation. In this case, habilitation or rehabilitation interventions are programmed together and the various parties act in concert, aiming at achieving the same goals by means of shared analogous modalities. Often this is the result of previous interactions characterized by reciprocal respect, high regard and cooperation.

Conclusion

For disability treatment and inclusion to work well, there are many requirements; among them convergence and cooperation, at least between professionals and families, are particularly important and significant. Although it may seem obvious, agreement and convergence cannot be taken for granted; often parents' goals and disability operators' goals are markedly different.

To diminish possible 'diffidence' and to increase the likelihood of reaching effective cooperation it is important that disability professionals, in line with Clarke-Stewart's (1988) suggestions, frequently reassure parents that:

- They will not be asked to modify their educational attitudes and behaviour towards their son or daughter unless they are fully convinced that it is necessary and they feel ready to do it
- They will be systematically informed of why some interventions and educational techniques are proposed
- If they have difficulties, they will always be able to count on the operators and services whether they accept their suggestions or not
- Changes will not be proposed or required that may turn out to be dangerous for their child or for themselves; any proposal for change will be accompanied by an explanation of the consequences associated with it

In other words, the 'contracts' between the operators in charge of habilitation or rehabilitation programmes should be able to be shared by the parents as well as being as explicit and as clear as possible.

References

Beckman PJ (1991) Influence of selected child characteristics on stress in families of handicapped infants. Am J Ment Def 88(2): 150–6.
Beckman PJ, Pokorni JC (1988) A longitudinal study of family of preterm infants: changes in stress and support over the first two years. J Spec Educ 22: 55–65.
Clarke-Stewart KA (1988) Parents' effects on children's development: a decade of progress? J Appl Dev Psychol 9: 41–84.
Cusinato M (1988) Psicologia delle Relazioni Familiari (Psychology of Family Relationships). Bologna: Il Mulino.
Cusinato M, Framba R (1988) La prevenzione nell'area delle relazioni familiari. (Prevention in the field of family relationships). In M Cusinato (ed.) Psicologia delle Relazioni Familiari. Bologna: Il Mulino, pp. 379–420.
Cusinato M, Tessarolo M (1993) Ruoli e Vissuti Familiari: Nuovi Approcci (Roles and Family Experiences: New Approaches). Firenze: Giunti, pp. 293–310.
D'Angela S (1990) Il Genitore Competente (The Competent Parent). Pordenone: Erip Editrice.
D'Angela S, Meazzini P (1990) L'incoerenza educativa: una proposta tassonomica. (Educational inconsistency: a taxonomic proposal). Psicologia e Scuola 51: 6–12.
Farber B (1960) Family organisation and crisis: maintenance of integration in families with a severely retarded child. Monogr Soc Res Child Dev 25: 1–95.
Friedrich WN, Friedrich WI (1981) Psychological assets of parents of handicapped and nonhandicapped children. Am J Ment Def 50: 10–19.

Gallagher J, Beckman P, Cross A (1983) Families of handicapped children: sources of stress and its amelioration. Except Child 50: 10–19.

Glidewell J (1971) Issues in Community Psychology and Preventive Mental Health. New York: Behavioral Publications.

Helm DT, Kozloff MA (1986) Research on parent training: shortcomings and remedies. J Autism Dev Disord 16(1): 1–22.

Milani P (1993) Progetto Genitori (A Project for Parents). Trento: Centro Studi Erickson.

Nota L, Soresi S (1997) Le Abilità Sociali: dall'osservazione all'intervento (Social Abilities: From Observation to Intervention). Pordenone: Erip Editrice.

Patterson GR (1986) Performance models for antisocial boys. Am Psychol 41: 432–44.

Ross AO (1972) Behavioral therapy. In BB Wolman (ed.) Manual of Child Psychopathology. New York: McGraw-Hill.

Shriver MD, Kramer JJ, Garnett M (1993) Parent involvement in early childhood: opportunities for school psychologists. Psychol Sch 30: 264–76.

Soresi S (1993) Sperimentazione di un programma di parent training con genitori di adolescenti handicappati (Experimenting a parent training program with parents of adolescents with disability). In M Cusinato, M Tessarolo (eds) Ruoli e Vissuti Familiari, Nuovi Approcci. Firenze: Giunti, pp. 293–310.

Soresi S (1995) Le disabilità secondo l'ICIDH: implicazioni per l'assessment e il trattamento (Disabilities according to the ICIDH: implications for assessment and treatment). In M Sala, M Pierri, A Campari, C Bianchi, A Russo, M Bonelli, L Moderato (eds) La Persona Adulta con Ritardo Mentale nelle Istituzioni: Cura e Riabilitazione. Milano: Ghedini Editore, pp. 74–9.

Soresi S (1998) Psicologia dell'handicap e della riabilitazione (Psychology of Handicap and Rehabilitation). Bologna: Il Mulino.

Soresi S, Meazzini P (1990) Prefazione (Preface). In S D'Angela (ed.) Il Genitore Competente. Pordenone: Erip Editrice, pp. 5–19.

Soresi S, Nota L (2003) Parent Training per Genitori di Figli Disabili (Parent Training for Parents of Children with Disability). Roma: Carocci Editore.

Chapter 23
Ageing in people with Down syndrome: educational, rehabilitation and social prospects

L. COTTINI

In the last few years, a new need has arisen due to increased ages of people with mental disabilities: that of preparing suitable social policies (calibrated services and support initiatives), which also take the needs of older people into account. Increases in the average survival age for mentally disabled people have been unequivocally documented by numerous research programmes in different countries, looking above all at people affected by Down syndrome (Richards and Sidiqui, 1969; Mulcahy, 1979, 1983; Bricarelli et al., 1984; Dupon, 1986; Fryers, 1986; Baird and Sadovnick, 1995; Eyman, 1991).

This increase in the average life span, which on the one hand is exciting and potentially full of positive implications, can pose new questions and problems. In fact, numerous studies have shown how mentally handicapped people develop signs of cognitive decline at an early age; to this, we can also add their regression in terms of autonomy and social integration.

In the light of these preliminary remarks, it is my aim in this chapter to recapitulate the data and research that are currently available, and also to formulate several operational proposals and considerations. More specifically, I will deal with the following aspects:

1. Analysis of the ageing-related processes in people with mental handicaps
2. Delineation of the inspiring principles (organizational, technical and scientific) behind educational, rehabilitation and social interventions
3. Presentation of initial data from an educational experiment still in progress

The effects of ageing on the mentally disabled: a brief analysis of literature

Literature about the effects of ageing in the mentally handicapped has particularly considered people with Down syndrome. Applying a (surely excessive) schematic format, this literature can be divided into three main areas.

Studies aimed at showing age-related deterioration processes

Numerous studies, generally conducted on a broad sample of people, aim to define and delineate precisely age-related deterioration processes (usually after 40 years) in mentally handicapped people. The skills most highlighted (Hewitt, 1985; Collacott, 1992; Rasmussen and Sobsey, 1994; Burt et al., 1995; van Gennep, 1995; Cooper and Collacot, 1995; Roeden and Zitman, 1995; Holland, 1999; Prasher, 1999; Krasuski et al., 2002) as being subject to deterioration are the following:

- Response rapidity
- Visual-spatial skills
- Memory skills
- Language skills
- Adaptation skills, considered as the possibility of living in an adaptive fashion within the social context of origin

It should be pointed out that, while all of the authors agree in finding a considerable deterioration in conditions as age increases in people with serious handicaps, it is not possible to say the same for subjects with less serious mental disabilities. On the contrary, in these people deterioration cannot be taken for granted (Devenny et al., 1992; Caltagirone et al., 1990), at least for many years and above all if they undergo suitable educational and rehabilitation training and maintain social relations. This, however, will be dealt with in a later section.

Studies in which the effects of ageing in people with Down syndrome are compared with the symptoms of Alzheimer's disease

In this area of study, the typical symptoms of Alzheimer's disease and other types of dementia are compared with the signs of cognitive deterioration recorded in people with Down syndrome aged over 40. A great deal of work exists on this subject (Ball, 1986; Patterson, 1987; Lai and Williams, 1989; Johanson et al., 1991; Haxby and Shapiro, 1992; Vicari et al., 1995; Brugge et al., 1994; Das et al., 1995; Thompson, 1994; Nadel, 1995; Evenhuis, 1996; Hyde and Crnic, 2001), analysing the relationship between Alzheimer's disease and Down syndrome from a neurophysiological viewpoint (comparisons between the degeneration modes in the central nervous system). Some findings seem to give credit to the existence of a degenerative pathology for people with Down syndrome of an advanced age; others invite the utmost caution and stress the need for further research, since it is not possible to arrive at a unified interpretation of the results obtained to date (Silverman and Wisniewski, 1998).

Studies which compare the ageing process in people with Down syndrome and in mentally handicapped people whose problems are due to other causes

There is a series of studies that seek to point out different behaviour, due to progressive ageing, in people with Down syndrome as opposed to people with mental handicaps caused by other factors (Saviolo and Trevisan, 1990; Gibson, 1991; Devenny et al., 1992; Dulaney and Ellis, 1994; Roeden and Zitman, 1995; Thompson, 1999; Nochajski, 2000). Research is at the initial stage and if the results are to be correctly interpreted, further experimentation is necessary. In fact, some studies point out increased age-related deficit conditions in sufferers of Down syndrome, while others do not; these latter, for example, stress an increased maintaining of skills. Such results lead us to believe that there are other variables besides those considered (the presence or lack of trisomy 21), which must be examined through further study.

Conclusions

Research carried out to date clearly reports ageing-related deterioration in the mentally disabled, even if such deterioration does not seem to be evenly distributed in some functions. However, careful analysis of the literature points out several grey areas that cannot be ignored concerning the methodological procedures used. More specifically:

- There is a vast difference in the evaluation tools used, which means that it is difficult to compare the results of different authors
- Cross-sectional research is the prevalent type used and this involves a high risk of group variability
- The effects of specific stimulation have not been greatly researched, with the exception of limited experimental studies (Devenny et al., 1992; Saviolo and Trevisan, 1990; Roeden and Zitman, 1995)

Guidelines for educational, rehabilitation and social interventions

The situation of increased life expectancy appears to be both exciting and worrying at the same time.

It is exciting because people with mental disabilities are now faced with the possibility of longer and potentially stimulating lives from both the personal and the social point of view. This prospect is in sharp contrast with the bleak prognoses that were formulated up until a few decades ago.

It is worrying because we need to recognize how poorly equipped we are to deal with ageing-related problems. The network of services that should support the mentally disabled person and his or her family still has insufficient means, especially in view of the fact that, at least in terms of parents, families are able to offer increasingly less effective support.

In the light of this, the planning of an assistance project should follow two main and closely linked paths:

1. The setting up of services and social initiatives that allow the person to maintain (and possibly to increase) his or her network of social relations as well as to supply families with a credible alternative to the forms of institutionalization that are often seen as the only possibility (especially in serious cases)
2. Focusing more attention on the technical and scientific aspects of educational, rehabilitation and social interventions, with reference to the vast experience that has allowed strategies for promoting skills and limiting forms of cognitive deterioration to be identified

These two lines of work are dealt with schematically in a later section.

Life in institutions: a prospective for development or for regression?

As already stressed, as a mentally handicapped person grows older, especially if the problem is serious, the response of the social services is to accentuate aid and all this does is accelerate functional deterioration. Only too often, institutionalization (in many cases, residential homes for the elderly) is seen as the easiest and most reassuring way out.

This occurs while a series of studies has shown how, on the other hand, this route leads to a reduction in any skill levels present. On this subject, the research programmes of Cohen et al. (1977), Hemming et al. (1981), Janicki and Jacobson (1986), Kleinberg and Galligan (1983), Fine et al. (1990) and Roeden and Zitman (1995) are most important and have pointed out that adaptation skills are clearly superior in people who have not been institutionalized (resident within the family, in shared housing, family units, etc.), compared to those people who spend all their time in institutions. These results have been traced back to environment, relationships and significant commitment to activities (e.g. running the home).

As Kleinberg and Galligan (1983) point out, the choice of a community living environment is certainly fundamental; however, to be effective, it must be accompanied by a series of systematic interventions and efficient training, above all of a cognitive nature.

Therefore, as well as residing in non-institutional contexts (in the family if possible, otherwise in small communities with home-like environments), the mentally handicapped person should attend daytime structures with specific characteristics. A model service that we are experimenting with in Urbino will be described below. It includes a wide range of activities with regard to the following:

- Cognitive skills which, as stressed more than once, are necessary to limit the bleak phenomena of cognitive deterioration
- Autonomy and integration skills, understood as personal care and care for one's living environment
- Social skills, seen as the ability to maintain relations with the social environment and to use community services autonomously
- Motor and recreational skills and management of free time activities
- Professional skills, understood as performance of some solidly based workshop activities (professional if possible)

Technical and scientific guidelines for suitable interventions

As already mentioned, the decline in skills connected with the onset of age does not seem to be such an incontrovertible and unchangeable event if we continue to invest resources, in human and professional terms, in education and rehabilitation, especially of a cognitive nature. In-depth research into the quality of interventions must be added to the network of services. In fact, these aspects, together with consideration of the seriousness of the mental disability, represent the most important prognostic indicators.

On this subject, the research carried out by Devenny et al. (1992) has much to say. It shows that in people with average mental disabilities (IQ above 35), who were active in workshops and lived with their families, perceptive, memory and adaptation skills did not decline over various years (the ages of the subjects ranged from 35 to 55 years).

Two aspects of the technical characteristics for designing educational and rehabilitation interventions are particularly important:

1. The possibility of using flexible and dynamic-functional assessment systems, that allow the individual's development to be monitored over time
2. The possibility of referring to specific strategies that have demonstrated their effectiveness on more than one occasion

I have already pointed out the significant diversity of the tools used in different studies to highlight changes in the skills and behaviour of mentally handicapped adults. Without dwelling upon the different diagnostic models and their theoretical presuppositions, it is important to point out that such tools should be sensitive towards the early indicators of cognitive deterioration that have been found by different authors.

To satisfy this need, we have devised an assessment system to monitor the development of older people with mental disabilities that can also be used for the early identification of cognitive deterioration indicators. The whole assessment system is currently available on CD-ROM (Cottini, 1999).

It is important to stress that initial applications show that there is a possibility of limiting cognitive deterioration. It is possible to cite, for example, different experiments conducted in Italy on visual-spatial and memory skills (Saviolo Negrin and Trevisan, 1990), on social and relational skills (Soresi and Nota, 1995), and on the ability to comprehend messages on film (Cottini and Meazzini, 1988).

As far as cognitive skills training strategies are concerned, as well as the classical cognitive-behavioural derivation procedures, there are also procedures for self-regulation (self-teaching, self-monitoring and self-reinforcement), the potential of which has already been stressed. The use of simple problem-solving situations and role-play has also been found to be important. Specific literature is able to supply more details (Cottini, 1993; Meazzini, 1998; Soresi, 1998).

Description of an educational experiment

Subjects involved

The experiment was conducted with three adults, all affected by organic mental disabilities (Zigler, 1984), one of which had Down syndrome. All three attend the Senior Facility of the 'Francesca' Social and Education Centre, Urbino.

The three were aged 44, 42 and 38 years respectively. Assessments of their Intelligence Quotients (IQ), performed by the centre's psychology staff using the WAIS scale (Wechsler, 1981), showed scores below the standard of 45 for all subjects.

Adaptive behaviour assessments were made using the following checklists, which are included in the Senior software package (Cottini, 1999):

* Autonomy skills
* Basic motor skills
* Social skills
* Integration skills
* Free time management skills

The results showed that the subjects had satisfactory skills for living in their surroundings in an adapted fashion, with good personal autonomy skills, basic motor skills (with the exception of the first subject) and social skills (with the exception of the third subject). Lower levels were found for integration skills and the ability to manage free time.

Table 23.1 shows the percentage scores obtained by the three subjects on the different adaptive behaviour scales.

Table 23.1 Percentage scores obtained on adaptive behaviour scales

Subject	Age	Autonomy skills	Motor skills	Social skills	Integration skills	Free time management skills
G.D.L.	44	59	26	63	31	34
L.C.	42	80	65	58	51	48
R.A.	38	74	63	33	41	36

Base assessment

As already emphasized, the development and conducting of educational and rehabilitation interventions requires a functional assessment system, whereby subjects' initial skill levels are found and the development of these skills is monitored over time.

In our case, to analyse the main cognitive processes flexibly and precisely, we used tests from our Senior software package (Cottini, 1999), which can be used to assess the following skills:

- Response rapidity (reaction times)
- Hearing discrimination
- Spatial memory
- Memory for numbers
- Memory for words
- Object naming
- Sequential comprehension
- Text comprehension

More specifically, the different tests, controlled directly from the software, both in terms of presenting and storing the results, include a series of tasks to which the subjects must respond differently. The following section summarizes the main features of the individual tests.

Test of reaction times

This test measures the subject's response rapidity, which, of all the different cognitive skills, represents one of the most important factors in assessing the effectiveness of the central nervous system. The test method is visual-motor since it requires visual discrimination and a motor response.

A first sample stimulus is presented and this must be memorized by the subject (for example, the colour red in the 'Colour on Colour' test). The stimulus remains in the centre of the screen for a certain amount of time; the computer then sends out a series of messages, such as: 'Warning: only press the bar every time you see this colour again. Do you understand? ... Now we will begin the test ...'. At this point, the programme shows a random series of different colours, including the sample one; it then records both the correctness of the response and the time required to enter it.

Hearing discrimination test

The computer presents a series of word pairs which may be the same (e.g. bread–bread) or different by several phonemes or syllables (e.g. winter–winner). The subject's task is to pay attention to the stimulus (word pair) and to say whether the words are different or the same.

The software records the number of correct answers (each list is formed by 10 identical word pairs and 10 different word pairs).

Spatial memory test

The subject is presented with a frame containing figures. He or she must carefully observe and memorize the position that each single figure occupies; a certain amount of time is allowed for this operation. The frame (stimulus) then disappears and reappears on the following screen display, this time with the figures placed outside and in random positions. The subject's task is then to indicate the position that each figure occupied within the frame.

In our assessment, we used eight figures to be repositioned spatially.

Number memory test

This test is part of the principal intellect assessments in evaluating a subject's ability to remember lists of numbers (short-term memory). The computer lists series of numbers that become increasingly longer, with the instruction to repeat them in the same order. The result stored in the memory is the length of the final series correctly repeated.

Word memory test

This test comprises two sessions: a different word list is presented in each one. The words in the first list are selected according to a criterion of highly frequent use and high image value. The words in the second list have low frequency use and low image value.

Each list is presented three consecutive times, with an interval of half an hour between the presentation, and in a different order each time. The task is that of repeating, each time, the words in the given list, in order to assess immediate memory and learning skills, subsequent to the successive presentations.

Object naming test

The object naming test consists of attributing a verbal label (noun) to the objects presented for very short periods in different areas of the screen. Attributing a name to an object means reactivating the existing link between the formal elements of the stimulus configuration (figure), which is presented and processed at a given time, and the formal elements of a second configuration (verbal label) which a subject has learned to associate with the first configuration during the experiment. In the first of the two tests, the subject is shown a series of 15 figures, selected according to a criterion of high frequency of use for the words themselves, as well as a high image value. In the second test, the subject is shown a further series of 15 figures whose frequency of use is lower than that of the first series. The software records the number of figures correctly named.

Sequential comprehension test

Subjects are shown three short stories, broken down and illustrated with pictures. The number of pictures is different for each of the stories (three, four and five). The pictures are laid out in a straight line in the centre of the screen and in a different order compared to the logical time sequence of events. Numbered spaces in which to fit the pictures appear below them.

The subject's task is to re-order the sequence of events for each story, following logical, causal and temporal criteria. Assessment of the test takes into consideration the number of cartoons placed in the correct order.

Text comprehension test

This test is used to analyse the subject's ability to comprehend a written text, after direct reading of it. Three passages of increasing difficulty are shown. After each passage has been read, the subject must answer questions, choosing from four alternative answers. In this case too, the number of correct answers is counted.

Results of base assessment

The results recorded for the subjects following evaluation of their assessment tests in the Senior Project are shown in Table 23.2, a summary table which compares the initial results with those obtained after 1 year.

Educational intervention

As already mentioned, the subjects in this study attended (and continue to do so) the Senior Facility of the 'Francesca' Social and Education Centre, Urbino. For each one, there was a personal organized schedule of activities, following the methods described previously. Figure 23.1 shows the summary prospectus for the person with Down syndrome (the scheduled activities for this person are those highlighted in italics).

For reasons of space, it is not possible to describe the activities developed as part of cognitive education in full detail. The subjects were involved in three lessons per week (approximately 1 hour each) and these activities included work on one of the following aspects:

• Response rapidity (reaction time)
• Hearing discrimination

- Spatial and temporal memory
- Problem solving and sequential comprehension

Readers who are interested in a description of the programme should refer to a recent paper on the subject (Cottini, 2002).

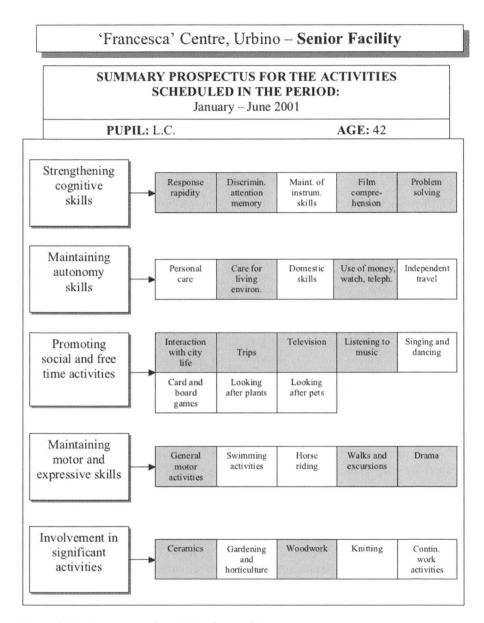

Figure 23.1 Programmed activities for a subject.

Results

The working period considered was from September 2000 to June 2001, when the evaluations used in the Senior Project assessment system were applied.

The full results of the cognitive group, including both the start-of-year assessments (pre) and final assessments (post), are shown in Tables 23.2a and 23.2b.

Table 23.2a Pre and post assessments of cognitive function indicators

Subject	Age	Response rapidity		Hearing discrimination		Spatial memory		Memory for numbers	
		Pre	Post	Pre	Post	Pre	Post	Pre	Post
G.D.L.	44	525	533	39	35	6	8	3	3
A.C.	42	559	662	31	38	6	8	2	3
R.A.	38	540	640	33	25	2	4	4	3

Table 23.2b Pre and post assessments of cognitive function indicators

Subject	Age	Memory for words		Naming objects		Sequential comprehension		Text comprehension	
		Pre	Post	Pre	Post	Pre	Post	Pre	Post
G.D.L.	44	5–6–6	10–11–13	16	15	8	7	N.A.	N.A.
A.C.	42	4–7–10	6–7–9	21	24	12	12	8	12
R.A.	38	5–5–6	7–6–8	19	18	5	7	8	5

As can be seen, the development of different cognitive function indicators shows an interesting and, on the whole, satisfactory situation.

In particular, deterioration in response rapidity tests (reaction times) was found for all subjects. As already mentioned, this skill is highly reflective of central nervous system function and this has certainly been affected by the passage of time. However, this deterioration has not involved worsening performances concerning discriminatory, memory and problem-solving skills. On the contrary, in many tests, these skills were found to have improved; a fact which seems to give a great deal of credit to the effectiveness of the cognitive interventions and of the organization of environments that are stimulating from every viewpoint.

As far as adaptive behaviour is concerned, reviews of the check-list have practically confirmed previous findings, with an increase in ability to manage social relations and long periods of free time (specific programmes have been conducted for these aspects, as can be seen from the prospectus of activities).

In conclusion, I would like to repeat that the positive developments found cannot merely be attributed to the cognitive interventions described above, but that they represent the results of an overall programme, which centres on the organization of an environment that is particularly rich in stimulating and relational opportunities. What is more, the participants lived and continue to live with their families and, as stressed in the previous section, this certainly plays a part in the extremely comforting developments we found.

I feel that I can affirm, within the limits of this simple pilot study, that the experiment described confirms the stance of those authors (Kleinberg and Galligan, 1983; Janicki and Jacobson, 1986; Saviolo Negrin and Trevisan, 1990; Devenny et al., 1992; Roeden and Zitman, 1995) who attribute great importance and influence to educational, rehabilitation and social activities in limiting forms of cognitive deterioration and in creating the necessary conditions to maintain high-level quality of life.

I hope that the continuation of this experimental programme will be able to supply further and more valid results at this level.

References

Baird P, Sadovnick A (1995) Life expectancy in Down syndrome. Lancet 2: 1354–6.

Ball MJ (1986) Neuropathological relationships between Down syndrome and senile dementia Alzheimer type. In CJ Epstein (ed.) The Neurobiology of Down Syndrome. New York: Raven Press, pp. 45–58.

Bricarelli DF, Inglese G, Moretti A, Rasore Quartino A (1984) Aspetti epidemiologici, genetici, clinici e sociali della sindrome di Down, CEPIM, Genova.

Brugge KL, Nichols SL, Salmon DP, Hill LR (1994) Cognitive impairment in adults with Down's syndrome: Similarities to early cognitive changes in Alzheimer's disease. Neurology 44: 232–8.

Burt DB, Loveland KA, Chen Y, Chuang A (1995) Aging in adults with Down syndrome. Am J Ment Retard 100: 262–70.

Caltagirone C, Nocentini U, Vicari S (1990) Cognitive function in adults with Down's syndrome. Int J Neurosci 54: 221–30.

Cohen H, Conroy J, Frazer D, Snelbecker G, Spreat S (1977) Behavioral effects of interinstitutional relocation of mentally retarded residents. Am J Ment Def 82: 12–18.

Collacott RA (1992) The effect of age and residential placement on adaptive behaviour of adults with Down's syndrome. Br J Psychiatry 161: 675–9.

Cooper SA, Collacot RA (1995) The effect of age on language in people with Down's syndrome. J Intell Disabil Res 39: 197–200.

Cottini L (1993) Strategie per l'apprendimento dell'handicappato mentale. Milano: Angeli.

Cottini L (1999) Progetto Senior. La persona con handicap avanza con gli anni: strategie per contenere il deterioramento cognitivo. Gorizia: Tecnoscuola.

Cottini L (2002) Bambini, Adulti, Anziani e Ritardo Mentale. Brescia: Vannini.

Cottini L, Meazzini P (1988) Quando H guarda la televisione. E' possibile migliorare la comprensione dei messaggi televisivi? Handicap e Disabilità 81: 3–12.

Das JP, Divis BA, Parrila RK (1995) Cognitive decline due to aging among persons with Down syndrome. Res Dev Disabil 16: 461–78.

Devenny DA, Silverman VP, Hill A, Patxot O, Wisniewski KE (1992) Aging in higher functioning adults with Down's syndrome: an interim report in a longitudinal study. J Intell Disabil Res 36: 241–50.

Devenny DA, Silverman VP, Hill A, Jenkins E (1996) Normal aging in adults with Down's syndrome: a longitudinal study. J Intell Disabil Res 40: 208–21.

Dulaney CL, Ellis NR (1994) Automatized responding and cognitive inertia in individuals with mental retardation. Am J Ment Retard 99: 8–18.

Dupon A (1986) Mortality and life expectancy of Down's syndrome in Denmark. J Ment Def Res 30: 112–20.

Evenhuis HM (1996) Further evaluation of the Dementia Questionnaire for Persons with Mental Retardation. J Intell Disabil Res 40: 369–73.

Eyman RK (1991) Life expectancy of persons with Down's syndrome. Am J Ment Retard 95: 603–12.

Fryers R (1986) Survival in Down's syndrome. J Ment Def Res 30: 101–10.

Fine MA, Tangeman PJ, Woodard J (1990) Changes in adaptive behavior of older adults with mental retardation following deinstitutionalization. Am J Ment Retard 94: 661–8.

Gibson D (1991) Searching for a life-span psychobiology of Down syndrome: advancing educational and behavioural management strategies. Int J Disabil Devel Educ 38: 71–89.

Haveman MJ, Maaskant MA, van Scrhojestein Lantman-de Valk HM, Urlings HFJ (1994) Mental health problems in elderly people with and without Down's syndrome. J Intell Disabil Res 38: 341–55.

Haxby JV, Shapiro MB (1992) Longitudinal study of neuropsychological function in older adults with Down's syndrome. In CJ Epstein, L Nadel (eds) Down Syndrome and Alzheimer Disease. New York: Wiley-Liss Inc, pp. 35–50.

Hemming H, Lavender T, Pill R (1981) Quality of life of mentally retarded adults transferred from large institutions to new small units. Am J Ment Def 86: 157–69.

Hewitt KE (1985) Aging in Down's syndrome. Br J Psychiatry 147: 58–62.

Holland AJ (1999) Down's syndrome. In M Janicki, AJ Dalton (eds) Dementia, Aging, and Intellectual Disabilities: A Handbook. New York: Wiley-Liss Inc, pp. 183–97.

Hyde LA, Crnic LS (2001) Age-related deficits in context discrimination learning in Ts65Dn mice that model Down syndrome and Alzheimer's disease. Behav Neurosci 115: 1239–46.

Janicki MP, Jacobson JW (1986) Generational trends in sensory physical and behavioral abilities among older mentally retarded persons. Am J Ment Def 90: 490–500.

Johanson A, Gustafson L, Brun A, Risberg J (1991) A longitudinal study of dementia of Alzheimer type in Down's syndrome. Dementia 2: 159–68.

Kleinberg J, Galligan B (1983) Effects of deinstitutionalization on adaptive behavior of mentally retarded adults. Am J Ment Def 88: 21–7.

Krasuski JS, Alexander GE, Horwitz B, Rapoport SI, Schapiro MB (2002) Relation of medial temporal lobe volumes to age and memory function in nondemented adults with Down's syndrome: implications for the prodromal phase of Alzheimer's disease. Am J Psychiatry 159: 74–81.

Lai F, Williams RS (1989) A prospective study of Alzheimer disease in Down syndrome. Neurology 46: 849–53.

McNellis CA (1997) Mental retardation and aging: mental health issues. Gerontol Geriatr Educ 17: 75–86.

Meazzini P (1988) Handicap: passi verso l'autonomia. Firenze: Giunti.

Mulcahy MT (1979) Down's syndrome in Western Australia: mortality and survival. Ir Med J 76: 71–5.

Mulcahy MT (1983) Census of the mentally handicapped in the Republic of Ireland. Ir Med J 16: 103–8.

Nadel L (1995) Neural and cognitive development in Down syndrome. In L Nadel, D Rosenthal (eds) Down Syndrome: Living and Learning in the Community. New York: Wiley-Liss Inc, pp. 107–14.

Nochajski SM (2000) The impact of age-related changes on the functioning of older adults with developmental disabilities. Phys Occup Ther Geriatr 18: 5–21.

Patterson D (1987) Le cause della sindrome di Down. Le Science 230: 32–8.

Prasher VP (1996) The effect of age on language in people with Down's syndrome. J Intell Disabil Res 40: 484–5.

Prasher VP (1999) Adaptive behavior. In M Janicki, AJ Dalton (eds) Dementia, Aging, and Intellectual Disabilities: A Handbook. New York: Wiley-Liss Inc, pp. 157–78.

Rasmussen DE, Sobsey D (1994) Age, adaptive behavior, and Alzheimer disease in Down syndrome: cross-sectional and longitudinal analyses. Am J Ment Retard 99: 151–65.

Richards BW, Sidiqui AQ (1969) Age and mortality trends in residents of an institution for the mentally handicapped. J Ment Defic Res 24: 99–105.

Roeden JM, Zitman FG (1995) Aging in adults with Down's syndrome in institutionally based and community-based residences. J Intell Disabil Res 39: 399–407.

Saviolo Negrin N, Trevisan E (1990) Contributo allo studio delle abilità percettivovisive in Down adulti. In D Salmaso, P Caffarra (eds) Normalità e Patologia delle Funzioni Cognitive nell'Invecchiamento. Milano: Franco Angeli, pp. 220–6.

Silverman W, Wisniewski HM (1998) Down's syndrome and Alzheimer disease: variability in individual vulnerability. In JA Rondal, J Perrera, L Nadel (eds) Down Syndrome: A Review of Current Knowledge. London: Tapper.

Soresi S (1988) Psicologia dell'handicap e della riabilitazione. Bologna: Il Mulino.

Soresi S, Nota L (1995) Ritardo mentale e abilità sociali: una proposta di intervento. Psicoterapia Cognitiva e Comportamentale 2: 13–18.

Thompson SB (1994) A neuropsychological test battery for identifying dementia in people with Down's syndrome. Br J Develop Disabil 40: 135–42.

Thompson SB (1999) Examining dementia in Down's syndrome (DS). Decline in social abilities in DS compared with other learning disabilities. Clin Gerontol 20: 23–44.

Vicari S, Carlesimo A, Caltagirone C (1995) Short-term memory in persons with intellectual disabilities and Down's syndrome. J Intell Disabil Res 39: 532–7.

van Gennep A (1995) Aging and quality of life. Br J Develop Disabil 41: 73–8.

Wechsler D (1981) Manual for the Wechsler Adult Intelligence Scale – Revised (WAIS–R). New York: The Psychological Corporation.

Zigler L (1984) On the definition and classification of mental retardation. Am J Ment Def 32: 215–30.

Chapter 24
The rehabilitation of adults with Down syndrome

A. MORETTI

The rehabilitation of adults with Down syndrome (DS) may appear contradictory in view of the models of early intervention and the rehabilitative theories developed regarding the newborn baby and child with DS.

We actually have to re-evaluate the general characteristics of the person with DS in the light of new knowledge that has developed in recent decades. In particular, we must consider average life expectancy, which today is about 55–60 years. There are the possibilities of social and educational interventions, developing different spheres of ability, which are gaining acceptance at international level (Baird and Sadovnick, 1987, 1988a; Eyman et al., 1991).

The concept of rehabilitation in the adult cannot merely involve the reproduction and continuation of those activities that are essential during development. Consequently the concept of continuity must be bound to the concept of adaptation and change, because of the emerging needs during the different phases of life of the person with DS. Models where there is constant reproduction of rehabilitative interventions for the whole life of a person have been justifiably criticized: these models do not have either a clinical or a social meaning. It is essential to identify needs and difficulties as they appear during the different phases of adult life, as DS exerts its influence. Intervention may be preventative.

The adult with Down syndrome

First of all we must stress the risks concerning the adult with DS. These risks are not due to social and economic integration, but are associated with a biological substratum which causes some aspects of deterioration present in almost all people with DS (Figure 24.1) (Zigman et al., 1995; Baird and Sadovnick, 1988b; Yang et al., 2002).

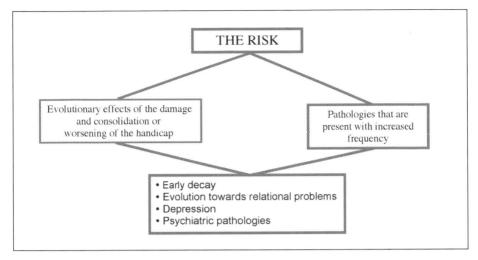

Figure 24.1 The adult with Down syndrome.

It is necessary to clarify that the adult with DS needs two different kinds of services: rehabilitation aimed at prevention and rehabilitation aimed at treatment of emerging problems. An evaluation of suitable services and the identification of a convenient model for the organization of effective and competent services should then be the next step.

Methods of intervention

Table 24.1. Methods of intervention

- Prevention
- Diagnosis
- Specific rehabilitation interventions
- Interventions of accompaniment
- Enhancement of autonomy
- Interventions for the maintenance of the acquired abilities

In prevention, we have to consider conditions that are the consequences of the evolution of DS in an adult person, especially situations which emerge in adulthood, as the DS adult could not have received significant intervention for these earlier in life.

Prevention can be developed in parallel with diagnostic, cultural and social methods during adolescence. The purpose will be to limit the pathological risk in an acceptable way.

Relational uneasiness, for example, and the consequent psychological risks, cannot be eliminated by prevention or conditioning because they are absent during pre-adolescence. On the other hand they become quite common in the adult who is uneasy in a situation of contact with the external environment. This obviously tends to amplify differences of abilities and competences. The adult with limited techniques of defence and of cultural integration tends to respond in a pathological way to a situation of uneasiness.

Preventive action needs to provide the right techniques to improve integration in specific environments.

Diagnosis is an essential instrument and must be able to recognize the presence of pathologies resulting from different situations. It must be developed using a cross- and multidisciplinary method by the team and should operate not only in diagnostic multidisciplinary terms, but also in rehabilitative, therapeutic and multidisciplinary ways. Rehabilitative interventions must be specific and personalized, to obtain the best recovery possible and to avoid possible risks of deterioration.

The rehabilitative intervention must take place in close connection with, but must not be mistaken for, social-cultural and social economic ones (Blackwood et al., 1988; Sung et al., 1997).

The rehabilitative intervention can assume different forms: several methods of rehabilitative intervention can have aspects in common with the methods used during early childhood, but they should be planned with attention to the specific social-cultural context of the person and to his or her age.

Psychomotricity in the adult, for example, cannot be interpreted, developed or in some way enhanced through the same methods used with children or babies, even if the abilities of the treated person are so poor that they appear similar to the competence levels of small children. It is impossible to make an adult work with material or with exercises designed for the newborn child. All the work must be modified according to the context of the adult, in order to maintain or to recover abilities that were lost or that never developed. In this sense, rehabilitation has a very important meaning. It must not be confused with charitable intervention. A fundamental aspect of this sector is neuropsychological rehabilitation. It is not comparable to parascholastic or didactic interventions in a traditional way, but it is essentially correlated to the development of abilities and capabilities bound to the concreteness of adult life. It is vital, in this sector, to maintain constant, active control and a capacity for intervention. The decline of intellectual abilities leads to a successive and more severe deterioration of relational competence and a high risk of development of dementia: these are often untreatable.

Since the average life span of people with DS is shorter than that of the general population, ageing in DS begins earlier. This fact does not represent a specific pathological element, but it is only part of a physiological situation of ageing that is shifted in temporal terms.

The general situation must be interpreted and bound to the life expectancy and to the specific biological situation of DS. In this way we avoid the mistake of considering a physiological aspect to be a pathological expression, and to respond to the emerging needs with inadequate methods.

Since the risk of appearance of early intellectual involution or physical decline is always possible, we have to pay great attention because these symptoms develop in the same phase of life in which the person with DS begins to grow old (Devenny et al., 1997; Cavani et al., 2000).

Prevention

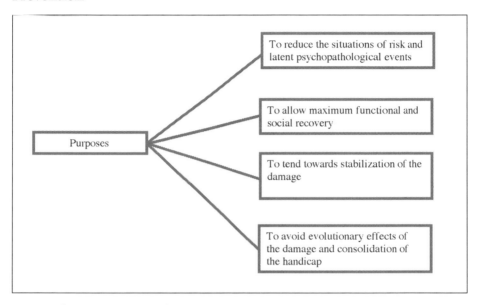

Figure 24.2 The purposes of prevention.

One of the most important aspects of prevention is to identify specific rehabilitative interventions for a particular person, detecting the general present clinical situation either in diagnostic or preventive terms. Obviously rehabilitative action cannot be just a clinical intervention, but it must include all the social and clinical aspects bound to social integration for that particular person. Therefore with the term 'rehabilitative' we should mean a series of actions combining to lead to maximum possible independence. It has to be considered as a fusion of the functional aptitude of a person and his or her social capabilities. The balance between these two aspects permits harmonious, even if restricted, integration and realization. The main purpose of rehabilitation in the adult with DS is to achieve these levels and to maintain them for as long as possible.

Correlation must exist during the different phases of pre-adolescence, adolescence and then adulthood in order to acquire the maximum possible autonomy connected with the initial endowment of the person and his or her social fulfilment. This is an extremely delicate task because it includes interdisciplinary skills that cannot operate individually; it is achieved by working in a group with a clear plan and with the capability of covering the different intersecting areas.

Specific rehabilitative interventions

Table 24.2 Diagnosis

- The use of specific protocols
- Constant monitoring
- Recording the acquired data
- Unique and personal clinical register
- Well timed identification of the difficulties that are subject to recovery
- Applications of methods that can obtain the maximum functional and social recovery
- Maintenance of the acquired abilities through interventions of secondary prevention
- Interventions of tertiary prevention consisting of the systematic application of methods necessary to avoid deleterious effects of the damage

---

Diagnosis

It is important to develop very accurate diagnostic techniques which avoid uncertain responses or responses which are not directed towards specific problems (Table 24.2). Diagnosis should involve the following features (Flórez, 1993):

- The use of specific protocols which indicate the level of maintenance of acquired abilities and possible evolutionary effects
- The evaluation of the presence of relational problems that can originate from the mental handicap, but can then develop towards psychiatric diseases
- The decline of psychomotor skills that can indicate the beginning of an early deterioration
- The loss of linguistic and communicative abilities that can also indicate a lack of environmental and cultural stimuli

Diagnostic data must be evaluated with great attention; they should be kept in a file and in a clinical register, to enable a complete view of the development of the situation. In this way it is easier to intervene at the right moment. It is also vital to correlate a clinical and rehabilitative diagnosis with a 'social' one, so that both preventive and corrective interventions can be activated. Unfortunately, social isolation is common and it can be the cause of disease or of deterioration, especially when one considers the substratum of mental handicap and of general weakness of the subject. Consequently, correlation between specific rehabilitative interventions and correct social monitoring is indispensable for achieving a rehabilitative project for the adult.

Table 24.3 Specific rehabilitative interventions

* Psychomotricity
* Kinesitherapy
* Neuropsychological re-education
* Psychology or psychotherapy
* Occupational therapy
* Social intervention
* Activity of 'accompaniment' towards formation and work
* Counselling and support for families
* Instrumental and laboratory exams
* Specialist examinations

Specific rehabilitative interventions can be of different kinds: some of them can be related to particular pathological situations of a functional type, as a consequence of a specific diagnosis. On the other hand, other specific rehabilitative interventions are thought to be needed by nearly all persons with DS. Some of these interventions are the logical continuation of earlier projects intended to maintain acquired abilities, others must be introduced as a response to specific situations of age-dependent deterioration. Interventions here may delay deterioration. One of the main aspects of intervention is related to the area of neuropsychology; this 'fragile' aspect of the system shows forms of deterioration earlier than other systems (Prasher, 1997).

Interventions of accompaniment

Table 24.4 Interventions of accompaniment

* Response to the specific pathology through validated methods
* Achieving greater possibilities of social integration
* Multidisciplinary interventions in the psychopedagogical, psychological and social sectors
* Needs of a unique multidisciplinary team for the rehabilitation and integration processes
* The establishment of abilities and competences, appropriate for the identified life project
* Reduction of the risks of deterioration
* Interventions of required competences (formation, autonomy), according to different periods of life

This kind of intervention is called 'social rehabilitative intervention' because it always aims to achieve the greatest possible social integration; it is therefore considered a real barrier towards early intellectual decline. Obviously social integration is not just exercising a right, but is the consequence of a series of actions. In order to achieve this purpose, it is important to evaluate the abilities and potentials that are present, and the person's social and cultural environment. In this way, it is possible to identify a life project as an indicator for the multidisciplinary team.

It is possible to use techniques for the fulfilment of the project, that might be considered useless in other situations. An example is insertion of a DS teenager into high school. This might appear disproportionate to the abilities of a person with DS but, on the contrary, it is extremely important from social and cultural aspects. It is even possible to achieve integration for an adult that could appear disproportionate to his or her abilities, but which can have important results, activating abilities and competences that were apparently lacking. This is the case with working integration and the project of independent life which help to establish the fulfilment of a person. It is clear that with advanced age, studied interventions for the maintenance of acquired abilities cannot be the same as those used in the early phases of life.

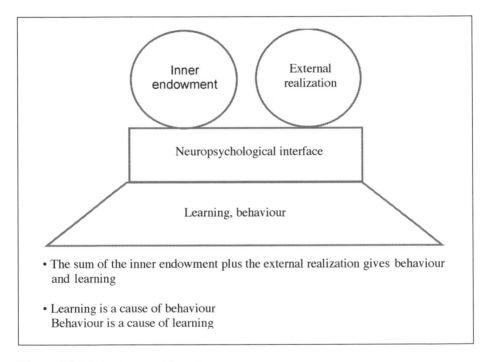

Figure 24.3 Behaviour and learning.

The adult with DS, despite limited inner endowment and external achievements, is nevertheless an adult who should be respected. It is important to be able to make interventions 'non-invasive', in order to avoid their rejection by the person with DS. The care-giving team should operate through continuous monitoring, avoiding direct action on the DS person. At the same time, the team must respect the life programming of that individual, including the factors of relationships and sociability (Zetlin and Turner, 1985; Haxby, 1989).

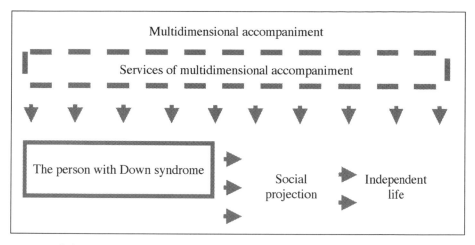

Multidimensional accompaniment

Services of multidimensional accompaniment

The person with Down syndrome

Social projection

Independent life

Figure 24.4 Interventions for the maintenance of acquired abilities.

References

Baird PA, Sadovnick AD (1987) Life expectancy in Down syndrome. J Pediatr 110(6): 849–54

Baird PA, Sadovnick AD (1988a) Life expectancy in Down syndrome adults. Lancet 10: 1354–5.

Baird PA, Sadovnick AD (1988b) Causes of death to age 30 in Down syndrome. Am J Hum Genet 43: 239–48.

Blackwood DHR, St Clair DM, Muir WJ, Oliver CJ, Dickens F (1988) The development of Alzheimer's disease in Down syndrome assessed by auditory event-related potentials. J Ment Def Res 32: 439–53.

Cavani S, Tamaoka A, Moretti A, Marinelli L, Angelini G, di Stefano S, Piombo G, Cazzulo V, Matsuno S, Shoji S, Furiya Y, Zaccheo D, Dagna-Bricarelli F, Tabaton M, Mori H (2000) Plasma level of amyloid 40 and 42 are independent from ApoE genotype and mental retardation in Down syndrome. Am J Med Genet 95: 224–8.

Devenny DA, Silverman WP, Hill AL, Jenkins E, Sersen EA, Wisniewski KW (1997) Envejecimiento normal en adultos con síndrome de Down: un estudio longitudinal. Rev Síndrome Down 14: 94–104.

Eyman RK, Call TL, White JF (1991) Life expectancy of person with Down syndrome. Am J Ment Retard 95: 603–12.

Flórez J (1993) Envejecimiento y síndrome de Down. ¿Alzheimer, sí o no? Rev Síndrome Down 10: 55–62.

Haxby JV (1989) Neuropsychological evaluation of adults with Down syndrome: patterns of selective impairment in non-demented old adults. J Ment Defic Res 33: 193–210.

Prasher VP (1997) Dementia questionnaire for persons with mental retardation (DMR): Modified criteria for adults with Down syndrome. J Appl Res Intellect Disabil 10: 54–60.

Sung H, Hawkins BA, Eklund SJ, Kim KA, Foose A, May ME, Rogers NB (1997) Depression and dementia in aging adults with Down syndrome: a case study approach. Ment Retard 35: 27–38.

Yang Q, Rasmussen SA, Friedman JM (2002) Mortality associated with Down's syndrome in the USA from 1983 to 1997: a population-based study. Lancet 359: 1019–25.

Zetlin AG, Turner JL (1985) Transition from adolescence to adulthood: perspectives of mentally retarded individuals and their families. Am J Ment Defic 89(6): 570–9.

Zigman WB, Schupf N, Sersen E, Silverman W (1995) Prevalence of dementia in adults with and without Down syndrome. Am J Ment Retard 100: 403–12.

Chapter 25
Evaluating treatment outcomes

S. SORESI

According to Fuhrer (1987), evaluating treatment outcomes should consist of specifying the goals rehabilitation services want to achieve, as well as the identification and assessment of actual results.

These procedures should be systematic and should aim towards evaluating treatment programme efficacy and efficiency, and clients' satisfaction for the results obtained. They should also allow us to observe differences over time in clients' abilities and performance. Thus, if we want properly to evaluate the efficacy of abilitative and rehabilitative programmes, we need to consider either the degree of decline in disability or the increase in the range of clients' activities. Therefore, it is the relationship between established, divulged goals and achieved results that should determine the degree of treatment programme efficacy.

Outcome evaluation and the choice of criteria for analysing the efficacy of programmes involve numerous and complex problems, especially for disabled persons, since the universe of the disabled is anything but uniform.

What generally leads disabled people or their families to turn to a service for treatment is the great need to see some sort of change take place, i.e. hope for potential improvement.

However, disabled persons may also, either in a straightforward or implicit manner, request intervention with the simple desire of maintaining their current situation or limiting the probability of experiencing greater problems and suffering in the future. Obviously, in cases such as these, programme efficacy cannot be evaluated in terms of easily observable, documented changes and improvement. Furthermore, when confronted with mild disabilities, we can realistically presume the feasibility of working at these individuals achieving significant levels of self-sufficiency in their daily activities. However, it would be quite naïve, when working with people with severe and progressive disabilities, to aim for complete self-sufficiency in, for example, personal hygiene, managing everyday problems, and work and community inclusion. Thus, for people with severe and multiple disabilities and with wide-ranging forms of comorbidity, it is considerably less likely that we will be able to set up multi-faceted and meaningful abilitative activities, such as the neuropsy-chological, cognitive, assertive, and social skills enhancement training that can increase disabled people's chances for participating in and achieving their own life projects. Moreover, given the enormous variability that exists within the same disability (e.g. intellectual disabilities or autism), it is not surprising to find that certain intervention programmes that succeed with some people do not work with others, even if clients belong to the same diagnostic category. Lastly, among the factors that can influence intervention outcomes, besides type and severity of disability, are clients' age and gender, as well as the characteristics of their environmental conditions, which may be more positively or less positively orientated towards including the disabled.

Hence, I share the conviction of those researchers, such as Lindsay and Gralton (1999) and McGill et al. (1996), who believe that the best predictor of abilitative and rehabilitative results is rigorous and meticulous assessment.

Why evaluate the efficacy of treatment?

There are many and diverse reasons for implementing specific evaluations of rehabilitative treatment:

- From a scientific perspective, it is important to evaluate the efficacy of rehabilitation procedures in order to decide if we should proceed with further intervention on the same person or replicate the treatment with people who have similar problems. These considerations should be kept in mind, above all, by anyone working in social and health services who has administrative, as well as scientific, responsibilities. Too often, as I have discussed elsewhere (Soresi and Nota, 2001), treatment programmes for the disabled seem to elude scientific control, 'in a kind of limbo that discourages serious researchers from approaching (the study) with adequate confidence' (Di Nuovo, 1995) and interest
- From an ethical perspective, it would undoubtedly be reprehensible for us not to reflect and verify if the results of our efforts to improve abilities or mitigate difficulties have been effective. In other words, it would be morally unacceptable to carry on with a programme without first evaluating the legitimacy and validity of what has already been accomplished. This is precisely why evaluation must be considered a crucial element of both rationalizing costs and improving service quality, and this goes for both public and non-profit sectors

- Also, from an economic perspective, evaluative considerations are growing ever more pressing. Let us not forget that, in the last few decades, there have been significant changes in rehabilitative services. According to Coulthard-Morris et al. (1997), we have gone from treating functional impairments to the long-term management of disabilities and handicaps. This has brought on a whole new series of extra costs, such that approximately 80% of Italian healthcare spending is now being funnelled into treating disabilities. At the same time, however, as Coulthard-Morris et al. (1997) maintain, more and more frequently, the managed care system requires keeping track of programme cost-effectiveness before reimbursing services for treatment costs; Herdon (1997) goes so far as to say that if a treatment cannot objectively be evaluated as efficacious, it will not be reimbursed and that certain therapies are bound to fall into disuse if their efficacy is not demonstrated by controlled clinical studies

Notwithstanding the 'good reasons' for evaluating abilitative and rehabilitative programmes, when we propose evaluation, the first people to experience confusion and reluctance to cooperate are rehabilitation workers and professionals themselves, who can feel controlled, as if they were 'under a microscope'.

However, it is important to note that, in any case, in our rehabilitation centres, 'Evaluation, consisting in judgments and attributions regarding clients, situations, co-workers, and episodes, goes on all the time, even if it is usually intra-personal with little awareness involved and is therefore not easily evident or accessible' (Scarlatti and Regalia, 2000). Such evaluative processes should eventually be brought to light, rationalized and channelled into improving the quality of service. This is why treatment outcome evaluations should never be conducted in secrecy, nor should they ever be directed 'against' anyone, since it can be beneficial or even necessary, to involve clients, as well as rehabilitation service providers, in the process (Simons, 1994). If personnel and clients are encouraged to cooperate in making choices or in formulating efficacy criteria, they can be more motivated, more cooperative, and more involved in the various stages of data gathering and analysis.

How to evaluate treatment outcomes

Now that we have established the importance of evaluation, it is time to expand upon the methodological problems anyone who intends to evaluate treatment effectiveness will be faced with solving.

The problems are complex, because evaluating treatment outcomes should be anchored, first and foremost, to a definition of efficacy, to the specification of the abilities or the performances to be examined, and to the stipulation of the conditions that are necessary for implementing evaluation.

To summarize Table 25.1, modelled on a study by Gori and Vittadini (1999), if we are to evaluate the efficacy of a programme or treatment, we must consider the following:

- The degree of correspondence between expected and obtained results: for example, a service provider might decide to get family members involved (in an awareness campaign, in meetings, or in an all-out parent training programme, etc.) with the aim of increasing their cooperation in a social interaction programme. Afterwards, however, the provider will have to ask, 'How many disabled clients did we actually manage to mainstream and how many did we do so with the cooperation of family members?'
- The discrepancy between achieved results and standards, which are either required or predicted by programme and treatment planners or by supervisory agencies. What is called for here is 'quality accreditation', which is indeed a compelling issue, considering how disabled people were treated in the past in locked institutions
- The significance of the effects a programme or service has on a problem, a target population, or a community. This is an important estimate for verifying the efficacy of prevention programmes or for setting up positive conditions concerning, for example, scholastic, vocational or community inclusion
- Comparing the efficacy of treatments or of different methods: the fact that there are many procedures and programmes that are similarly legitimate from a scientific perspective means they must be compared in order to estimate their 'relative efficacy'; i.e. to identify the most

Table 25.1 Types of efficacy, areas, and evaluation conditions

Operational descriptions of efficacy	Evaluation areas	Necessary conditions
Discrepancy between expected and obtained results	Have rehabilitative goals been achieved?	Goal disclosure (operational description and prognosis)
Discrepancy between predicted and achieved standards	Are the implemented procedures and techniques top quality?	Existence of an easily implemented, accredited standard
Significance of effects	Presumable severity of deterioration and hardship had the programme not been carried out	Availability of criteria regarding the 'natural' evolution of impairment and disability
Clients' satisfaction ratings	Are facilities valued and easily accessible?	Knowledge of clients' expectations and satisfaction

beneficial procedures and programmes (e.g. those that entail fewer costs, are easier to implement, are best in agreement with a service provider's philosophy or available expertise, etc.)

- Users' satisfaction ratings: although it is not a true measure of efficacy, I believe that the degree of clients' satisfaction with a service should also be assessed. Indeed, I think that it is extremely unlikely that rehabilitation service providers will ever be able to pursue their goals, which, with disabled people imply enhancing abilities, participation, and empowerment, if they cannot even manage to gain their clients' trust, respect, or agreement regarding their work

Once we have defined an evaluation area, procedures can be selected and, based on the meaning of 'treatment efficacy', it is generally preferable to rely on functional measures, e.g. those concerning scholastic, vocational and social tasks, thereby reducing the risks of even strong disagreement developing between clients and abilitation-rehabilitation experts. For example, as Scherer (1993) points out, rehabilitation service providers might consider even minimal improvements in some cognitive functions or in some areas of motor functioning as marginal success indicators. Conversely, clients or their families might consider similar gains irrelevant, since they are not associated with significant improvement in self-sufficiency, independence or psychosocial participation.

The selected success indicators should also be properly communicated and agreed upon with disabled people and their family members, to avoid them, for example, paradoxically considering any gains in self-sufficiency as negative. In fact, such gains will eventually lead to a reduction in relief support assistance and, even if they clearly represent a client's progressive improvement, can be a source of anxiety and worry. Clients should therefore be involved in establishing efficacy evaluation criteria, and as Scherer points out (1993), results should always be measured in terms of both change and clients' satisfaction.

Evaluating abilitative-rehabilitative intervention efficacy

It is known that the disabilities that are associated with different types of impairment are many, diverse, and can vary greatly with respect to severity. Nonetheless, I believe that a rehabilitation worker's task is primarily the following: to help clients achieve their utmost capacities, within the limits of their own unique problems.

Learning, and the conditions that favour it, play a decidedly crucial role here, because disabilities essentially refer to what people are not able or are no longer able to do: a person who has suffered a spinal injury, for example, must modify certain behaviours (e.g. deambulation). They have to modify what they must do, as well as what they are able to do; but they will not be able to do the new things they need to and are potentially able to do, until they have learned to do them. Frequently, we must start from the ground up and design a complete relearning programme. For example, for a person who has suffered severe brain damage or who has had a stroke, we may need to set up exercises to work on balance and deambulation just to get them walking again, or perhaps we will organize speech therapy sessions to help them regain the use of speech, or we may even need to teach them other complex methods of communication. We might also have to teach a client new skills, like those required for moving around inside or outside the home with a wheelchair or some other type of prosthesis.

Gordon (1987) maintains that if we are to assert that treatment has been effective, we must proceed with thoroughness and precision, taking cues from neuropsychological treatment evaluation criteria. We should therefore proceed with three types of verification:

- Evaluating if the improvements observed during the course of a training session transfer to other sessions and if they can be observed when other, similar conditions, situations and tasks are proposed
- Verifying if changes are also evident with the re-administration of the same assessment instruments that had originally served to diagnose the problem (cognitive and neuropsychological tests, ability or disability evaluation scales, etc.)
- Ascertaining if the observed improvement pertains to the quality and quantity of a client's daily activities. This last criterion begins a new chapter – that of the quality of life and of the impact that any planned abilitative and rehabilitative practices must have on it (Soresi et al., 2003)

Together with the current need for controlling abilitative and rehabilitative practices and with the ever-more insistent demand for the efficiency and efficacy of social and health services, there has been enormous growth in the availability of evaluation measures. They go from very simple and clear-cut scales, which directly measure a particular function, e.g. the deambulation index, to scales that are quite removed from any type of pathology, like those measuring quality of life. Some of these are well structured and accurately validated, but others are administered without keeping track of the measure's efficiency and reliability, or the validity of the scale itself (Herdon, 1997). In this regard, there are several criteria that must be considered for selecting an instrument.

As Herdon (1997) stated in the introduction of a book presenting the most frequently used scales in neurology, our instruments must be:

- Appropriate to the task
- Valid
- Reliable
- Efficient, easy to use and require little training

- Sensitive to changes in a particular situation but also relatively insensitive to the random fluctuation of symptoms

I think it is appropriate here to expand on just some of the requisites evaluation scales should have, especially when used for analysing programme efficacy.

1. They must be efficient and easy to use. Some very valid and reliable tests end up never being used in rehabilitative services or even in research, because their administration and scoring take too much time, and this is probably what happens in best case scenarios. Unfortunately, it is not unheard of, as Herdon (1997) says about the Kurtzke scale (1983), for a 'busy' physician to try to speed up the evaluation process, and instead of observing a client walk as the test requires, the doctor may simply ask the client how far he or she can walk. Furthermore, a scale's efficiency is important not only for healthcare and social assistance professionals. Indeed, none of us like spending lots of time filling out forms and questionnaires, even when we need therapy or treatment. We will be more likely to maintain a properly high level of concentration if we perceive that questions are important for us and, especially, if the whole process does not take too much time and effort
2. They must be sensitive to change. A scale should allow us to reveal if a person has a specific disability and if so, to differentiate him or her from another person with the same disability. Therefore, since it is now widely accepted that programmes need to be personalized, sensitivity to change, in addition to being a desirable assessment criterion, has become a prerequisite for planning abilitative and rehabilitative programmes. Such programmes cannot be prepared without specific evaluations and personal profiles, which highlight a person's strengths and weaknesses. Moreover, the benefits of treatment usually become slowly evident, with changes occurring over time, and sometimes, almost imperceptibly. Hence, it is crucial to have instruments available that can reveal even slight, but significant progress. This same requisite is also important for certain other cases in which we must settle for considering efficacious any intervention that helps prevent what Trexler and Sullivan (1995) call 'the spiral of deterioration', i.e. the gradual decline of neurological functions and behavioural and relational conditions. At the same time, however, we must not forget that a scale's excessive and apparent 'sensitivity' can indicate that it lacks stability and therefore, reliability

Regarding the choice of measures and tests to evaluate intervention efficacy, I have already affirmed that they should be 'practical' and should pertain to a person's particular problem areas. Functional impairment (e.g. symptoms such as diploplia, ataxia, tremor or spasticity) may vary or not after treatment, which is why functional impairment indicators are not generally considered valid for evaluating outcomes. These measures, as Johnston et al. (1993) also maintain, are not very sensitive to change with respect to evaluating disabilities and limitations in daily functioning. Bowling (1991) also maintains that tests assessing the range of a person's activities (e.g. grasping strength or limb movements) are generally considered the most valid indicators of a person's abilities and, therefore, of treatment outcomes.

Evaluating efficacy: methodological aspects

From a scientific perspective, as is well known, the chosen procedure for verifying the existence of significant outcomes consists in carrying out group comparisons, most often between what are called control groups and experimental groups. This type of procedure is practically obligatory for anyone who engages in experimental research, because it enables us to single out effects and determine the possibility of generalizing results. However, it is not easy to establish this condition when working with the disabled, because of any number of methodological 'hitches', which, although they are encountered in other psychological domains, are particularly frequent and difficult to solve in this one. These risks include those listed below.

- Even if treated and compared groups present the same impairment and disability, they have a high incidence of internal variability, which, methodologically speaking, makes it hard to be sure of the adequacy of any applied statistical procedures and, consequently, of the legitimacy of any conclusions drawn
- It is unlikely that treated and compared groups will be sufficiently equivalent. Indeed, research studies frequently do not provide information on service providers' characteristics and preferred procedures. For example, new treatment programmes are usually conducted by people who are enthusiastic about the programme, while control groups, as Dunn (1996) reminds us, may end up being assigned to poorly motivated and disenchanted personnel, who are often aware of being used for the sole purpose of making comparisons. Moreover, participants in different experimental groups are not isolated, but they interact with each other and with personnel. The nature of these relationships can be just as influential on outcomes as any particular therapy, but there is little mention of this in most published studies
- Concerning participant pairing, researchers often use miscellaneous and not always universally accredited criteria. For example, when conducting research on participants with intellectual disabilities, as Tampieri et al. (1988) point out, comparisons can be based on mental age (ME), chronological age (CE), or on measures of cognitive development (IQ) and will consequently have varied and hard-to-compare results (Baumeister, 1984)

- Most researchers in this field usually base their observations on a very small number of participants. On the one hand, this can reduce within-group variability, because participants are usually selected according to a limited number of common attributes, but on the other hand, it makes it harder subsequently to generalize any conclusions reached on a particular treatment's efficacy
- Selection procedures for choosing experimental groups are not always clearly described and, accordingly, we cannot always consider samples as representative of a particular population of disabled persons. Indeed, often, one is left with the impression that participants are chosen merely because they frequent institutions to which researchers have access

If we are interested in verifying hypotheses of treatment efficacy and if we want to reduce the previously described risks, we should bear in mind some of Greene and D'Oliveira's (1982) recommendations. First of all we have to remember that the choice of a suitable statistical test ultimately depends on the experimental design chosen to verify a hypothesis.[1] For example, we might be interested in verifying if the scores of certain variables are related to each other, that is, if they are correlated (e.g. if the social skills of some clients are related to their self-determination skills). In this case, we would have a correlational study, which, however, cannot demonstrate causal relations between variables. More specifically, we cannot suppose that one variable causes any variations observed in another variable. Correlational studies require the application of specific data analysis procedures.

We might otherwise be interested in measuring the differences induced by a particular treatment. For example, we might want to verify if there are differences in performance before and after a treatment programme, or if there are differences between clients who have received treatment and others who have not or who have undergone another type of treatment (treatment vs. no treatment; treatment 'A' vs. treatment 'B', etc.). We must rely on specific data analysis procedures here, as well.

It must be noted that analytical procedures, in addition to depending on research objectives, also depend on the test and survey methods employed. These can pertain to three different types of scales: nominal, ordinal and interval.[2] In order to choose statistical tests properly, the number of independent variables and experimental conditions in our experimental design must be also considered.

In fact, there are two types of statistical tests: parametric and non-parametric. Non-parametric tests are used when data are of a nominal or ordinal level, while parametric tests are usually for interval measurement scales and when other conditions are satisfied (e.g. normal distribution of data, and uniformity of variance).

It is also crucial to distinguish between repeated and non-repeated measures experimental designs. If we want to assess the effectiveness of a treatment programme, we can examine differences between different participants, by employing a between-subjects experimental design. In this situation, we compare the performance or scores of people in two different groups, which are presumed to be unrelated. Conversely, if we want to compare the performance of the same participants in different conditions (e.g. pre- and post-treatment), we prepare what is called a within-subjects experimental design. In this case, the comparison is made within the same group of participants, by examining their scores at two or more different times (e.g. disability severity, IQ, self-determination ratings, or quality of life), which therefore cannot be considered independent.

Another possibility is the matched-subjects experimental design (matched by age, sex, or types of institutionalization or treatment received, etc.); although these can present their own problems in the study of disabled persons, they have the advantages of both the above-described procedures. The data can be treated as if they pertain to a within-subjects design, and there is a lower incidence of inter-individual variance, due to learning effects. Unfortunately, and frequently as well, in the study of disability, the possibility of arranging balanced groups through meticulous pairing procedures is small: the variables that need to be considered here are many and hard to measure and often include other intervening factors, pertaining to anamnesis, context and environment.

Evaluating treatment in N = 1 experimental designs

In the last few years, much effort has been channelled into conferring scientific legitimacy to single case studies. The reasons are linked to the limits and problems of carrying out comparisons between groups and their ensuing costs, but the recourse to the analysis of case studies is also due to the fact that there are syndromes which, fortunately so, from another perspective, are so rare as to make it extremely difficult, if not impossible, to conduct group comparison studies on them (Wilson, 1985). The advantages of single case studies would not be such, however, without 'the support of statistical-inferential stratagems, which in the last few years, have conferred the requisite methodological rigor to the analysis of single case studies' (Pastore et al., 2003).

Furthermore, if we are dealing with numerically small groups and one subject, we can also rely on time-series designs, which call for analysing a set of data gathered longitudinally and which help us analyse the clinical significance of data (Hersen and Barlow, 1976; Jacobson, 1988; Di Nuovo, 1992). In cases such as these, if we want to demonstrate a decline in disability or a gain in adaptive behaviour, we can rely on specific statistical tests, endowed with particular power, e.g. the calculation of linear trends with the minimum squares method, the chi square for trends, the rho for trends, or the C test. Obviously, there are other, more complex experimental designs available: it is possible, for example, to analyse several time-series associated with the simultaneous monitoring of more than two variables and conditions (between series) or we can use what are referred to as multiple baseline experimental designs.

If pursued rehabilitation activity were supported by similar controls, no one could ever make the claim that working with people with severe disabilities means either providing relief help or passing off treatment programmes as rehabilitative, when they are anything but that.

Quality of service

As we have seen, the theme of analysing treatment efficacy is particularly intricate and raises several methodological problems, which further cloud the picture if we consider that they usually occur among services with different quality standards. More specifically, the considerations I propose here, regarding evaluating treatment efficacy, challenge the quality and evaluation of services.

In fact, quality of service and evaluation are interlinked and interdependent concepts, and they require conferring meaning and legitimacy to intervention, to organizational choices and to the monitoring of results. Hence, the need for proper evaluation procedures goes hand in hand with the prerequisite of quality of service.

It is precisely for this reason that in recent years, the issue of service quality is becoming more and more a topic of discussion. According to Dalley (1989), I cannot settle for just setting up and implementing services; they must be systematically based on verification procedures suited to evaluating the quality and improving standards. On this subject Clifford et al. (1989) suggest carefully examining:

- The goals a determined service has chosen or is in the process of choosing
- The initiatives undertaken to promote quality of service, improvement in personnel and staff performance, the evaluation of results and the correct use of abilitative and rehabilitative practices

More recently, Dickens (1990, 1991) illustrated these ideas by proposing an analysis of:

- The quality of a service's environmental conditions, management style, organizational structure, as well as its philosophical tenets and values and the resources it makes available to clients. All of these aspects can be surveyed with structured questionnaires and direct observation
- The quality of care, which pertains to personnel–client interaction, the systems and methods employed in order to provide the service and personnel expertise. These evaluations can be made by relying on

direct and indirect observational methods, but the analysis, however, should privilege the clients' perspective
- Clients' quality of life, which can be assessed with satisfaction measures and the achievement of abilitative and rehabilitative goals

In the same vein, Bradley (1991) advises examining at least four important areas:

1. *Input*: the structural aspects of a service, such as ease of access, type of client, number of workers, personnel expertise, and the facilities where the service is provided. This information is relatively easy to obtain, and it comprises the basic ingredient for developing a quality evaluation system
2. *Procedure*: the interactions between clients and the organization
3. *Output*: the 'results', in terms of the number of clients assisted or discharged. Output is also relatively easy to measure
4. *Results*: the 'finished product' or culmination of service, intended as surveying a service's effects or impact on clients

Since maintaining high quality standards is an arduous task, in conclusion of our reflections on evaluating treatment efficacy and in reference to the works of Berwick (1992), Berwick et al. (1990) and Maxwell (1992), I list below some important factors and conditions that must be satisfied to best promote an improvement in the quality of service:

1. *The will to change* must be palpable in a service provider. In any organization, improvements that are to be implemented and, hopefully, achieved, must obviously be hoped for and desired. Too often, in our opinion, social and health service providers, administrators, and management seem chiefly concerned with maintaining the status quo, as if in the sphere of abilitation and rehabilitation, nothing can be done better than it is already being done, and as if research in this field provides no incentive and stimulus
2. Each organization must formulate and divulge its own *definition of quality*, in such a way as to encourage participation and to make verifying quality standards feasible internally as well as externally. Both users and professionals will be more likely regularly to refer to the definition of quality if they have originally concurred on operationally specifying its indicators, and if they do not perceive results and evaluations as clinging to administrative standards
3. Every service should periodically reintroduce *quality survey measures*, in order to facilitate improvement in quality and its maintenance. This obviously requires valid and reliable instruments, together with sophisticated surveying skills. These monitoring activities will benefit quality of service if the analysis includes personnel, all available and utilized (material and financial) resources, treatment, and organizational and administrative processes. In fact, we must not forget that in healthcare

and rehabilitation, improvement relies on the entire curative, abilitative and rehabilitative system. The elements that help foster it or, sadly, hinder it are many and interdependent. If we adopt this perspective, the quality of service will be perceived as depending on the entire system, so that even when problems do arise, analyses will not be focused solely on individual responsibility

4. *The need to invest in professional training.* A continually improving service is one that wants to keep learning all the time, not only in order to improve its 'practices', but also with the goal of greater organizational efficiency in mind. Consequently, if a service proposes training programmes for the various professions involved in rehabilitation, this can be considered a good indicator of interest in maintaining and improving the quality of service

5. Paying *attention to costs.* Clearly, the quality of a service cannot be considered solely in terms of how much it does or does not cost. Anyone who thoroughly analyses and evaluates their own endeavours in this field will also carefully examine the economic aspects, by attempting systematically to reduce any waste, duplication of effort, or overlaps in the system, because improving quality also means saving energy and resources

6. *Transforming good ideas into action.* All too frequently, services' 'theories and guiding principles' are undoubtedly noble, but things are easier said than done. In our opinion, it is management's responsibility to ensure that grand-sounding propositions and good intentions are transformed into specific operations and activities, which are constantly verified with informed, interpersonal and easily replicable procedures. Creating opportunities for the collaborative deliberation and planning of treatment is therefore of crucial importance, provided, however, that the quality of interpersonal dynamics and productiveness is also properly managed

7. Responsibilities should be assigned openly, rationally and sensibly, so that each employee, in relation to his or her own capacity and expertise, is inspired to contribute efficaciously to maintaining and improving the quality of service

Evaluating efficacy: some final considerations

At this point it must surely be evident that selecting methodologically correct procedures for evaluating treatment programme efficacy is not the only aspect involved. Treatments are usually introduced and conducted by services whose quality standards end up influencing, often decisively, the results obtained. The considerations that I have proposed here, in addition to encouraging the use of more rigorous evaluation procedures, attest to the advisability and need for a sweeping 'organizational and cultural reorientation, which does not stop at the mere proposition and utilization of more-or-less sophisticated monitoring instruments and the compilation of operational handbooks ...' (Orsenigo, 1999). Quality and evaluation are interlinked concepts, deriving, all things considered, from the need to confer meaning to the choices we make in our efforts to mitigate the problems of ever larger numbers of people.

Recently, Green (1999) has argued that it is time for social programmes to justify what they introduce into people's lives, and not the simple fact that they provide services, and that the time has come to stop settling for procedural rules as adequate indicators of the efficacy and quality of treatment programmes.

Notes

1   An experimental hypothesis describes an expectation a researcher formulates concerning the predicted relations between two or more variables, i.e. between an *independent* variable (in our case, a treatment programme) and observed, or *dependent*, variable or variables (e.g. disability severity; social skills, self-determination, etc.).

2   We use the first level of measurement, the *nominal* level, when we want to classify research participants into mutually exclusive categories (e.g. people with different types of disabilities or impairment, with distinct characteristics, male vs. female, institutionalized or mainstreamed, etc.).

The second level, the *ordinal*, is used whenever it is possible to specify participants' attributes or performances by ranging them (e.g. mild, moderate, severe, intellectual disability, etc.)

The third level of measurement, the *interval* level, is usually employed when one is working with numerical scores (e.g. the number of correctly recalled items, reaction times to a stimulus, etc.), which lets us assume that the distances between the scores are equal and are therefore equally interpretable. This type of measurement is called 'interval' because it is based on the supposition that there are equal intervals between the data, and these intervals comprise a continuous numerical scale. It is assumed, for example, that remembering two vs. three items represents the same interval that exists between remembering three vs. four items (Greene and D'Oliveira, 1982). Data gathered with self- or hetero-evaluation, including five- or seven-point Likert scales, which actually function on an ordinal scale, are often used as if they were interval scales, because it is presumed that the numerical differences on these types of scales are equal.

We must not forget that there is also a measurement level called *proportional*, which, like the interval level, refers to numerical-type scales, but requires the existence of an absolute zero. Proportional-level scales, however, are unlikely to figure among those used for assessing treatment programme efficacy.

References

Baumeister AA (1984) Some methodological and conceptual issues in the study of cognitive processes with retarded people. In P Brooks, R Sperber, C McClauley (eds) Learning and Cognition in the Mentally Retarded. Hillsdale, NJ: Lawrence Erlbaum Associates.

Berwick DM (1992) Heal thyself or heal thy system: can doctors help to improve medical care? Qual Health Care 1(Suppl): S2–S8.

Berwick DM, Godfrey A, Roessner J (1990) Curing Health Care. San Francisco: Jossey-Bass.

Bowling A (1991) Measuring Health: A Review of Quality of Life Measurement Scales. Philadelphia: Open University Press.

Bradley VJ (1991) Conceptual issues in quality assurance. In VJ Bradley, HA Bersani (eds) Quality Assurance for Individuals with Developmental Disabilities: It's Everybody's Business. Baltimore: Paul H Brookes Publishing.

Clifford P, Leiper R, Lavander A, Pilling S (1989) Assuring Quality in Mental Health Services. The QUARTZ System. London: RDP.

Coulthard-Morris L, Burks JS, Herdon RM (1997) Misure di esito della riabilitazione (Outcomes in rehabilitation). In RM Herdon (ed.) Scale di Valutazione in Neurologia. Torino: Centro Scientifico Editore, pp. 225–64.

Dalley G (1989) On the road to quality. Health Serv J 99: 150–80.

Di Nuovo S (1992) La Sperimentazione in Psicologia Applicata (Experimentation in Applied Psychology). Milano: Franco Angeli.

Di Nuovo S (1995) I metodi della ricerca in psicologia clinica (Research methods in Cinical Psychology). In L D'Odorico (ed.) Sperimentazione e Alternative di Ricerca Milano: Raffaello Cortina Editore, pp. 153–210.

Dickens P (1990) Aiming for excellence in mental handicap services. Int J Health Care Qual Assur 3(1): 4–8.

Dickens P (1991) 'Aiming for excellence' – the evaluation of quality of life and quantity of services for people with a mental handicap. In National Perspectives on Quality Assurance in Mental Health Care. Geneva: World Health Organisation.

Dunn G (1996) Statistical methods for measuring outcomes. In G Thornicroft, M Tansella (eds) Mental Health Outcome Measures. Berlin: Springer-Verlag.

Fuhrer MJ (1987) Rehabilitation Outcomes: Analysis and Measurement. Baltimore: Paul H Brookes.

Gordon W (1987) Methodological considerations in cognitive remediation. In M Meier, A Benton, L Diller (eds) Neuropsychological Rehabilitation. New York: Guilford.

Gori E, Vittadini G (1999) Qualità e Valutazione nei Servizi di Pubblica Utilità (Quality and Evaluation in Public Facilities). Milano: Etas.

Green J (1999) The inequality of performance measurement. Evaluation 5: 160–72.

Greene J, D'Oliveira M (1982) Learning to Use Statistical Tests in Psychology: A Student's Guide. Philadelphia: Open University Press.

Herdon RM (1997) Scale di valutazione in neurologia. Torino: Centro Scientifico Editore.

Hersen M, Barlow DH (1976) Single Case Experimental Design: Strategies for Studying Behavior Change. New York: Pergamon Press.

Jacobson NS (1988) Defining clinically significant change. Behav Assess 10 (Special Issue): 2

Johnston MV, Wilerson DL, Maney M (1993) Evaluation of the quality and outcomes of medical rehabilitation programs. In JB DeLisa, BM Gans, D Currie (eds) Rehabilitation Medicine: Principles and Practice. Philadelphia: Lippincott Williams & Wilkins Publishers, pp. 240–68.

Kurtzke JF (1983) Rating neurological impairment in multiple sclerosis: an expanded disability status scale (EDSS). Neurology 33: 1444–52.

Lindsay ML, Gralton E (1999) Measuring the outcomes of services. In N Bouras (ed.) Psychiatric and Behavioural Disorders in Developmental Disabilities and Mental Retardation. Cambridge University Press, pp. 412–26.

Maxwell RJ (1992) Dimensions of quality revisited: from thought to action. Qual Health Care 1: 171–7.

McGill P, Clare I, Murphy G (1996) Undestanding and responding to challenging behavior: from theory to practice. Tizard Learning Disability Review 1: 9–17.

Orsenigo A (1999) Per una critica della qualità degli interventi di prevenzione e dei servizi socio-sanitari (The quality of interventions and social services). In P Ugolini, FC Giannotti (eds) Valutazione e Prevenzione delle Tossico-dipendenze. Teoria, Metodi e Strumenti Valutativi. Milano: Franco Angeli.

Pastore M, Dell'Acqua R, Seregni S (2003) Teoria e metodi per lo studio di casi singoli neuropsicologici (Single case in neuropsychology). In S Soresi (ed) Disabilità, Trattamento e Integrazione. Pordenone: Erip Editrice, pp. 55–86.

Scarlatti G, Regalia C (2000) Approcci metodologici alla valutazione dei servizi (The evaluation of services). In C Regalia, A Bruno (eds) Valutazione e Qualità nei Servizi. Una Sfida Attuale per le Organizzazioni. Milano: Unicopoli, pp. 43–84.

Scherer M. (1993) Living in the State of Stuck: How Technology Impacts the Lives of People with Disabilities. Cambridge, MA: Brookline Books.

Simons K (1994) Enabling research: people with learning difficulties. Research, Policy and Planning 12: 4–5.

Soresi S, Nota L (2001) La Facilitazione dell'integrazione Scolastica (School Inclusion). Pordenone: Erip Editrice.

Soresi S, Nota L, Sgaramella T (2003) La Valutazione delle Disabilità. Volume secondo (The Evaluation of Disabilities. Second volume). Pordenone: Erip Editrice.

Tampieri G, Soresi S, Vianello R (1988) Ritardo Mentale. Rassegna di Ricerche (Mental Retardation). Pordenone: Erip Editrice.

Trexler LE, Sullivan C (1995) Prospettive neuropsicologiche del trauma cranico-encefalico (Brain injury and perspectives). In M Zettin, R Rago (eds) Trauma Cranico. Torino: Bollati-Boringhieri, pp. 36–52.

Wilson BA (1985) Single-case and small group design. Paper presented at the Cognitive Neuropsychology Meeting, Venezia.

Chapter 26
Vocational guidance for persons with intellectual disability

L. Nota, S. Soresi

Premise

Given that the ability to cover a professional role is an established evaluation criterion for the efficacy of any treatment conducted on behalf of impaired and disabled persons (Nota et al., 2002b; Scoretti, 2002), work inclusion, and the services that must be implemented to promote it, is indeed an important 'issue'. As evidence for this, we cite that:

- According to Wilson (1990), the purpose of rehabilitation is to take patients to the highest possible degree of physical, psychological and social adjustment, by aiming to mitigate a disability's impact and to work toward achieving the best level of inclusion possible
- The World Health Organization considers rehabilitation as the sum of actions and interventions targeted at mitigating impairment and disability as well as at improving people's lives within all possible limits (OMS, 1997)
- Liberman (1997) holds that the most important rehabilitation outcome indicator is not so much a presumed improvement in the quality of behaviour, but rather the most positive impact possible in patients' social lives

From this perspective, we believe that vocational guidance forms a basic premise for any type of employment placement and re-instatement project.

When people think of vocational guidance, what usually comes to mind is the attempt to measure the degree of correspondence between people's attributes and the demands that specific job sectors and work environments place or will place on them. Nonetheless, we prefer to refer to a process, proposed by the Vocational Evaluation and Work Adjustment

Association, with the main goal of helping people develop their own vocational projects, by drawing on medical, psychological, social, vocational and economic information (Dahl, 1980).

There are inherent difficulties in the search for this correspondence, which are in part due to the fact that people, and especially disabled people, have their own 'peculiarities' and 'differences' and are the products of their own states of health and experience. Another source of difficulty lies in the fact that work environments are extremely varied and diverse. This renders any attempt to predict the success of a person–environment match particularly problematic and full of risks. Let it suffice to mention that some studies have described more than 12,000 different occupations, which require quite distinct abilities, knowledge, skills, and motivations (Herr and Cramer, 1992; Farr, 1993; Isaacson and Brown, 1993; Mayall, 1994). When faced with such a variety of jobs and requirements, calculating a correspondence index is not feasible. If, for example, we use Lewin's formula (1935) to determine work behaviour, $B = f(P, E, P \times E)$, intended as a function of the person (P) and of the environment (E) and interaction between the two ($P \times E$), the above-mentioned problems immediately emerge in all their complexity.

Moreover, we should not overlook the fact that each personal factor can have different interactions with the work environment, thereby creating other specific influences (Fitzgerald and Betz, 1994). To complicate the picture even further, people, jobs and work environments are becoming more flexible and dynamic, and are in rapid transition.

Therefore, although it may be tempting to believe that environmental features and personal traits can easily be identified as good predictors of career success, the idea is misleading, especially if considered in the absence (as frequently occurs) of specific school-career guidance training (Parker and Schallar, 1996).

Vocational guidance phases for persons with intellectual disability

Those who devote themselves to the work inclusion of disabled persons usually intervene after a series of treatment programmes, which, more often than not, were carried out by other social service providers and professionals. Therefore, if we want to implement job placement and work inclusion properly, we need to start from an analysis of what has already been done in terms of assessment and intervention. This may seem obvious at first glance but, all too frequently, because of the common 'divide' among service providers, memoranda, records and information on what has already been done are often missing or incomplete. Planning work inclusion should therefore be preceded by an analysis of what a disabled person has achieved at school, during the course of scholastic inclusion, of activities conducted at rehabilitation centres, of a person's previous experience, and so on.

All of this should be followed up by specific assessment activities, instrumental to organizing guidance and work inclusion programmes. These should aim at:

- Analysing people's actual ability to make choices concerning limitations imposed by their impairments and disabilities and, possibly, concerning the preconceptions and cultural barriers that exist in their living situations
- Emphasizing their strengths, their remaining functional abilities and skills and their cognitive, physical and emotional resources
- Analysing their potential to learn job search and job performance skills

As we have discussed more extensively elsewhere (Soresi et al., 2003), anyone who works in career guidance and placement should proceed following a sequence of phases, in order to confer continuity to their intervention. The four most important, and we think ineluctable, phases are described below.

Phase one: analysing desires, career expectations and strengths

Disabled people, just as we all do, nurture expectations and aspirations regarding their professional futures (Soresi and Nota, 2000; Nota and Soresi, 2000). As Hagner and DiLeo point out (1993), these are often rather vague and confused hopes and desires, so that obtaining precise indications on preferences for a particular career can be an arduous task: it is the guidance and placement specialist's task to transform this uncertainty into precise professional objectives.

Even when faced with unrealistic expectations, counsellors should proceed with thoroughness and care. For example, in the case of a severely disabled person who wants to be a firefighter, a singer or a pilot, we can inquire into the interests that underlie these clues and the meaning that this person attributes to the job. We can then highlight the most appealing aspects of the job, such as the work environment, the chance to wear a uniform, the equipment or tools the job requires, and so on. Then, we can single out work tasks with at least some of the desired characteristics and attempt to have the client pursue decidedly more realistic job goals.

It is also important to try to pinpoint the root sources of persons' expectations: professional identification and modelling processes, which originally contributed to the structuring of their expectations, and how, over the course of clients' lives, these have evolved and changed. By so doing, we can also work at clarifying people's social networks, the models to which they aspire, and also any available cooperation that can be relied on to get clients to 'change their minds'. We can also propose training and placement courses that are more in accordance with clients' characteristics and abilities.

There are specific survey methods available for assessing interpersonal interests. For example, the Audio-Visual Vocational Preference Test (AVVPT), recently developed by Wilgosh (1994), can be used with adolescents and young people who have mild and moderate intellectual disabilities. The test is presented using a video cassette and computer-generated images, and it asks people to choose between pairs of scenes portraying work environments and therefore does not require reading skills or particular verbal abilities.

After having assessed persons' values, hopes and expectations, counsellors should ask them to estimate their chances of success in undertaking an activity. An analysis of their skills, aptitudes and abilities can be useful to this end. These terms are often used interchangeably as if they were synonyms. However, Walsh and Betz (1990), maintain, for example, that 'aptitude' essentially refers to the capacity for learning, and it corresponds in large part to innate and hereditary attributes, which characterize a person's potential for learning. These researchers also use the term 'ability' to indicate cognitive or physical capacities (mental, cognitive, mechanical). Lastly, the word 'skill', denotes the capacity to do something (be a carpenter, solve problems, do arithmetic calculations, etc.).

Just as for the assessment of values and interests, specific tests are available, which should obviously be selected with a client's characteristics in mind, for analysing aptitude, skills and abilities.

Although aptitude tests are designed to be used in group as well as individual settings, people with impairments should receive individual administration. It will then be easier to verify if instructions have been understood, if the client accepts the test and, therefore, if there is a sufficient degree of cooperation. It is important to note that even if a standardized approach cannot be used with certain persons to create a normative profile, we can still use items to help us reflect on their actual capacities and possibilities. This 'qualitative' method of investigation, as affirmed also by Goldman (1990), can produce significant effects in a person's comprehension and self-exploration.

With analysis of this type, it is important to remember that the work skills people demonstrate in a certain job can also be transferred, either entirely or in part, to other tasks. This phenomenon assumes even more importance with intellectually disabled people, and counsellors need to ensure that their clients understand the potential for this type of transfer.

Phase two: analysing training and work environments

In order to conduct realistic vocational counselling and eventually to scale down a person's expectations, it is necessary to verify opportunities for job placement and work inclusion in the community (Moon et al., 1990). Such an analysis requires knowledge of the local labour market (in order to obtain information on skills that need to be taught in vocational training courses), the social characteristics of workplaces, the sequence of required tasks, expected production levels, a job's 'physical' require-ments, architectural and social barriers, required and available assistance, reinforcements, and so on.

This type of information can be gathered by means of a job analysis, which currently represents the bedrock of most human resource man-agement systems (Butler and Harvey, 1988; Morgenson and Campion, 1997). The term generally refers to processes aimed at the systematic analysis of a job, by gathering detailed information on it.

McIntire et al. (1995) suggest that a job analysis can be conducted for many different purposes: for personnel selection, to make performance evaluations, to set up specific training programmes, to plan career devel-opment, to increase job security, and to determine forms of incentive.

Job analysis procedures are varied and depend upon jobs' and workers' characteristics. Gottfredson and Holland (1991) developed a test for this purpose, the Position Classification Inventory, which analyses and classifies occupations according to Holland's classification of interests (realistic, inves-tigative, artistic, social, enterprising and conventional). For each grouping, the cognitive requisites necessary for performing job tasks are identified in such as way as to match job requirements and personal characteristics.

When interested in the work inclusion of disabled persons, we should first examine, as McIntire et al. propose, the knowledge, skills, abilities, and other, more specifically psychological, characteristics (Knowledge, Skills, Abilities, and Other characteristics – KSAOs) that workers should have in order to pursue a vocational goal successfully. To this end, guid-ance counsellors should adhere to the following six distinct and interdependent phases:

1. Planning job analysis: the job must be precisely defined, along with counsellors' goals, other people involved and available resources
2. Surveys and observations: this phase consists primarily of interviewing people who are experts in a particular job and in organizing the direct observation of people performing the job. The 'experts' must be peo-ple who have experience and knowledge of the job, such as managers and supervisors. During interviews, experts are first asked to identify the job's main functions and roles and then the job tasks associated with them (see below). Concerning the observation of workers, we must record their actions, tasks and the people they interact with and why, as well as the instruments, tools and materials they use. The most important objective of these observations is to specify in detail what the job consists of and the conditions in which it is performed
3. Describing functions and tasks: functions and tasks should be synthe-sized by analysing the information gathered in the previous phases. *Functions* represent the interrelated activities, which, all together, enable workers to accomplish job goals. One way to identify functions is to inquire about the reasons for the existence of that particular job or what would happen if that 'position' in that company were vacant. *Tasks*

are elements of functions; they describe the activities workers engage in order to carry out a determined function. A task is adequately described when it includes an action, an object and a goal. For example, one function of a gardener might be that of 'keeping the lawn in good condition', and one of his or her tasks might be: 'fertilizing the golf course in order to grow green grass, by watering it and using a small tractor and fertilizers'. In this task, the action is made up of the verb 'fertilize', the object is the 'golf course' and the goal is 'to grow green grass'. Dividing the function into small tasks helps describe the job and identify the knowledge, skills, abilities and other characteristics it requires

4. Identifying KSAOs: this phase is dedicated to describing the knowledge, skills, abilities, and the psychological characteristics that are required for successfully performing a job. *Knowledge* refers to the concepts that are usually acquired through specific vocational training and are required for ably handling a specific job. *Skills* are observable behaviours that workers implement when they perform specific tasks. They are acquired and improved through practice and work experience. *Abilities* refer to physical and cognitive elements that are instrumental in carrying out specific functions (Table 26.1).

Table 26.1 Examples of abilities

a. The ability to understand and follow verbal instructions
b. The ability to understand and follow written instructions
c. The ability to read at third middle school grade level, at least
d. The ability to read at high school level, at least
e. The ability to lift at least 13 kg
f. The ability to go up stairs or steps
g. The ability to bend over or to bend forward
h. The ability to coordinate arm and leg movements
i. The ability to distinguish colours, especially between red and green
j. The ability to listen to verbal messages
k. The ability to physically restrain a 60 kg adult

Lastly, the *other characteristics* concern aspects of a more psychological nature, such as interests, motivation and attitudes that workers should have in order to adapt to work conditions adequately (Table 26.2)

Table 26.2 Examples of other characteristics

a. Willingness to work outside, as well as inside
b. Willingness to work shifts, if necessary
c. Willingness to work in close contact with other employees
d. Willingness to work in group, as well as individual, settings
e. Willingness to work with co-workers, who are different from the usual ones
f. Willingness to participate in training and updating activities
g. Partiality for jobs requiring thoroughness and precision
h. Willingness to follow co-workers' directions and instructions

5. Evaluating the job analysis: after having identified the KSAOs, McIntire et al. (1995) suggest preparing a questionnaire to submit to a group of experts. Experts should evaluate the importance of the selected tasks, knowledge, skills, abilities, and other characteristics and the frequency with which they are required
6. Analysing the results: the analyses can go from the very simple (analysis of frequency, percentages, etc.) to more advanced types of verification, e.g. the calculation of expert agreement indexes and significance of differences between KSAOs associated with different functions and job performances

After having completed a job analysis, in order to foresee any potential problems people might encounter in performing a job, guidance counsellors should proceed with a performance assessment in simulated and real work environments:

1. Job simulation. We can overcome the many limits of psycho-vocational tests if we simulate work requirements, especially practical-manual ones. Observing how people use the tools and materials required in various work environments affords information that traditional tests usually cannot provide. At the same time, especially if simulations are organized in such a way as to 'recreate' real work environments faithfully, we can take the opportunity to observe other, not necessarily task-related abilities and difficulties (communicative, relational and motor) (Nota and Soresi, 1997; Soresi et al., 2003). To avoid organizing potentially invalid and unreliable activities, we should carefully observe and precisely record people's reactions, their performance, and their accuracy and speed of execution. If clients' disabilities and impairments allow it, we can also rely on 'group discussion' and self-reports. To maximize the probability that the information obtained can be 'generalized' to real settings (ecological validity), we recommend simulating activities, which, on the one hand, actually take place in work environments and which on the other hand, require skills that have been specifically taught during previous vocational training courses.
2. Evaluating vocational skills in real work environments. Observations conducted directly in the work environment generally have three important advantages:

   • The information obtained has greater validity than information on people's performances in specially prepared 'artificial settings'
   • People are generally more motivated by the outcome of the evaluation itself, and we can examine their interest in and liking for specific work environments
   • We can identify the expedients, modifications and adaptations that might be required of a 'work environment' in order to mitigate any problems a disabled person might encounter in performing efficiently and effectively

After having identified the work tasks a client is capable of handling and his or her abilities and skills, we should verify what changes will have to be made in the workplace in order better to meet his or her capacities and to facilitate his or her adaptation. To this end, we can analyse workplace noisiness, quality and quantity of expected productivity, type and closeness of supervision, quality, type and closeness of relationships with co-workers.

Lastly, after job task analysis, we need to consider the interference that other people's life 'systems' can have on a particular job choice, such as the family system (what more or less positive impact might this job have on a client's family atmosphere, on his or her role as a parent, a spouse, or child?) or the 'transportation' system, by trying to identify architectural barriers that might limit access to school buildings, work departments, restrooms or cafeterias. It may therefore be necessary to check hallway widths, the availability and location of elevators, lighting, the presence of functioning ventilation systems, noisiness, desk and workbench heights, and so on.

It is also crucial that employers receive intervention and support, since, as Greenwood and Johnson (1985) point out, they can harbour misgivings about the job placement and work inclusion of disabled people and be hesitant to hire them.

To this end, it can be expedient to:

- Provide suggestions for job reorganization
- Set up training to eliminate any cultural barriers and preconceptions
- Set up on-the-job training with disabled persons to encourage the better acquisition of new skills
- Guarantee assistance to co-workers of the included person
- Conduct monitoring and follow-up activities

Phase three: decision-making support

Since career and educational conditions vary, the vocational guidance counsellor must be able to help clients identify, reconsider, comprehend and interpret available information. The literature, although largely North American, provides guides, which career service providers can consult when they are interested in analysing jobs with a disabled person. Some of the most well known among these are:

1. The *Dictionary of Occupational Titles* (US Department of Labor, 1991) lists almost all of the jobs in the American economy (more than 12,000). In addition to offering a detailed description of job activities, it also provides information pertaining to the physical force and educational level each job requires and the time required for apprenticeship
2. The *Occupational Outlook Handbook* (US Department of Labor, 1994) examines the most common occupations in the American economy (225), describing:

- Job type
- The conditions in which various duties are usually performed
- Current employment opportunities
- Required training
- Wages
- Other associated occupations

3. The *Guide for Occupational Exploration* (US Department of Labor, 1979) contains 2,500 job descriptions, which are classified according to Holland's (1985) interest areas, thereby enabling its users to 'visit' the areas they find most interesting

In addition to career information, vocational guidance counsellors should also be able to provide information on possible training activities. For example, some computerized guidance systems, like the Guidance Informational System (Patterson, 1996) and DISCOVER (McCormac, 1988) list public and private schools, vocational schools, university courses and apprenticeship regulations. Also, more and more now, university, local public agency, and high school guidance centres are preparing and distributing their own brochures and informative materials. A word of caution is advised, however: counsellors should examine this type of material carefully, since the information schools, universities, newspapers, magazines and television networks publicize is not always objective. Indeed, the chief interest is usually that of attracting new students, and to avoid these risks, we must verify that the information provided is:

- Updated, objective and reliable
- Pertinent to the geographical area in which the person lives or where he or she wants to complete training
- Complete and coherent

People who are aware of their own values, needs, interests, abilities and motivations, and who understand the rules of the world of work and of the other environments in which they live, will be better prepared to make 'good' decisions and to stick with them. Nonetheless, people can find it hard to make choices, especially if they have impairments and disabilities that drastically reduce the number of options they can actually take into consideration. Counsellors should therefore favour a logical and rational decision-making approach (Isaacson and Brown, 1993; Zuncker, 1994). In this regard, Harren (1979) describes at least three styles by means of which people make decisions:

- Rational: a logical, step-by-step approach, in which a person who is preparing to choose between several options, gathers and weighs information concerning the self and the alternatives considered
- Intuitive: this style focuses mainly on analysing personal aspects and an alternative's impact on one's state of mind. Decisions of this type are often reached rapidly, because they are considered 'right' for oneself

- Dependent: a person who relies on this style is strongly influenced by the opinions and expectations of peers and of people who are perceived to have a certain authority. Here, the adequacy of a choice is interpreted in terms of the perceived amount of approval and agreement obtained

Nota et al. (2002a) in reference to Janis and Mann's (1997) decisional conflict theory, prefer referring to adaptive and maladaptive decision-making styles. Adaptive decision-making styles concern *vigilance*, that is, the ability to set personal goals, to examine various solutions, to seek out accurately and select information, to analyse it while keeping preconceptions and stereotypes in check, and to foresee and carefully evaluate the probable consequences of various courses of action. This style is associated with moderate levels of stress and represents a premise for making 'rational' and effective decisions. Maladaptive styles are *procrastination*, the tendency to postpone the moment for facing a decision; *defensive avoidance*, the tendency to avoid conflictual situations, and to leave decisional responsibility to others; and *hypervigilance*, excessive focus on information and 'details' of secondary importance, or impulsively seizing onto the first solutions identified, without considering their medium- and long-term consequences.

The *Melbourne Decision Making Questionnaire* by Mann et al. (1997) can be used to analyse the decision-making styles of adults and adolescents (from age 15 and up) (Nota and Soresi, 2000). Analyses conducted on the instrument confirm its reliability and validity and its potential for gathering information on people's particular decision-making patterns.

If we are interested in analysing decision-making styles in young adolescents (11–14 years old), it is preferable to use the *Adolescent Decision Making Questionnaire* by Mann (see Mann et al., 1988; Soresi et al., 2001). It measures people's tendencies to put off decisions and to delegate this task to others (*avoidance*); the degree of discomfort experienced during decision-making (*worry*); the tendency to invest little effort in decision-making and proceeding cursorily (*superficiality*); and the tendency to use rational decision-making processes and self-confidence in this ability (*vigilance*). Since the questionnaire helps shed light on people's adaptive or maladaptive decision-making styles, it can also identify certain at-risk persons. For example, because of their tendency to put off decisions until the last minute, some people end up reducing their chances of proceeding carefully and rationally; or, because they tend to delegate decision-making to others (to parents, teachers or friends), other people miss opportunities for analysing and achieving their own desires and aspirations; or, lastly, because some people make superficial and hurried decisions, they have greater chances of making inappropriate ones.

We maintain, furthermore, that vocational guidance counsellors for disabled persons should be familiar with their clients' decision-making styles and, if necessary, encourage clients to learn more adaptive decision-making methods. Having ascertained that often disabled, as well as non-disabled, persons have a hard time working out advantageous school-career choices, we mention that:

• Guidance should focus on the cognitive, affective, behavioural and relational processes involved in what are commonly known as 'career problems' (Soresi, 2000)
• Vocational guidance counsellors should provide all assistance necessary to support people in the process of gathering, processing and using school-career information and in making decisions and planning the realization of the choices
• Should it be necessary, career service providers should arrange and organize training aimed at helping clients learn efficient decision-making strategies as well as professional problem-solving (Nota et al., 2002a)

Phase four: planning work adaptation

Counsellors who work in vocational guidance and school and work inclusion tend to consider their task complete when they have managed to help people realize their educational and career choices. However, we believe that counsellors should also provide follow-up operations, which, on the one hand, help disabled people adapt satisfactorily to a job, and, on the other, help them deal with job insecurity and job market flexibility and, eventually, with retirement, i.e. the experience of ending work.

Regarding work adaptation, we must consider, as McMahon proposed 20 years ago (1979), a vast array of worker attributes, which are crucial for obtaining and maintaining a job. Among these are:

• Behaviour skills (stable on-the-job presence, punctuality, good grooming)
• Social-personal skills (knowing how to moderate emotions, to use job parlance, to establish proper relationships)
• Work readiness skills (understanding work concepts, using job information, showing interest in a job) (McMahon, 1979)

Obviously, McMahon's model, but also the more recent ones of Hershenson (1981) and Dawis and Lofquist (1984), place special emphasis on analysing interactions between workers and their work environments. Thus a research trend is evoked, which in recent years has begun highlighting the importance of the quality and quantity of relationships that disabled persons establish with their co-workers in competitive, as well as supportive, work environments (Chadsey-Rusch, 1992; Nota and Soresi, 1997; Soresi and Nota, 2000; Rondal et al., 2003).

References

Browder D (1991) Assessment of Individuals with Severe Disabilities: An Applied Behavior Approach to Life Skills Assessment. Baltimore: Brookes.

Butler SK, Harvey RJ (1988) A comparison of holistic versus decomposed rating of position analysis questionnaire work dimensions. Personnel Psychol 41: 761–71.

Chadsey-Rusch J (1992) Toward defining and measuring social skills in employment settings. Am J Ment Retard 96: 405–18.

Dahl P (1980) Mainstreaming Guide-book for Vocational Educators Teaching the Handicapped. Denton: East Texas State University.

Dawis RV, Lofquist LH (1984) A Psychological Theory of Work Adjustment. Minneapolis: University of Minnesota Press.

Farr JM (1993) The Complete Guide for Occupational Exploration. Indianapolis: JIST Works.

Fitzgerald JM, Betz N (1994) Career development in cultural context: the role of gender, race, and sexual orientation. In M Savickas, R Lent (eds) Convergences in Career Development Theories. Implications for Science and Practice. Palo Alto, CA: Consulting Psychologists Press, pp. 207–14.

Goldman L (1990) Qualitative assessment. The Counseling Psychologist 18: 205–13.

Gottfredson GD, Holland JL (1991) The Dictionary of Holland Occupational Codes. Odessa, FL: Psychological Assessment Resources.

Greenwood R, Johnson VA (1985) Employer Concerns Regarding Workers with Disabilities. Hot Springs: Arkansas Research and Training Center in Vocational Rehabilitation.

Hagner D, DiLeo D (1993) Working Together: Workplace Culture, Supported Employment, and Persons with Disabilities. Cambridge, MA: Brookline Books.

Harren VA (1979) Research with the assessment of career decision making. Character-Potential: A Record of Research 9: 63–9.

Herr E, Cramer S (1992) Career Guidance and Counseling through the Lifespan: Systematic Approaches. New York: HarperCollins.

Hershenson DB (1981) Work adjustment, disability, and the three R's of vocational rehabilitation: A conceptual model. Rehab Couns Bull 25: 91–7.

Holland J (1985) The Self-directed Search: Professional Manual – 1985 edition. Odessa, FL: Psychological Assessment Resource.

Isaacson L, Brown D (1993) Career Information, Career Counseling, and Career Development. Boston: Allyn & Bacon.

Janis IL, Mann L (1997) Decision-making: A Psychological Analysis of Conflict, Choice and Commitment. New York: Free Press.

Lewin K (1935) A Dynamic Theory of Personality: Selected Papers. New York: McGraw-Hill.

Liberman RP (1997) La Riabilitazione Psichiatrica (The Psychiatric Rehabilitation). Milano: Raffaello Cortina Editore.

Lofquist LH, Dawis RV (1969) Adjustment to Work: A Psychological View of Man's Problems in a Work-oriented Society. New York: Appleton-Century-Crofts.

Mann L, Burnett P, Radford M, Ford S (1997) The Melbourne Decision Making Inventory: an instrument for measuring patterns for coping with decisional conflict. Journal of Behavioral Decision-Making 10: 1–19.

Mann L, Harmoni R, Power C (1988) GOFER: Basic Principles of Decision Making. Woden, ACT: Curriculum Development Centre.

Mayall D (1994) The Worker Traits Data Book. Indianapolis: JIST Works.

McCormac ME (1988) The use of career information delivey system in the States. Journal of Career Development 14: 196–204.

McIntire S, Bucklan MA, Scott DR (1995) Job Analysis Kit. Odessa, FL: Psychological Assessment Resources.

McMahon BT (1979) A model of vocational redevelopment for the midcareer physically disabled. Rehab Couns Bull 23: 35–47.

Moon M, Inge K, Wehman P, Brooke V, Barcus J (1990) Helping Persons with Severe Mental Retardation Get and Keep Employment: Supported Employment Issues and Strategies. Baltimore: Brookes.

Morgenson FP, Campion MA (1997) Social and cognitive sources of potential inaccuracy in job analysis. J Appl Psychol 82: 627–55.

Nota L, Mann L, Friedman IA, Soresi S (2002a) Decisioni e Scelte (Decision and Choice). Firenze: Giunti-Organizzazioni Speciali.

Nota L, Rondal JA, Soresi S (2002b) La Valutazione delle Disabilità. Volume primo (The Evaluation of Disabilities. First volume). Pordenone: Erip Editrice.

Nota L, Soresi S (1997) Le Abilità Cociali: Dall'Osservazionc all'Intervento (Social Abilities: From Observation to Intervention). Pordenone: Erip Editrice.

Nota L, Soresi S (2000) Adattamento italiano del Melbourne Decision Making Questionnaire di Leon Mann. Giornale Italiano di Psicologia dell' Orientamento 3: 38–52.

OMS (1997) ICIDH-2: International Classification of Functioning and Disability. Geneva: WHO.

Parker RM, Schallar JL (1996) Issues in vocational assessment and disability. In EM Szymanski, RM Parker (eds) Work and Disability. Issues and Strategies in Career Development and Job Placement. Austin TX: Pro-Ed, pp. 127–64.

Patterson JB (1996) Occupational labor market information and analysis. In EM Szymansky, RM Parker (eds) Work and Disability. Issues and Strategies in Career Development and Job Placement. Austin TX: Pro-Ed, pp. 209–54.

Rondal JA, Hodapp R, Soresi S, Nota L, Dykens E (2003) Intellectual Disabilities. London: Whurr Publishers.

Scoretti C (2002) Valutazione delle disabilità e reinserimento lavorativo e sociale (Evaluation of disabilities and social and work inclusion). In S Soresi (ed) Disabilità, Trattamento ed Integrazione. Pordenone: Erip Editrice, pp. 449–79.

Soresi S (2000) Orientamenti dell'Orientamento (Vocational Guidance and Career Service Providers). Firenze: Giunti-Organizzazioni Speciali.

Soresi S (2001) Riflessioni a margine della seconda edizione della Classificazione Internazionale delle menomazioni, delle Disabilità degli Handicap (The second edition of International Classification of Impairments, Disability and Handicap). Giornale Italiano delle Disabilita 1: 5–22.

Soresi S (2003) Disabilità, Trattamento ed Integrazione (Disability, Treatment, and Inclusion). Pordenone: Erip Editrice.

Soresi S, Nota L (2000) A social skills training for persons with Down's syndrome. European Psychologist 5: 34–43.

Soresi S, Nota L, Mann L (2001) Adolescent Decision Making Questionnaire. In S Soresi, L Nota (eds) Optimist: Autoefficacia e Decison Making. Firenze: Iter-Organizzazioni Speciali, pp. 43–68.

Soresi S, Nota L, Sgaramella T (2003) La Valutazione delle Disabilità. Volume secondo (The Evaluation of Disabilities. Second volume). Pordenone: Erip Editrice.

US Department of Labor (1979) Guide for Occupational Exploration. Washington, DC: US Government Printing Office.

US Department of Labor (1991) Dictionary of Occupational Titles. Indianapolis: JIST Works.

US Department of Labor (1994) Occupational Outlook Handbook. Washington, DC: US Government Printing Office.

Walsh WB, Betz N (1990) Tests and Assessment (2nd edition). Englewood Cliffs, NJ: PrenticeHall.

Wilgosh L (1994) Assessment of vocational preferences for young people with intellectual impairments. Develop Disab Bull 22: 63–71.

Wilson B (1990) Metodi innovativi di riabilitazione della memoria. In L Caldana (ed.) Atti del Corso di Aggiornamento Teorico-Pratico. Roma: Editore Marrapese.

Zuncker VG (1994) Career Counseling: Applied Concepts of Life Planning. Pacific Grove, CA: Brooks Cole.

Chapter 27
People with Down syndrome at work: experiences and considerations

A. CONTARDI

The Associazione Italiana Persone Down (the Italian Association for People with Down Syndrome) is an association for people with Down syndrome (DS) and their families. It is a reference point in Italy for parents and for all who are involved in this field. Its aim is to provide information and to promote initiatives to improve the situation of people with DS. In recent years it has increasingly devoted more attention to the problems of adults.

The increase in life expectancy in recent years has drawn attention to new issues. One consequence of this has been that the association has changed its name from Associazione Bambini Down (the Down Children Association) to Associazione Italiana Persone Down and has started up projects and is providing services with this in mind.

We have begun, therefore, to work on the concept of developing social autonomy (for example, the ability to handle money, find one's way, use public transport and public services) convinced that this is important for two reasons: firstly to have people with DS included in a normal social context, and then to have the means for them to be accepted in the workplace, a possibility that does not apply to all people with DS but certainly applies to many.

When, in 1992, we analysed the few existing experiences of work inclusions (Danesi and Sampaolo, 1993) we saw that the basis for success in these inclusions was, on the one hand, a good level of personal autonomy for each worker, and, on the other, certain characteristics of the training period, which have since become the key formulae in recent years, i.e. in-service training and care in choosing a job.

The Association has thus concentrated on promoting autonomy in adolescents and young adults with DS and on trying wherever possible to encourage new job placements where autonomy was possible.

It was clear that many companies did what they could to avoid employing a person with a mental disability, whether out of concern for problems of inclusion or because they believed that such a person would not be productive. To a large extent this was due to prejudice, but also to the fact that the law, L.482/68, which was in force until 1999, did not provide for a specifically aimed employment scheme to ensure that the worker chosen for the post had the requirements and training necessary for that job.

For this reason, and with a view to fostering the inclusion of young people with DS in the workforce, our Association has tried to contact companies directly to work with them to find an inclusion procedure that satisfies both sides.

Working with Food Italia

With these aims in mind the Association has been working since 1993 with Food Italia, a company which runs five McDonald restaurants in Rome. Food Italia is a company which is obliged by law to employ workers with disabilities, but it often experienced difficulty at the inclusion phase with the people who were sent by the Employment Office of the Province, an office which deals with unemployed groups.

We decided together to prepare a number of people with DS for work in McDonald's restaurants, aiming to make this a genuine work experience of mutual interest.

Selecting employees

The first problem we faced here was that of selecting potential employees, bearing in mind the specific job involved.

In the case of a specifically chosen job, the first step is an evaluation of the work and a resulting evaluation of the candidate's ability to do it.

The job description is 'fast food operator' and it includes a variety of tasks which range from the preparation of food, to cleaning, and to serving members of the public. In creating a profile of the worker the following characteristics were kept in mind:

• The need for personal cleanliness. This is particularly important when there is contact with food and with the general public. Hair must be short or tied back, men must be clean-shaven
• The ability to reach the work-place independently because the work involves different shifts
• The capacity to ask for help in case of difficulty
• The capacity to carry out simple instructions
• The ability to read and write was considered useful, but not essential

As we can see, almost all these characteristics involve personal or social autonomy.

The second issue we faced was that of the organization of the job.

We decided together that the contract should be a part-time training contract (20 hours per week). This type of contract was already used by the company for other workers, as indeed was the part-time contract. The latter is ideal for many people with DS as it eliminates the problem of their becoming excessively tired. Work in a fast-food restaurant is considerably more tiring than in other work situations.

The only concession made that other workers do not have was that the daily working hours and the day off were fixed. This was to ensure that the worker with DS was as independent as possible as far as work was concerned. Other workers change shift on a regular basis. There was no difference in salary compared with other workers doing similar jobs.

It is worth pointing out that the training contract implies a certain amount of in-service training and that McDonald's has produced a manual and has a well structured training scheme which can also be used with people with DS. Each work station, such as 'Salads', 'Drinks' etc. has a specific work procedure which everyone follows in every McDonald's restaurant.

Within the McDonald's organization, moreover, there are other characteristics which helped contribute to the success of the experience:

- The fact of wearing a work uniform helped our young people to feel that they belonged to the company and to identify with the role of worker
- The fact that there is a clear hierarchical order, where the roles of manager, director etc. are very clear, giving very solid points of reference

As part of the agreement with the company, the Association undertook to select potential candidates in order to have a pool every time a post became vacant. Given the requirements mentioned above, we felt it was important that the candidates should have taken part in the Association's acquisition of autonomy course. Almost all the young people selected had attended these courses, which proved extremely useful both because they had acquired specific abilities and because they had developed an ability to interrelate with colleagues and managers.

Starting work

Almost immediately the company felt the need for someone to deal specifically with the training of workers with special needs and so the position of 'job coach' was created. The characteristics considered necessary for this role were a good knowledge of the work and of the training schemes, a basic knowledge of psychology, and the ability to listen and to observe. The choice of person for this job was made jointly by Food Italia's Head of Personnel and the staff member of the Association who was following the project. A young manager was chosen who was subsequently given a short course at the AIPD and who continues to refer to the Association staff member for supervision and help in specific areas.

The procedure followed for each appointment is the following:

- Notification by the company of a job vacancy
- Identification by the Association of a possible candidate (one or more than one)
- Job interview at the company. This normally takes place together with normal job interviews for people without problems but in this case the job coach and the representative of the Association are also present
- Completion of the necessary bureaucratic procedures
- Employment with a training contract

In the initial period the job coach is often present to supervise the training procedure and help the individual with DS to carry out the tasks they have been assigned and help in his or her role as worker. The training period provides the worker with DS with the possibility of gradually learning all the tasks that the job involves, although the time necessary for learning and the order in which the tasks are taught may vary.

Initially the simplest tasks are dealt with: cleaning, the drinks station, stacking the shelves, etc. in order to increase self-confidence and, with this, the desire to work. The next stage is the learning of more complex tasks, from the various kitchen tasks to working at the cash desk, although the time scale and the methods used vary from case to case according to the individual and the needs of the company. Our young people use all the machinery, including high temperature fryers.

This is the story of one worker with DS:

My first day of work was on Monday at 4 o'clock. I saw the restaurant and the manager and I tried on the uniform and met my colleagues. I was nervous.

On Monday, Thursday, Friday and Sunday I work from 3 o'clock until 7 o'clock. On Wednesday I work from 10 to 2 (because in the afternoon I go swimming), and Tuesday and Saturday are my free days. Every day I clock in when I arrive and I clock out when I finish work, before I go away.

With my colleagues everything's fine. They work different shifts, the night shift too.

I do my job by myself and they help me when I need it. I prepare all the kinds of burgers, and I do the training till – the manager helps me and explains how the till works. I prepare the drinks, the chips, the ice-creams, the apple pies and I make the milk shakes and the sundaes, which is a kind of ice cream, and I do the cones with cream. When I work in the morning I do the salad bar, where the salads are sold, I take the orders, I put them on the plates, I take the money at the till.

After the initial period, which varies with each individual case, the job coach steps back, spending only 1 day a week in the same McDonald's as the young person to encourage greater autonomy, while at the same time remaining a point of reference. From the first day the young person is expected to consider the job seriously, to arrive punctually, to show respect for the rules and towards his or her colleagues, to take orders from superiors, to be polite to the public and generally to carry out the different tasks efficiently. That is to say, they are expected to perform the job in the same way as other workers.

Results of the project

From 1994 to 1998, eight workers with DS between the age of 23 and 31 were given jobs. Two left the job after more than 2 years' work, because they found another job closer to their homes. All those who completed the 2 years of training contract were given a permanent contract. The six people currently employed work in five different restaurants, with the two who are in the same restaurant working different shifts.

All eight of the young people had a good level of autonomy and they quickly learnt how to reach work on their own, taking one or two forms of public transport.

As far as learning the different tasks is concerned there have been no particular problems, although not all have yet learned to use the till. The job coach has worked in particular to help with comprehension of the particular requests and with understanding why the various actions are necessary.

The Association was involved primarily in the early phases to help colleagues to understand that the worker with DS was first and foremost a worker like the others and to understand any specific difficulties that they might have. At the beginning the colleagues were given this short note:

A new colleague is going to start work here. Because it is someone with Down syndrome and we want this new experience to be positive both for them and for the restaurant we would like you to pay attention to the following points:

Use simple language that is easy to understand, both in conversation and when you are making a specific request. Often when a person with a mental handicap does not respond to a request it may be because they have not understood and not because they are not able or willing to do it. A request may be too vague, for example 'Clean the place up as quickly as you can'. Here we expect the person to understand the underlying message (clean the tables, clean the floor, do the work quickly, but at the same time do it well, etc.). At other times we may make 2 or 3 requests in a single sentence or use a negative form to indicate an affirmative message ('You don't want to come to the cinema, do you?' to ask 'Do you want to come to the cinema?') All these things make understanding difficult.

Learn to observe and to recognize your new colleague's successes by notic-
ing small changes in behaviour and give credit for them. It is important to
praise them for these successes and also to analyse with them the reasons
for failure. This is what will help them to be aware of their capabilities and
increase their desire to learn.

Try to develop a relationship with your new colleague which is based on
truthfulness. This means always giving real and easily comprehensible reasons for what you are asking them to do. Take your colleague seriously and
help them not to avoid reality but to face it. For example, if they say to you
'I'm in love with you and I want to marry you', tell them 'No, I'm not in love
with you, but we can be friends.' Another example is not to accept without
question any tales of impossible experiences. Behave as naturally as possible.

Try to involve your new colleague actively in choices and in the running of
the business, and even when this is not wholly possible get them to express
their opinion ('Do you like this?', 'Why don't you like this?'). While you are
working together never take over the task they are doing and avoid trying
to help too much.

Recognize explicitly the fact of their 'being grown-up' and use this awareness to reinforce their development towards further autonomy. Consider
them as what they actually are, that is, adults, and avoid behaviour that
treats them as children, like, for example, taking them by the hand or using
language that is not appropriate for their age.

We hope you find these suggestions useful and that you enjoy working
together.

The relationship with colleagues today is generally good, and in some
cases excellent. In a recent report a company manager has written, 'My
impression is that the arrival of these new employees has widened the
general consciousness, brought more understanding and harmony, and
an appreciation of other colleagues that was difficult to find before...
Many of their colleagues have become friends. They go out together for a
pizza or to celebrate someone's birthday or just to chat about boyfriends,
girlfriends, clothes or football.'

The company has recently carried out an evaluation of productivity and
has found that the productivity of these workers is between 70 and 80%
of that of other workers. We believe that this is a very important result and
that it fully justifies the methodology chosen for the inclusion procedure.
It also refutes the idea that employment for a person with special needs
is a form of social assistance.

When we observe the behaviour of the young people involved in this
scheme we can see how their new status as a worker has had a positive
effect on their self-confidence. The fact that they feel grown-up and are
recognized as such and that they are bringing home a salary, has meant

that their behaviour both at home and with their friends is more adult and more responsible. This is still more evident in the cases where the families have allowed them to be responsible for the money they have earned, although this is always under supervision. One young person has opened a bank account and uses a cash-point card, another has bought a mobile telephone, which he uses intelligently. Most have started to do new things, such as going to a beautician's or organizing evenings with friends.

Gloria says this about her job:

> My salary is paid into the bank so when I need money I use the cash point. I buy myself things – smart clothes, shoes with high heels, jackets and shirts, and I go to the theatre and to the cinema or have a pizza with my friends. Since I've been working my life has got better – I've changed as a person, I've grown up, become an adult. I've become a woman.

I believe our experience can be a template for a procedure for specific work placements and at the same time a means of collaboration between companies and social services.

Legislation

In recent years the legislation regarding work placements for people with special needs has changed radically as a result of the approval of the law 68/'99 'Ordinances for the right to work of people with special needs'.

The central principle around which the new law has been constructed is that of *specific job placements*, which are defined as 'series of technical and support strategies which allow for the evaluation of people with special needs regarding their capacity to work and for their inclusion in a suitable job training scheme'. This is achieved by analysing the job itself, and the forms of support, by positive action and the solution of problems relating to the work environment, the help available and interpersonal relations both in the workplace and socially.

In this way the need for coordination of the different interventions and the relative instruments of support is stressed in relation to the individual situations of handicap and more generally of life for people with special needs.

The choice the law has made is to overcome a restrictive legislation and it aims to involve all those dealing with the inclusion, starting with the employer, by means of incentives for those who employ people with 'severe' special needs and by organizing a network which will provide support for the inclusion.

Although 3 years have passed since the law was approved, in many regions it is still in the initial phases of its application. Further legal steps need to be taken and offices and services need to be organized at local level.

I feel, however, that when we consider specifically the inclusion of people with DS in the workplace or workforce it is important to underline the importance of:

- The possibility of specific work placements and for the employer to select a specific individual for a given job
- Incentives for employers, particularly in the case of intellectual handicap
- The availability of posts in small companies which are present throughout the territory and more 'livable' for the worker
- The use of the Special Agreement (undersigned by the Employment Office), which allows for specific training to be carried out at a later stage in those cases where it was not done at the beginning

Experience has taught me, moreover, that many companies also felt the need to pass from an approach to work placements that involved assistance to a productive approach. In this way the possibility of developing 'good projects' to allow for a positively viewed inclusion of people with DS will find allies and help us to break down prejudice.

Workers with Down syndrome

In Italy there are no data available to say how many people with DS work, and registers kept by the Employment Offices do not include information regarding the various pathologies. We know, however, from the direct experience of our local branches throughout Italy, that the number of those who work is certainly lower than the number of those capable of working, although it should be remembered that not all people with DS are capable of working or could easily find placements in the free market. We must certainly be aware that when considering adults with DS a number are capable of working, a number will be able to express and realize themselves in the context of protected employment and a third group will require appropriate assisted solutions.

I would like to concentrate, however, on those who work or could potentially do so, and make certain points which have emerged from studies carried out by the AIPD, particularly, but not exclusively, in the Rome area.

A recent study in Rome, which is still partially underway, has identified, out of 249 people with DS between the ages of 18 and 50 who are in contact with the Association, 43 who are regularly employed (26 cases were verified in the last month and 17 had already been recorded in 1992). A further 14 are in the process of having their contracts formalized. Of those already employed, 27 work full-time and 16 part-time.

As other studies have underlined, the kind of work carried out is not particularly relevant, as this is principally determined by the work market. Consequently most of those employed in Rome are in the tertiary sector.

The elements which determine the success or difficulty of the inclusion and the level of productivity reached are: simple and well organized tasks; clearly defined roles and a clear hierarchical structure; and the consideration of the employee with DS as a genuinely productive worker.

As a result of the absence of services for work inclusion at a local level, excluding the experience conducted in Rome by a few professional training centres, in the last 8 years the Association has started to follow some inclusions directly. In the last 2 years it has set up a specific service, which works in three main directions:

- With a campaign to promote awareness and provide information for companies and institutions
- To provide profiles and CVs
- To provide support during the inclusion period

I feel it is important to underline that treating the theme of work means treating the theme of adulthood for people with DS.

It is not possible to talk about inclusion in the work-place without talking about training, but neither is it possible to interpret training merely as the learning of tasks and skills. In order to go to work the person must feel adult, and through work they continue to build up their individual adult identity.

We have reflected on this theme a great deal, both as operators and with the families and the young people with DS, and there is still much to do. The paths towards autonomy, which the Association has been following for many years, have contributed towards this process, but unless the reality of this importance is understood within the family, the problem of finding a job is a secondary one.

The theme of social autonomy has, therefore, particular importance in the elaboration of profiles to present the young people to their potential employers.

At the same time it is necessary to reflect on the above with the parents; although, on the one hand, there are parents who are aware of, and respect, the new condition of adulthood of their sons and daughters, on the other, we are often faced with two types of attitude: those who give up, and those who are uncertain. The former are afraid of losing benefits and give up from the beginning, while the latter group see the experience of working only as a form of rehabilitation, without truly believing in their productive capabilities. On occasion these parents make requests to the employers ('Please don't tire him out', 'Can she have longer holidays?'...) which destabilize their sons and daughters as workers and alter their image in society.

Workers in this field are well aware that today there is still a social image of people with an intellectual disability who are too often seen as eternal children, which hinders their potential ability to express themselves.

Unless we work on this image with the testimonials of those who are working today, it will continue to be difficult to convince an employer of what they can expect from a worker with special needs.

Fabrizio, a 16 year-old boy with DS recently wrote, in answer to the question 'What job would you like to do?', 'I'd like to drive, collect wood, do things by myself, do grown-up things.' Italo, who works at McDonald's, writes, 'I enjoy my work because I've had good advice about working in the kitchen and so I don't find it difficult. At the moment I'm working in the restaurant and I do the cleaning, but my job changes every week and next week I'll be in the kitchen. The fact that I work and that I get a salary gives me a lot of satisfaction and it gives me the feeling that I can do a lot of things.'

These are two people with DS who are expressing their awareness of who they are and are growing up fully aware of being teenager and adult.

If these considerations can help us to understand how to support people with DS and their families in their progress towards work, there are other considerations which emerge from the relationship with employers and which provide further points for discussion.

In the past year several work placements have been carried out in different productive sectors, with the help of Special Agreements.

Aiming for quality and successful inclusion, we have always proposed working weeks of 21–25 hours over 5 days, although this has meant a lower salary. This has allowed us to aim for higher productivity by reducing the problems of tiredness and help the in-house tutor to identify the tasks and responsibilities involved. In this way employers carry out their legal obligations and at the same time, rather than finding this a burden, are able to appreciate the strengths of the new employee.

In some situations employers have preferred an initial training period prior to offering a contract, while in others this has not been necessary. In both cases, however, there has been an obvious need for support for the company and the worker in the first few months, which has been guaranteed by the Association, given that the Social Services do not have the means to provide such a service. The nature of this support varies from case to case, according to a project which is defined together and which may be modified during the course of the placement.

Various types of intervention are possible:

1. In the workplace
- Observation and analysis of the workplace in order to identify the various tasks by a social worker from the AIPD
- Discussions with colleagues and managers regarding both general organization and particular problems which may emerge
- Hidden observations for the purpose of verification
- Periodic verifications with managers

2. In the Association
• Support interviews and the analysis of problems with the worker
• Interviews with the family

The most active phase of support varies from six months to one year from the start of the placement. However, the Association continues to be available to help the employers, the workers and their families where this is necessary. Where a Special Agreement has been set up with the Employment Office, the Association is presented as a training organization. In the other cases the agreement is set up directly with the company. At present the costs of this activity fall completely on the Association, although in some cases there is a contribution from the families.

Conclusions

• Inclusion in the workforce of people with DS in Italy is possible and can give good results both for the worker and for the company
• A worker with DS is a worker and an adult, who has Down syndrome, and their personal growth in terms of identity and of ability must be promoted
• It is essential to proceed with specific job placements. Local support services must be developed with this in mind
• Flexibility is an important element in order to work out specific projects tailored to the needs of the workers
• Steps should be taken to integrate the salary, in the case of part-time work, or to make this compatible with benefits

I believe there is still a great deal of prejudice, as a result of which, work placements for people with special needs, particularly those with an intellectual disability, are viewed only as a burden for the company. This is a problem that must be faced and resolved. In our opinion it must be faced not simply by expecting companies to be 'kinder', but by each one of us being better at creating the conditions that enable people with special needs to express their full capacities.

The law 68/'99 has introduced many innovations, among them the principle of specific job placements and incentives for companies. As a result, today we have many more means at our disposal, but it is now up to us to roll up our sleeves and get to work.

Bibliography

Biolchini E, Liverani M, Valgimigli C (1986) Handicappati Psichici e Lavoro. Un'integrazione Possibile. Pisa: Del Cerro.
Contardi A (1992) Libertà Possibile. Educazione all'autonomia dei Ragazzi con Ritardo Mentale. Roma: La Nuova Italia Scientifica.

Contardi A, Vicari S (1994) Le Persone Down. Aspetti Neuropsicologici, Educativi e Sociali. Milano: F. Angeli.

Danesi P, Sampaolo E (1993) Un Posto per Tutti. Analisi di Esperienze Lavorative di Adulti con Sindrome di Down. Pisa: Del Cerro.

Fabrizi G, Vulterini P (2000) Orientamento e Inserimento al Lavoro di Persone in Condizioni di Svantaggio. Manuale per gli Operatori. Milano: F. Angeli.

Lepri C, Montobbio E (1993) Lavoro e Fasce Deboli. Strategie e Metodi per l'inserimento Lavorativo di Persone con Difficoltà Cliniche e Sociali. Milano: F. Angeli.

Lepri C, Montobbio E, Papone G (1999) Lavori in Corso. Persone Disabili che Lavorano. Pisa: Del Cerro.

Montobbio E (1994) Il Viaggio del Signor Down nel Mondo dei Grandi. Pisa: Del Cerro.

Montobbio E, Lepri C (2000) Chi Sarei se Potessi Essere. La Condizione Adulta del Disabile Mentale. Pisa: Del Cerro.

Index

sex and contraception 169, 172–3
sexuality 180, 181–3, 184–6, 189, 193
siblings 196–202
work 265, 273
partial trisomy 18, 19–23, 41
peptides 100, 102, 103, 106, 116
personal hygiene 236, 266
pharmacology 112–20
Alzheimer's disease 105–6
unconventional therapies 119–20
phonology 151, 162–3
phospholipase C 21
phosphorus 59
Piracetam 119–20
pituitary-gonadal axis 58
placental growth hormone (PGH) 59
pneumonia 7, 8, 44
Portugal 6–7
Position Classification Inventory 255
potassium 90
Prader Willi syndrome 64
precardiogenic misoderm 34
pregnancy 57–9, 172
sex and contraception 170, 171, 172,
173
terminations 3–6, 9
vitamin A 118
presbiacusis 68
prevalence
CHD in Down syndrome 39–41, 46
coeliac disease 83–4, 85, 114–15
Down syndrome 3, 4–7, 9–10, 51–2
epilepsy 54, 55
thyroid disorders 54, 62
prevention 227–8, 229, 230, 238
problem-solving 217, 221, 222, 254, 261
progesterone 57–8, 171, 174
proteins 16–17, 35–6, 119
ageing 95
Alzheimer's disease 99–100, 102, 103,
105
CHD 32–3, 35–6
coeliac disease 114
proteomes 16
pseudoarthrosis 78, 79
pseudodementia 148
psychiatric disorders 55, 176, 227, 230
psychomotricity 228, 231
psychoses 177, 180, 181
psychotherapy 231
puberty 57, 61–2, 114

pulmonary atresia 42
pulmonary disease 43–4, 45–6
vascular 39, 42–3
pure-tone audiometry 67, 69, 91
pyramidal cells 24

quality of life 55–6, 207, 223, 240, 244,
246

radiography 75–80
reactive astrocytes 102, 103
reading ability 155, 163–4, 208
language 161–4
vocational guidance 254, 256
work 164, 266
Registry of Congenital Malformations 52
rehabilitation 226–33, 239–42
ageing 212–23, 228–9, 231, 232
evaluation of treatment outcomes
235–7, 239–42, 245–7
family involvement in treatment
205–10
long-term memory 142, 143
sexuality 178, 180, 184
vocational guidance 251, 253
work 231, 232, 273
relationships 169–74, 176–93
evaluation of treatment outcomes
241, 242
rehabilitation 227, 228, 230, 232
vocational guidance 257–8, 261
work 270–1
religion 169, 186, 187–8
REM sleep 93–4
repetition priming tests 143, 144–6
reproduction 57–9, 187–8
resentment 199–200
respiratory disease 52
response rapidity 213, 218, 220–2
retinoblastomas 83, 116
risks 4–5, 226–9, 231, 242–3
Robertsonian chromosomes 18
role-play 217

seizures 8, 99, 119, 126
see also epilepsy
selenium 117, 118
self-confidence 268, 270
self-determination 243, 244, 248
self-esteem 164, 194
self-sufficiency 235–6, 239